Orthopaedic Practice

Orthopaedic Practice

Edited by

P. M. Yeoman MA, MB, BChir, MD, FRCS
Emeritus Consultant Orthopaedic Surgeon, The Royal United Hospital and The Royal National Hospital for
Rheumatic Diseases NHS Trust, Bath, UK

and

D. M. Spengler MD
Chairman, Department of Orthopaedics and Rehabilitation, Vanderbilt University, Nashville, Tennessee, USA

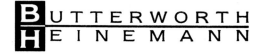

Butterworth-Heinemann
Linacre House, Jordan Hill, Oxford OX2 8DP
225 Wildwood Avenue, Woburn, MA 01801-2041
A division of Reed Educational and Professional Publishing Ltd

A member of the Reed Elsevier plc group

OXFORD   BOSTON   JOHANNESBURG
MELBOURNE   NEW DELHI   SINGAPORE

First published 1996
Paperback edition 1998

British Library Cataloguing in Publication Data
Orthopaedic Practice
  I. Yeoman, Philip   II. Spengler, Dan M.
  617.3

Library of Congress Cataloguing in Publication Data
Orthopaedic practice/edited by P. M. Yeoman and D. M. Spengler
p. cm.
Includes bibliographical references and index.
1. Orthopaedics. I. Yeoman, P. M. (Philip M.) II. Spengler, Dan M.
[DNLM: 1. Musculoskeletal Diseases-therapy. 2. Orthopaedics-
methods. WE 168 C97631995]   94-44573
RD731.C87   CIP

ISBN 0 7506 4206 8

Printed and bound in Great Britain by The Bath Press plc, Bath, Avon

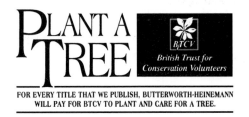

PLANT A TREE

British Trust for
Conservation Volunteers

FOR EVERY TITLE THAT WE PUBLISH, BUTTERWORTH-HEINEMANN
WILL PAY FOR BTCV TO PLANT AND CARE FOR A TREE.

Contents

List of contributors   vii

Foreword   ix
J. Goodfellow

Preface   xi

1 Problem solving in orthopaedics   1
D. M. Spengler

2 Club foot   5
A. Catterall

3 The surgical treatment of congenital displacement of the hip joint   20
J. A. Wilkinson

4 Orthopaedic management in spina bifida   32
E. A. Szalay

5 Perthes' disease   40
G. Hall

6 Slipped upper femoral epiphysis   49
W. E. G. Griffiths

7 Spinal deformities   64
R. A. Dickson

8 Lengthening of limbs by the Ilizarov method   105
R. Cruz-Conde Delgado and J. C. Marti Gonzalez

9 The multiply injured patient with musculoskeletal injuries   115
M. F. Swiontkowski

10 Traumatic shock and the metabolic responses to injury   128
R. A. Little and M. Irving

11 Reconstructive orthopaedic surgery: skin cover following injury to a limb   138
P. L. G. Townsend

12 Arthroscopy of the knee   153
J. L. Pozo

13 Flexor tendon surgery   170
C. Semple

14 Musculoskeletal trauma: nerve   177
D. Marsh and N. J. Barton

15 External skeletal fixation for the treatment of fractures   189
J. Kenwright

16 Brachial plexus injuries   200
A. O. Narakas, P. M. Yeoman and C. B. Wynn Parry

17 Rotator cuff injury   240
M. F. Swiontkowski

18 Osteoarthritis of the hip   246
C. H. Wynn Jones

19 Management of unicompartmental arthritis of the knee   279
J. H. Newman

20 Mechanical and degenerative disorders of the lumbar spine   286
J. S. Denton

21 Surgical management of the cervical spine in rheumatoid arthritis   321
P. M. Yeoman

22 **Surgical treatment of rheumatoid arthritis of the shoulder**   329
P. J. M. Morrison

23 **Rheumatoid arthritis of the elbow**   338
P. M. Yeoman

24 **Rheumatoid arthritis of the wrist and hand**   342
D. R. Dunkerley

25 **Surgical treatment of rheumatoid arthritis of the knee**   359
P. Bliss

26 **Rheumatoid arthritis of the ankle and foot**   367
J. R. Kirkup

27 **Correction of posture in ankylosing spondylitis**   380
P. M. Yeoman

28 **Musculoskeletal sepsis: current concepts in treatment**   387
R. H. Fitzgerald

29 **Osteomalacia and osteoporosis**   401
D. J. Baylink and M. R. Mariano-Menez

30 **Physics and technology of bone-mineral content measurements**   422
R. R. Price and M. P. Sandler

31 **Limb salvage surgery for primary bone tumours**   431
R. S. Sneath and R. J. Grimer

32 **Chemotherapy and radiotherapy in sarcoma of bone and the musculoskeletal system**   443
J. Bullimore

Index   455

Contributors

Barton, N. J. FRCS
Consultant Hand Surgeon, Nottingham
University Hospital and Harlow Wood
Orthopaedic Hospital, Civilian Consultant in
Hand Surgery to the Royal Air Force, UK

Baylink, D. J. MD
Jerry L. Pettis Veterans Hospital and Loma
Linda University, Loma Linda, California, USA

Bliss, P. MB FRCS JP
Emeritus Consultant Orthopaedic Surgeon,
Royal United Hospital and The Royal
National Hospital for Rheumatic Diseases,
Bath, UK

Bullimore, J. MB BS DMRT FRCR
Consultant Clinical Oncologist, Bristol
Oncology Centre, Bristol Royal Infirmary,
Bristol, UK

Catterall, A. MChir FRCS
Children's Unit, Royal National Orthopaedic
Hospital, London, UK

Cruz-Conde Delgado, R. MD
Head of Orthopaedic Department, Asepeyo
Orthopaedic Hospital, Coslada, Madrid, Spain

Denton, J. S.
Department of Orthopaedic Surgery,
University of Liverpool, Liverpool, UK

Dickson, R. A. MA ChM FRCS DSc
Professor of Orthopaedic Surgery, University
of Leeds, St James's Hospital, Leeds, UK

Dunkerley, D. R. FRCS
Consultant Orthopaedic and Hand Surgeon,
Royal United Hospital NHS Trust, Combe
Park, Bath, UK

Fitzgerald, R. H. Jr MD
Professor and Chairman, Wayne State
University, School of Medicine, Detroit, USA

Griffiths, W. E. G. FRCS Eng FRCS Ed
Consultant in Orthopaedics, Queen Alexandra
Hospital, Cosham, Portsmouth, UK

Grimer, R. J. FRCS FRCS Ed (Orth)
Consultant Orthopaedic Oncologist, The
Orthopaedic Oncology Service, The Royal
Orthopaedic Hospital, Northfield, Birmingham,
UK

Hall, G. MD FRCS
Consultant Orthopaedic Surgeon, West Dorset
Health Trust, Dorset, UK

Irving, Sir M. MD ChM FRCS
Professor of Surgery, University of
Manchester, Hope Hospital, Manchester, UK

Kenwright, J. MA MD FRCS
Nuffield Professor of Orthopaedic Surgery,
University of Oxford, Nuffield Orthopaedic
Centre, Headington, Oxford, UK

Kirkup, J. R. MA MD FRCS
Emeritus Consultant Orthopaedic Surgeon,
Royal National Hospital for Rheumatic
Diseases, Bath, UK

Little, R. A. PhD FRCPath FFAEM
Head MRC Trauma Group, Director North
Western Injury, Research Centre, University of
Manchester, Manchester, UK

Mariano-Menez, M. R. MD
Jerry L. Pettis Veterans Hospital and Loma
Linda University, Loma Linda, California,
USA

Marsh, D. MD FRCS
Senior Lecturer in Orthopaedics, University of
Manchester, Hope Hospital, Manchester, UK

Marti Gonzalez, J. C. MD
Unit of External Fixation, Asepeyo
Orthopaedic Hospital, Coslada, Madrid, Spain

Morrison, P. J. M. FRCS
Consultant Orthopaedic Surgeon, Royal
National Hospital for Rheumatic Diseases,
Bath, UK

Narakas, A. O. MD FRCS EngHon
(Deceased)
Associate Professor at the Medical School and
Consultant at the University Hospital of
Lausanne, Lausanne, Switzerland

Newman, J. H. MA MB BChir FRCS
Consultant Orthopaedic Surgeon, Bristol Royal
Infirmary and Avon Orthopaedic Centre,
Southmead, Bristol, UK

Pozo, J. L. MA FRCS
Consultant Orthopaedic Surgeon, Royal
United Hospital and The Royal National
Hospital for Rheumatic Diseases, Bath, UK

Price, R. R. PhD
Professor of Radiology, Director, Radiological
Sciences Division, Department of Radiology
and Radiological Sciences, Vanderbilt
University Medical Center, Nashville,
Tennessee, USA

Sandler, M. P. MD
Professor and Vice-Chairman, Radiology and
Radiological Sciences, Director of Nuclear
Science, Vanderbilt University Medical Center,
Nashville, Tennessee, USA

Semple, C. FRCS
Hand Surgeon, 79 Harley Street, London, UK

Sneath, R. S. FRCS
Consultant Orthopaedic Surgeon, Formerly
Director, The Orthopaedic Oncology Service,
The Royal Orthopaedic Hospital, Northfield,
Birmingham, UK

Spengler, D. M. MD
Chairman, Department of Orthopaedics and
Rehabilitation, Vanderbilt University,
Tennessee, USA

Swiontkowski, M. F. MD
Professor, Department of Orthopaedics,
University of Washington, Chief of
Orthopaedics, Harborview Medical Center,
Seattle, Washington, USA

Szalay, E. A. MD
Paediatric Orthopaedics and Scoliosis,
Beaumont Bone and Joint Clinic, Beaumont,
Texas, USA

Townsend, P. L. G. BSc FRCS(c) FRCS
Consultant Plastic Surgeon, Department of
Plastic and Reconstructive Surgery, Frenchay
Hospital, Bristol, UK

Wilkinson, J. A. BSc MCh FRCS
Senior Consultant Orthopaedic Surgeon
(Emeritus), Southampton University Hospitals
and The Lord Mayor Treloar Hospital, Alton,
UK

Wynn Jones, C. H. MBBS FRCS
Consultant Orthopaedic Surgeon, Hartshill
Orthopaedic Hospital, Stoke-on-Trent, UK

Wynn Parry, C. B. MBE MA DM FRCP
FRCS
Formerly Director of Rehabilitation, Royal
National Orthopaedic Hospitals, London and
Stanmore, UK

Yeoman, P. M. MD FRCS
Emeritus Consultant Orthopaedic Surgeon,
Royal United Hospital and The Royal
National Hospital for Rheumatic Diseases,
Bath, UK

Foreword

There are many problems in orthopaedic surgery 'upon which it is difficult to speak, and impossible to be silent'. Difficult to speak, because at this stage in our learning no one fully understands them; impossible to ignore, because they make up a large part of daily practice. The subjects discussed in this book are mainly those for which no complete solution has yet been found. The list of chapter headings might serve as a student's guide to areas in which research is most needed and most likely to prove rewarding.

Not that these subjects have been overlooked in the past. On the contrary, they have been the very stuff of orthopaedics ever since our speciality was born. There has hardly been a major orthopaedic meeting without papers on Perthes' disease and club foot, but the best protocol for the treatment of talipes is not yet agreed and doubts remain about the efficacy of any of the procedures devised for Perthes' disease. Similarly, in the field of traumatology, although there is consensus on how to treat many types of fracture, the challenge of the multiply injured patient is still debated. Our knowledge of these subjects, like the knowledge that underpins most surgery, has accrued over the years mainly from experience in the field and from retrospective analysis. Very little of it has resulted from prospective study or structured research. The time may now have come for surgeons to start to build on this vast and incoherent legacy by submitting their theories to better informed criticism and their practices to the test of controlled prospective trials. The 'difficult' subjects dealt with in this book might then become easier to write about.

Practising surgeons, however, cannot wait for the last word to be said. They need to make decisions here and now, and they will find in this collection of essays an authoritative review of our current understanding (and present ignorance) of several of the most testing areas in which they are called upon either to take action or, what is just as important, to withhold it.

John Goodfellow MS, FRCS
Sometime Consultant Surgeon,
Nuffield Orthopaedic Centre,
Oxford UK

Preface

The intention of this book entitled *Orthopaedic Practice* is to highlight many of the more difficult conditions which affect the musculo-skeletal system and not to encompass all orthopaedic disorders. Although our text is not a comprehensive volume we believe it will appeal to those houseofficers and registrars who seek knowledge to prepare for higher qualifications, or indeed to those consultants who are already in practice yet still searching for sound information.

A team of contributors from the USA, the UK, Spain and Switzerland were purposely selected because of their special knowledge and interest in their particular subject. Each chapter provides a reasoned account without entering into too many detailed operative techniques.
The chapters provide sufficient detail to allow acceptable discussion during Socratic/oral examinations and to provide selected references for further reading.

Where advances have been made, the specialists have risen to the challenge which is very evident in the chapters on shock, multiple injuries, scoliosis, nerve injuries and the fairly wide coverage on rheumatoid arthritis. Osteoporosis and mineral content of bone is one of the topics in the forefront of research today. In addition, the combined management of bone tumours is related to the team on the Bristol Bone Tumour panel.

Sadly, since the book was almost in the proof stage, we have to announce the death of Algy Narakas from Lausanne who was a great pioneer in the understanding of brachial plexus injuries. He was an international expert and ran a stimulating course each year which attracted surgeons from far and wide. His chapter is published almost unabridged and comes as a token of the high regard we had for him. The detail of his operative findings and the results of his surgery are remarkable and should be appreciated by all even if they had not the privilege of knowing him.

On a happier note we send congratulations to Miles Irving who received a knighthood in the recent Honours List for his great contribution to surgery in general.

We wish to thank all our contributors who have written memorable chapters in spite of difficulties; their forbearance is much appreciated. Finally we also wish to thank Susan Devlin at Butterworth-Heinemann for her help and guidance through some rough patches, and also Alison Duncan for her patience and efficient work at the editorial desk.

Philip M. Yeoman
Dan M. Spengler

1

Problem solving in orthopaedics

D. M. Spengler

Introduction

All of us in medicine realize the importance of rendering a precise and accurate diagnosis [1]. All too often, however, we falter and recommend a treatment approach which, although appropriate for our perceived diagnosis, may be seen to be unwarranted in light of the proper diagnosis. For example, many patients undergo surgical intervention for a lumbar disc herniation, when in fact many of these patients do not demonstrate a herniation at surgery [2]. Thus, for whatever reason, the preoperative assessment was faulty. The most common source of error is misinterpretation of the classic straight leg raising test [3]. Unless distracting signs are employed, symptom amplifiers will also appear to have positive straight leg raising signs, indicative of sciatic tension. Other possible causes for a faulty assessment include inappropriate intervention because of the prevalance of 'asymptomatic' extradural lesions on most imaging studies, including the computed tomographic scan, myelography and magnetic resonance imaging [4,5].

Numerous other sources of error in assessment of the musculoskeletal system could be described. Since many of these errors involve benign processes, the orthopaedist often dismisses an error of intervention as 'a rational attempt to help the patient with little downside risk.' Although a certain level of false negative explorations may be

very reasonable when treating patients for acute appendicitis, this is not the case in other instances. For example, an unwarranted surgical intervention for a benign process such as a lumbar disc herniation has been shown to result in a markedly decreased likelihood for a good outcome. This fact has been clearly demonstrated by Spangfort; patients who undergo lumbar spine surgery, but who have no evidence of a pathological process, have poorer outcomes than would be predicted by the natural history for the symptom complex [8].

These unfortunate clinical realities provide a strong incentive to develop a logical, consistent approach to clinical decision-making. Such an approach can range from the pragmatic algorithms developed by individual clinicians to sophisticated formal decision analysis strategies devised by theoreticians [5–7]. The main objectives for all organized approaches to this problem-solving process include: 1) to quantify uncertainty, 2) to select the most efficient and consistent approach to manage patients, and 3) to minimize risk and to optimize benefit or outcome [5–7].

This chapter will review some of the interesting and potentially useful data which are relevant to decision analysis. In addition, the author hopes to challenge orthopaedists to continue to design scientifically sound clinical studies to fill the many gaps in our knowledge, so that in the future we will improve our diagnostic and therapeutic accuracy with resultant improved outcomes for our patients.

Process of problem solving

Any process which analyses clinical judgement is inevitably complex. The traditional medical assessment described by Weed, which includes subjective, objective, assessment and plan (SOAP), can be used to summarize a clinical approach for the evaluation and treatment of patients. The subjective phase of this process begins with the medical history and review of the presenting complaint. This process requires a large data base. The sophisticated clinician probably recognizes important patterns of symptoms which will enhance both retention and recall of important information. Such knowledge is essential to recognize unusual presentations of common clinical entities, as well as to raise the index of suspicion for symptoms consistent with uncommonly encountered clinical entities, such as Gaucher's disease. The subjective evaluation merges into the objective phase in the physical examination. However, certain observations in the physical examination are definitely subjective. Consider the analysis of range of motion of the spine. The examiner determines that the patient can forward flex only 20°, clearly a marked restriction. Does this restriction of motion reflect a limitation imposed secondary to a pathological process, or does the limitation reflect a decrease in effort on the part of the patient to exaggerate symptoms? Such questions are not trivial. Indeed, they deal with a fundamental principle of medicine – proper diagnosis = proper treatment. Although this is a clear-cut example of 'subjective' information, we routinely use such data to assess impairment! [1].

Examples of objective measures which can be identified on the physical examination include the presence or absence of a reflex, circumferential atrophy of an extremity, deformity and Horner's syndrome. Presumably, the ideal physician considers the degree of subjectivity/objectivity of various data and prioritizes this information during data synthesis.

Following completion of the history and physical examination, the examiner next considers additional diagnostic studies to reaffirm or refute the tentative diagnosis. In most situations, the need for a particular diagnostic test is based on the likelihood of usefulness combined with the relative risk of the study. Thus, a physician would seldom recommend a lumbar myelogram for a patient who has had only mild low back pain for less than 24 hours. The same clinician, however, may well recommend an emergent myelogram in a patient who presents with a progressive neural deficit. Once laboratory data and relevant imaging studies have been reviewed, the differential diagnostic possibilities are again considered to determine the specific diagnosis. If the diagnosis can be validated by the data available to this point, treatment is instituted and an optimal outcome will probably result. If the diagnosis cannot be validated, additional, more invasive tests may be required (e.g., arteriography, myelography, biopsy).

Once all necessary studies have been obtained and the appropriate diagnosis has been formulated, many tasks remain before treatment is instituted. For example, the clinician will probably inform the patient of the diagnosis and the natural history of the pathological process. Both the short-term consequences and the long-term implications should be discussed. The risks or complications that may be encountered should also be reviewed. This communication with the patient and family is of primary importance to develop and maintain a good patient–physician relationship. Honesty is always the best policy. If you do not have the data available to accurately detail all implications, tell the patient, 'I do not know . . .' Often doctors have been advised not to say those four simple words, but rather to say 'idiopathic . . .', even though 'I don't know' is more honest. Once a pathological process or lack of such a process has been elucidated, the next task requires an appraisal of the goals and expectations of the patient. These goals are then integrated into the various treatment options available. Clearly, the patient must play a major role in this process. For example, if total hip replacement, hip arthrodesis, and extra-articular osteotomy comprise three viable alternatives for management, the orthopaedist should present these options and discuss the relative advantages and disadvantages with the patient. The patient will usually ask pertinent questions, followed by the inevitable 'What would you do, Doctor, if it were your hip?' This question, although perceptive, is usually not relevant unless the patient is close in age to the physician. The patient must be permitted adequate time to reflect and gather additional data, or to seek other consultations, before reaching a final decision. Treatment options must also take into account multiple factors, including the patient's age and gender as well as occupation and general health. In the field of orthopaedics, we are presently experiencing a technological frenzy. Many new surgical techniques and implants are being rapidly developed and implemented. Indeed, long-term outcomes for most of these approaches remain unknown. Although newer strategies may improve on previous failures in certain situations, in other conditions they may only increase the risk side of the risk–benefit ratio. Approaches which offer risk without any enhanced benefits must be eliminated from general application. If necessary, such approaches can be evaluated through proper prospective studies which include a comparable control group. Classic marketing objections to evaluations, such as '. . . this study would be unethical since my product is so good, etc., etc. . . .', must be dismissed as non-persuasive.

Background noise

Now that we have considered the general process used to solve clinical problems, we must consider factors which impede our ability to render a proper diagnosis and to proceed with treatment. The major problems can be divided into two categories: biological variation and inadequate data [5,6]. These problems must be considered throughout the entire decision analysis process, not just during the treatment phase. Thus, biological variation may affect the subjective (clinical history) portion of decision analysis as well as the plan (response to treatment).

We are all overwhelmed with data. How can I then suggest that inadequate data represent a major hurdle to proper patient evaluation and treatment? Easy: quantity does not reflect quality. Most of us receive every week five or more throw-away journals containing articles espousing the latest and greatest treatment approaches for most orthopaedic conditions. We also subscribe to several journals which may or may not submit to a rigorous peer review process. In addition, the lay press continuously subjects our patients and us to reports of extraordinary medical progress which emphasize the successes, and downplay the risks or failures, of the treatment being presented. These articles usually represent marketing efforts rather than good science. Depending on the circulation of the journal in question, we will be certain to receive a large number of phone calls requesting the new 'super surg procedure' reported in the local 'Enquirer'. In these situations, an impatient and demanding public attempts to short circuit the complex problem-solving approach herein described through the 'aunt Minnie' logic scenario. The 'aunt Minnie' syndrome works in this way: 'I have the same symptoms as the patient in the magazine. "Super surg" worked for that person. Therefore, I need "super surg"!'

Likewise, the tremendous proliferation of the printed word through the publication of meeting abstracts, case reports and review articles creates significant background noise which may easily confuse us when we attempt to call into focus articles which relate to a specific problem. Deyo has persuasively shown that the vast majority of articles which deal with the common clinical phenomenon of low back pain are worthless [2]. Since all clinicians are not as thoughtful as Deyo, many may accept the written word as fact, and ignore the validity or reproducibility of the information presented.

Finally, most of us are constantly approached by sales representatives who offer us even more articles and advice attesting to the brilliant performance of their company's product in contrast to the miserable record of that of their competitor. Alas, a veritable minefield appears when we attempt to pursue additional knowledge. If we are not critical, we may attempt problem solving with an outmoded or insufficient data base. When such major deficiencies are present in our data base, the entire process of decision analysis becomes invalid.

Relevant data

Given the above problems which may adversely affect our desire to provide quality care for our patients, what should we do? Where should we turn? I hope to formulate data and challenges which may result in enhanced knowledge over the long term.

One of the most important characteristics of the ideal clinician is his or her unparalleled knowledge of the natural history for the clinical entity to be managed. If one has a good grasp of the outcome of a particular pathological process, one is in an excellent position to compare the natural history of the disorder with the course noted with newer treatment approaches, and thus to determine if an improved outcome results. One must be careful, however, to ensure that a different outcome is related to the different treatment approach. In addition, one must ascertain how well the new approach works over time. For example, assume that a manufacturer has developed a new widget to cure a common clinical symptom complex such as backache. The company then lines up several clinicians to evaluate the widget. Following an exhaustive 3 month study, the company reports on a major TV program that the widget cures low back pain in 70% of the patients who were treated and followed for this length of time. Moreover, the widget also permits the patient to be managed as an outpatient, eliminating the need for costly hospital admissions. Sounds good? Indeed, you would have to be extremely sceptical not to rush out and buy the widget. But sceptical you must be, or you will add to the ever burgeoning cost of health care.

If the performance of the widget is carefully evaluated, we quickly realize that a control group of patients treated for backache with untuned diathermy also responded with a 70% success rate. Moreover, with longer follow-up, we discover that 50% of the patients treated with the widget require additional hospitalization and treatment. Thus, the widget is not only ineffective, but fuels the increasing health care cost spiral in an upward direction. This is a hypothetical story, but one does not need to look very far to find widgets throughout our field. The important point is that as concerned physicians, we must critically analyse our approaches to patients and we must always insist on proper information to allow us to formulate logical conclusions. To do less is to abrogate the trust and responsibility which have been placed on us by our patients.

All of us can help meet the ongoing need for data. We must meticulously follow our patients so that we recognize early problems with our treatment approaches. We can then appropriately modify our strategies to decrease complications and optimize outcome. Only through the establishment of large multi-centre trials will we ever be able to fill in all of the gaps in knowledge, and thus be able to identify the ideal treatment approach for a specific patient! We must persevere – after all, that patient will some day be us.

Summary

This presentation has reviewed some of the more important aspects of clinical problem solving. We can all benefit by being thorough in our approach to the evaluation and treatment of patients. Approaches which have been validated and which are logically consistent should be emphasized. We must continually seek additional data to improve our ability to quantify human performance, which will help us to better understand biological variation. Finally, our biggest challenge will be to focus on objective outcome criteria to reaffirm that careful decision analysis does indeed make a positive difference in patient care.

References

1. AMA (1984) *Guides to the Evaluation of Permanent Impairment*. AMA, Chicago.
2. Deyo, R. A. (1983) Conservative therapy for low back pain: Distinguishing useful from useless therapy. *JAMA*, **250**, 1057–1062.
3. Hitselberger, W. and Witten, R. (1968) Abnormal myelograms in asymptomatic patients. *J. Neurosurg.*, **28**, 204–206.
4. Lippert, F. G. and Farmer, J. (1984) *Psychomotor Skills in Orthopaedic Surgery*. Williams and Wilkins, Baltimore.
5. Pauker, S. and Kassirer, J. (1987) Decision analysis. *N. Engl. J. Med.*, **316**, 250–258.
6. Pauker, S. and Kassirer, K. (1980) The threshold approach to clinical decision making. *N. Engl. J. Med.*, **302**, 1109–1117.
7. Sisson, J., Schoomaker, E. and Ross, J. (1976) Clinical decision analysis. *JAMA*, **236**, 1259–1263.
8. Spangfort, E., (1972) The lumbar disc herniation. *Acta Orthop. Scand. (Suppl.)*, **142**, 1–95.
9. Spengler, D. and Freeman, C. (1979) Patient selection for lumbar discectomy: An objective approach. *Spine*, **4**, 129–134.
10. Wiesel, S., Tsourmas, N., Feffer, H. *et al.* (1984) A study of CAT. *Spine*, **9**, 549–551.

2

Club foot

A. Catterall

Introduction

There are now many texts which deal with the problems of children born with club foot deformities. The majority of these deal comprehensively with the whole subject and explain the failures of previous series on the lack of a sufficiently radical operation to correct the deformity. Few, however, define in simple terms the deformities with which they are dealing or the indications for minor and major procedures during the course of treatment. Most authors recognize a postural deformity of good prognosis; but are there other forms of this condition for which minor surgery will produce a satisfactory outcome? Main *et al.* [1] and Green *et al.* [2] report

that a simple posterior release alone produced a satisfactory result in one-third of cases. Assessment must, therefore, be the major key to a solution of this condition and must be made with the knowledge of the way the normal foot moves in dorsiflexion together with the site of any fixed deformities which are to be found in the club foot. This chapter will not, therefore, deal with the topic in the standard way but will concentrate on a method of assessment made by a common language of 'Observer independent observations' and will define a protocol of treatment, the object of which is to convert a tendon or joint contracture into the resolving pattern of deformity.

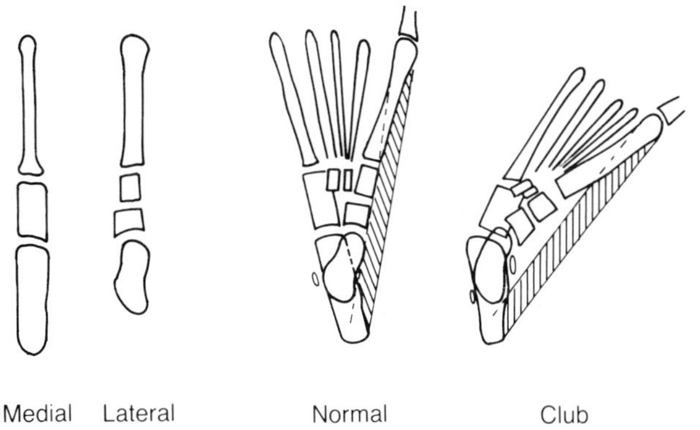

Anatomy

A hypothesis of foot movement

In thinking about the way the normal foot moves, it is suggested that functionally the foot consists of a medial and lateral ray with a number of link mechanisms (Fig. 2.l). The medial ray consists of the talus, navicular, medial cuneiform and first metatarsal while below it the lateral ray consists of the calcaneum, cuboid and fifth metatarsal. Connecting these two rays are three link mechanisms. At the talo-calcaneal level there is the interosseous ligament which permits rotation of the talus on the calcaneum and therefore divergence of the medial and lateral rays. Anterior to this is a bony link mechanism comprising the

Medial   Lateral   Normal   Club
ray   ray   foot   foot

Fig. 2.1 Drawing of the rays of the foot.

remaining bones of the tarsus stabilizing the two rays but allowing rotatory movement. Beyond this the middle metacarpals act as spacers connected anteriorly by the intermetatarsal ligament. This latter ligament should be looked on as a restraining check ligament to the normal spreading of the foot which would occur in inversion and eversion if such a ligament was absent. There is one other structure which links these two rays, namely the plantar fascia, which starting from the posterior surface of the lateral ray reaches forward to pass underneath the anterior end of the medial ray in an oblique direction. By doing so it maintains the medial arch. Being attached to the great toe, dorsiflexion of the M-P joint will depress the first metatarsal. The movements of inversion and eversion, pronation and supination are in essence rotatory with one ray moving over the other, and the movement limited by the natural tension in the three link mechanisms. In eversion a space forms between the navicular and cuboid and a tether in this region will hold the foot in supination, a position commonly encountered in the club foot.

Ossification centres

Not all the foot bones are fully ossified at birth and it is important to realize where the ossifica-tion centres within the individual bones lie, particularly in the talus and calcaneum. In the talus the centre lies in the anterior body and the neck. This means it will lie anterior to the tibia in full equinus (Fig. 2.2) and moves back to become parallel to the lower margin of the tibia as dorsiflexion proceeds. The centre for the calcaneum is centrally placed but square in shape and a globular appearance commonly seen in the club foot is a rotated, oblique view. The navicular is seldom ossified in the first few months of life but its position may be identified by extending the line of the first metatarsal proximally where it should cross the ossification in the talus. By contrast, the cuboid is normally ossified early in life and its position on the lateral ray is easily identified and assessed on plain radiographs.

The anatomy of the normal dorsiflexion in the infant child

From the position of full equinovarus the movement of dorsiflexion occurs mainly at two sites: the ankle and the subtaloid joint [3,4]. At the ankle joint there is a posterior movement of the talus on the tibia with the fibula and lateral malleolus rotating around its curved lateral border. For this movement to occur relaxation of the calf and Achilles tendon is required. At the subtaloid joint the calcaneum and lateral ray rotates under the talus and medial ray with the centre of rotation being the interosseous ligament. For this second phase of dorsiflexion to occur, relaxation of both the Achilles tendon and the tendon of the tibialis posterior is required. If dorsiflexion proceeds without relaxation of the tibialis posterior from the position of equino-varus the foot will reach a right angle (Fig. 2.3) but it will be noted that the lateral malleolus is remaining posterior and that the forefoot is seen in oblique rather than lateral projection. A lateral radiograph of the foot (Fig. 2.4b) in this position confirms the clinical appearances and shows a position very similar to the relapsed club foot in which a supination deformity is present. Release of the tendon of the tibialis posterior at this stage allows the second phase of dorsiflexion to proceed normally so that the forefoot is seen in lateral projection and the lateral malleolus moves forward to cover the anterior margin of the lateral border of the talus. A lateral radiograph

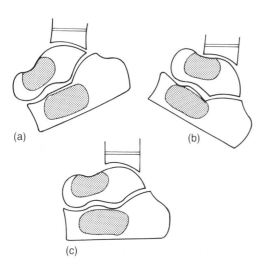

Fig. 2.2 Drawing of the ankle with the hind foot. (a) In plantar flexion. (b) Plantargrade position. (c) Dorsiflexion to show position of the ossification centres. Note that the talus moves forward on the calcaneum in plantarflexion and backwards in dorsiflexion.

the anterior portion of the body of the talus is forward out of the mortice and inclined downwards and medially with the calcaneum lying directly below it. In full dorsiflexion the body of the talus has moved backwards into the mortice and its direction now points laterally with the calcaneum lying lateral to it. It may be concluded that for every 10° of dorsiflexion from the position of full equinus 10° of external rotation of the

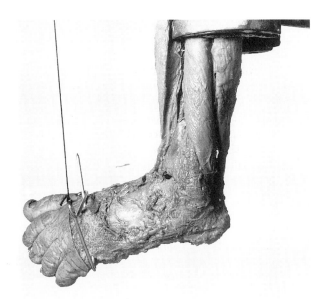

Fig. 2.3 Lateral view of an infant foot with the foot dorsiflexed but with tethering of the tibialis posterior (Fig. 2.4b).

(Fig. 2.4b) of the foot at this stage confirms the true nature of the process. The rotatory aspect of dorsiflexion is most easily observed with the forefoot removed (Fig. 2.5a and b). In full equinus

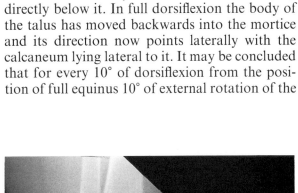

(b)

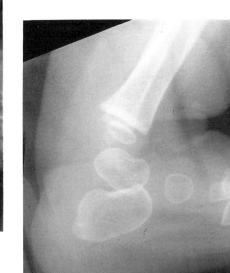

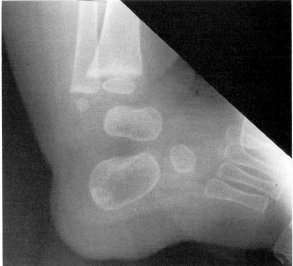

(a)

Fig. 2.4 Lateral radiographs of the infant foot in (a) full equinovarus. (b) dorsiflexion without relaxation of the tibialis posterior. (c) in full dorsiflexion. Note that in (b) the lateral malleolus is remaining posterior and the forefoot is seen in oblique projection.

(c)

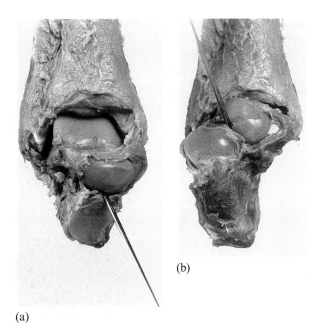

(b)

(a)

Fig. 2.5   Anterior view of the hind foot and tibia with the forefoot removed through the talo-navicular and calcaneo-cuboid joint. (a) Plantarflexion. (b) Dorsiflexion. Note the backward and rotatory movement of the talus. The calcaneum also rotates laterally on the interosseous ligament.

foot on the tibia occurs [3]. This means that if the foot is placed in full dorsiflexion without external rotation a spurious position is being produced.

Pathology

The untreated infant foot

In terms of the normal anatomy which has already been described there are a number of deformities present in the infant with a club foot deformity.

1. Investigations by Irani and Sherman [5], Carroll *et al.* [6], Bensahel *et al.* [7] and others have demonstrated that the neck of the talus is short and is more medially deviated than normal. The talus lies in equinus and the navicular articulates with the medial surface of the head, being itself tethered to the medial malleolus in a position of medial subluxation. The tissues between the navicular and medial malleolus have been shown to be abnormal and contain an excess of myofibrils and elastic fibres, allowing continuing contracture of this tissue to occur [8].

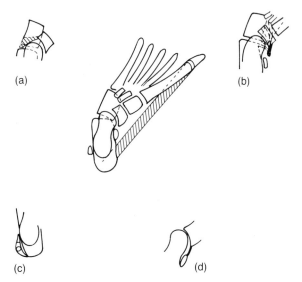

(a)

(b)

(c)

(d)

Fig. 2.6   The tethers of the club foot. (a) Antero-lateral, (b) distal attachment of tibialis posterior, (c) postero-lateral, (d) medial malleolus-navicular.

2. The calcaneum is normal in shape, but in full equinus. In this position the body of the talus moves forwards on the tibia and also on the calcaneum at the posterior talocalcaneo facet (Figs 2.2 and 2.7). There is adaptive shortening of the posterior capsule of the ankle, the Achilles tendon and lateral ligamentous structures. As a result, the body of the talus is displaced forwards out of the mortice and comes to lie so that its greatest vertical height is in front of the anterior part of the mortice. The talus, therefore, cannot move back into the mortice until this posterior space has been increased. In essence the talus is being driven forward out of the anterior aspect of the mortice as an orange pip (Figs 2.2, 2.4 and 2.7)

3. There is a medial subluxation of the cuboid on the calcaneum. In addition, a knot of tissue lying lateral to the head of the talus tethers the navicular to the calcaneum and cuboid, preventing independent movement of the medial and lateral rays of the foot (Figs 2.1 and 2.6a).

4. The tibialis posterior is abnormal [9]. The excursion of its muscle fibres is reduced and its attachment distal to the navicular to the cuboid, calcaneum and metatarsals is shortened. By contrast, the flexor digitorum and flexor hallucis are capable of normal movement in the majority of cases if they are progressively stretched. They are, however, functionally short. The long plantar

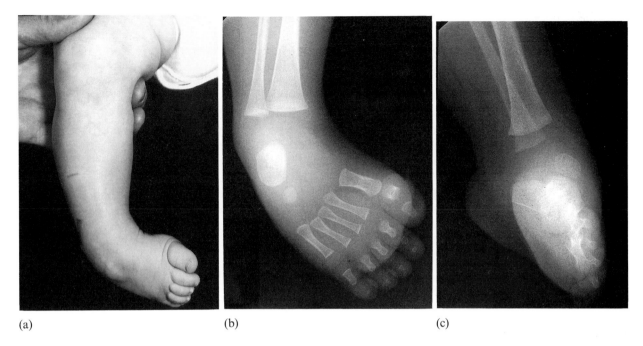

(a)   (b)   (c)

Fig. 2.7 The uncorrected club foot. (a) Photograph. (b) Lateral radiograph of the foot. (c) True lateral radiograph of the ankle. Note the anterior displacement of the talus outside the mortice and the cavus deformity of the forefoot.

ligament lying between the distal attachment of the tibialis posterior and peroneus longus is adaptably short, as is the plantar fascia. The effect of shortening of these tissues within the sole of the foot produces a cavus deformity and tethering of the medial and lateral rays at the level of the bony link mechanism. Scott *et al.* [3] have shown that tethering in this site reduces the ability of the foot to dorsiflex by preventing the second stage of rotation from occurring.

Late or relapsed cases

Following surgical release of the posterior, medial or more radical type, a number of secondary changes may be noted. These will depend on the severity of the surgical procedure, the duration of the remodelling and the presence of avascular necrosis in centres of ossification within the foot bones.

1. The talus. The neck of the talus remains short and points medially. In addition, the body of the talus loses height, particularly posteriorly, and becomes wedge shaped [10]. This results in an apparent equinus position of the talus and will

make the results of posterior release very unpredictable.

2. Fixed forefoot supination. Soft tissue tethering of the bony link mechanism has already been discussed. If this has not been corrected at the time of soft tissue release, apparent correction of the deformity can be achieved by a dorso-lateral subluxation of the navicular on the talus. Such a correction elevates the first ray which can only be brought to the ground by eversion of the hind foot and flexion of the MP joints. This produces a dorsal bunion and prominence of the navicular which can be seen laterally in the region anterior to the ankle. Clinically, fixed forefoot supination is recognized by noting a prominence of the head of the first metatarsal dorsally, a hallux flexus and varus deformities of the lateral toes. In addition, there is a persisting subluxation of the calcaneo-cuboid joint with adaptive remodelling of the joint surface which will result in an incongruous joint if it is released. Calcaneo-cuboid fusion (Dilwyn-Evans procedure [11]) is required for such cases.

3. The talo-calcaneal joint. Radical release of the talo-calcaneal joint may result in a valgus subluxation with over-correction. This has been

documented by Fahrenbach *et al.* [12] and Ghali *et al.* [13], and in the majority of cases this valgus deformity compensates for forefoot supination.

Clinical assessment of the fixed deformities

Swann *et al.* [4] were the first to report the presence of a concealed external rotation deformity in a number of feet with a relapsed club foot deformity (Figs 2.8, 2.9 and 2.10). This concealed external rotation deformity demonstrated by palpation of the medial and lateral malleoli represents the end of the first phase of dorsiflexion where the second phase is blocked by the effect of tight tissues. In addition to the concealed external rotation deformity, a number of other fixed deformities may be present and concealed. Fixed equinus is masked by recurvatum in the knee and often recognized by a slight apparent valgus deformity in the knee (Figs 2.8 and 2.9). When the child stands this valgus is also associated with external rotation of the leg, confirming that it is compensating for deformity of the forefoot. Turning the knee and ankle forward reveals the full extent of the forefoot deformity. Fixed fore-

foot supination is best observed with the foot off the ground when with the heel in the neutral position there is a rotatory supination of the forefoot. When the child stands, however, the heel goes into valgus and the great toe flexes to compensate for the elevation of the first ray producing a dorsal bunion and a compensatory varus deformity of the lateral toes (Fig. 2.8). This deformity is seldom seen in the untreated foot. Where there has been previous extensive soft tissue release the supination deformity may be masked by fixed valgus in the hind foot secondary to lateral displacement of the calcaneum on the talus. The cardinal sign in such cases is fixed valgus of the hind foot with the heel outside the line of weight bearing when the child stands. Fixed cavus which has already been described in relation to the untreated foot may be observed and grossly exaggerated in the treated or relapsed foot (Figs 2.9 and 2.10).

A method of examination

With a working knowledge of the anatomy of dorsiflexion and where to find the concealed rota-

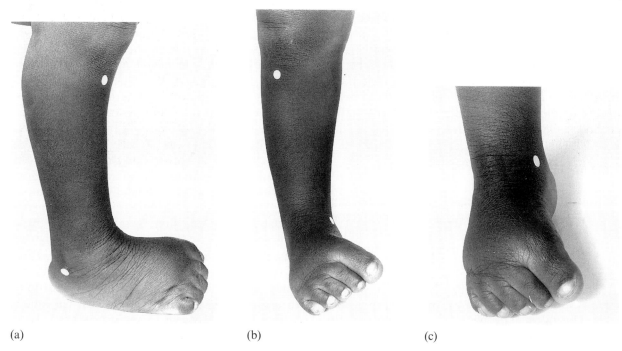

(a)   (b)   (c)

Fig. 2.8   (a–c) Photographs of a child's foot with residual deformity. Note the anterior position of the medial malleolus; posterior position of the lateral malleolus; and the external position of the leg and knee are shown. Fixed forefoot supination is also present with flexion of the great toe.

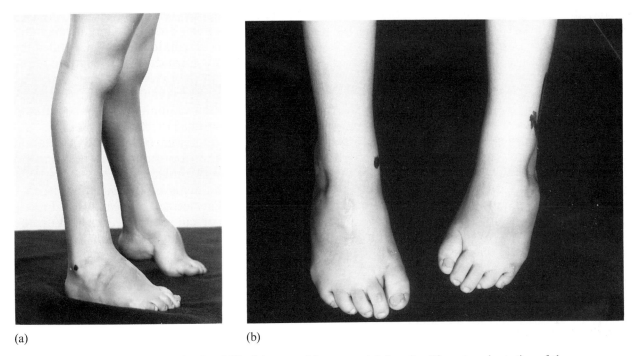

(a) (b)

Fig. 2.9 (a,b) Clinical photograph of a child of 4 years with recurrent deformity. The external rotation of the hindfoot, recurvature of the knee is noted compensating and the fixed equinus is observed.

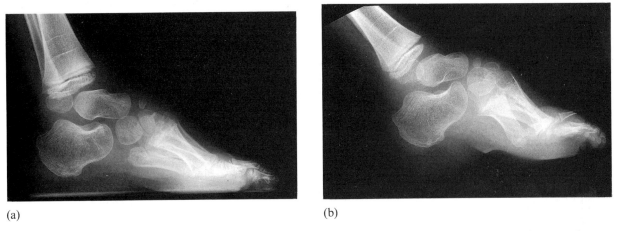

(a) (b)

Fig. 2.10 Lateral radiographs of the child in Fig. 2.9. (a) As the child stands, (b) true lateral of the ankle. Note that the 'flat topped talus' in (a) became normal in (b) revealing the rotatory deformity present.

tory deformities it is now possible to establish a method of examination for a child, initially at presentation and subsequently at follow-up. Implicit in this method of examination must be the production of observations which are 'observer independent' (Table 2.1) [30,31]; these are signs which may be made without observer bias and provide a language for discussion of cases. They are therefore reproducible.

Assessment should begin with the child in general and only later proceed to the feet. Is there a generalized anomaly or a recognized syndrome (Tables 2.2 and 2.3)? Specific attention should be paid to the spine for evidence of spinal dysraphism which would suggest a neurological cause for the foot deformity. The hips must be carefully examined for instability in the neonatal period and for restriction of abduction in flexion in the

Table 2.1 The observer-independent observations

1. Fixed equinus

2. Lateral malleolus
   – position
   – mobility

3. Creases
   – medial
   – posterior
   – anterior

4. Foot
   – lateral border curved or straight?
   – correctable in equinus

5. Changes on dorsiflexion

6. Fixed forefoot deformity
   – cavus
   – supination

Table 2.2 Congenital syndromes with CTEV

Arthrogryposis multiplex congenita
Diastrophic dwarfism
Spina bifida and spinal dysraphism
Larsen syndrome

Table 2.3 General assessment of CTEV

1. Is there a congenital anomaly?

2. The spine
   – scoliosis?
   – dysraphism?

3. The hips – congenital dislocation?

4. Generalised joint laxity?

older child. Restricted hip movements may be associated with congenital dislocation of the hip but are also seen in children with a neurological deficit. It is convenient at this stage to note the general laxity of the joints, as if this is marked it is often associated with the problem of false correction during treatment.

Examination of the leg

Examination is now turned to the feet. In the baby, the feet should be examined with the hips and knees flexed in order to orientate the tibia. In the older child this is more easily assessed with the child sitting. The tibia is orientated by palpation of the tibial tubercle, and medial and lateral malleoli (Fig. 2.11a). Having identified the plane of the ankle joint and the orientation of the tibia, the head of the talus is now palpated (Fig. 2.11b) and the posterior tubercle of the calcaneum. This will establish the position of the hind foot and the presence of fixed equinus.

Having identified the position and orientation of the hind foot the foot should now be examined to establish the relationship of forefoot to hind foot. This is best achieved by observing the foot from below. The lateral border of the foot is either straight or curved (Fig. 2.11c). With the foot in full equinus and the tendons relaxed can the lateral border of the foot if curved be brought straight by gentle manipulation (Fig. 2.11d)? If this does occur the head of the talus should be palpated to see if it becomes covered by the navicular and the space between the navicular and medial malleolus felt to be sure that there is movement of the navicular away from the medial malleolus (Fig. 2.11e). The presence of these signs implies a mobile and reducible mid-tarsal joint.

Only at this stage should an attempt be made to dorsiflex the foot. As the normal foot dorsiflexes from the position of a full equinovarus three observations are recorded. The lateral malleolus moves forward, a gap appears between the navicular and the medial malleolus, and the posterior border of the ankle changes from bulbous to straight.

Failure of these signs to be present implies that normal dorsiflexion is not occurring and the point at which this block occurs is noted (Fig. 2.11f). On occasions the foot appears to reach the plantarflexed position but the shape of the heel does not change and a crease appears on the anterior aspect of the ankle. This foot is breaking in the mid-tarsal joint with the hind foot remaining in the plantargrade position, producing the so-called 'rocker bottom foot'. An X-ray taken of the foot in maximal dorsiflexion will confirm this. Finally, a general neurological examination is performed looking for evidence of neurological abnormality particularly in the lower limb.

Gait

Only after this detailed examination of the foot should the child be observed walking and run-

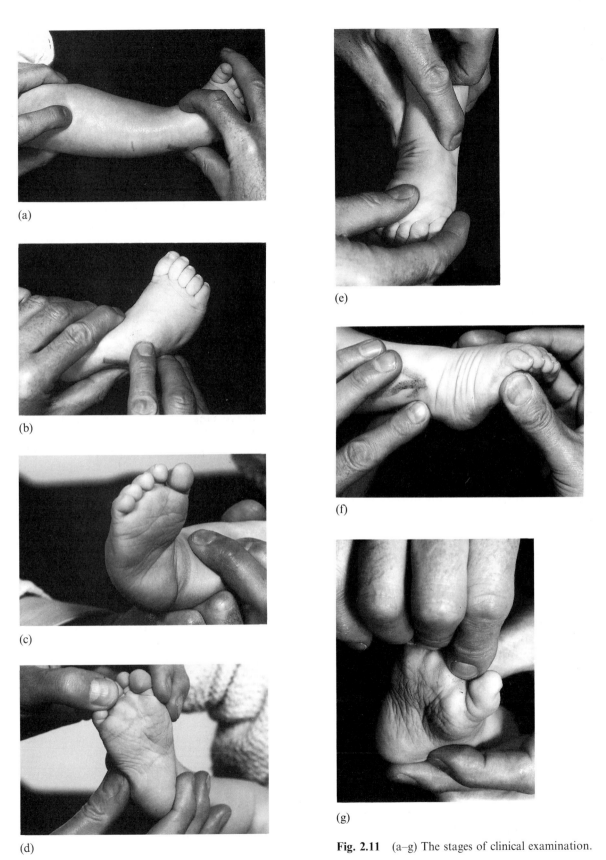

Fig. 2.11 (a–g) The stages of clinical examination.

Table 2.4   Reproduced with permission from *Clinical Orthopaedics*

Type of foot	Resolving pattern	Tendon contracture	Joint contracture	False correction
Observation				
Fixed equinus	No	Yes	Yes	Yes
Lateral malleolus				
– position	Anterior	Anterior	Posterior	Posterior
– mobility	Yes	Yes	No	Yes
Creases				
– posterior	No	Yes	Yes	Yes
– medial	No	No	Yes	No
– anterior	±	No	No	Yes
Lateral border				
– curved or straight	Straight	Curved	Curved	Rooker Bottom
– correctable	Yes	Yes	No	Yes
Cavus	No	±	Yes	No
Supination	No	No	±	No

ning. The position of the knee in walking will show the degree of the fixed or postural external rotation of the leg and the recurvatum describes the degree of concealed equinus. Commonly, the forefoot varus increases with exercise but will reduce as the child stands. Simple muscle testing will establish whether the child can stand on its toes and heels.

Conclusions

At the end of this examination which has included a careful assessment of any neurological deficit the clinician should be able to identify four types of foot deformity (Table 2.4); resolving pattern, tendon contracture, joint contracture and a false correction. The last variety is a form of tendon contracture and is an absolute indication for a posterior release in view of the hypermobility of the joints in the mid tarsal area. In a tendon contracture the hind foot remains locked by tightness of the tibialis posterior and Achilles tendon and tethering of the lateral malleolus; the forefoot is mobile with the foot in full equinus. Such a foot is suitable for a posterior release. The presence of fixed deformity in the forefoot will require a more extensive posterior and medial release if all the tethers present are to be corrected.

Management

Traditionally, the primary management of the club foot deformity at birth is conservative by the use of manipulation and either plaster of Paris or strapping splintage. If the results of this primary management are, however, reviewed [13–15], it will be found that some form of operative procedure will be required during treatment in between 40% and 90% of cases (Table 2.5). With this high failure rate of primary treatment the question has to be asked as to whether this primary treatment does more harm than good.

Table 2.5

	No. of feet	Operations
Harrold *et al.* [14]	129	52
Lavaage *et al.* [15]	104	57
Ghali *et al.* [13]	$\frac{94}{327}$	$\frac{74}{183}$ (56%)

An additional factor in this consideration is the observation that when a child comes without previous treatment after the walking age, although the foot is still in the position of full equinovarus it is seldom stiff, being mobile within the position of deformity. It must be questioned, therefore, whether the stiffness commonly seen in the later stages of treatment is acquired as the result of inadequate treatment.

Few series consider the results of primary treatment in relation to the initial severity. Where this is done [14] three types of primary deformity may be recognized.

1. *A postural deformity*. Here the deformity is mild and the foot can be brought to the plantargrade position by gentle manipulation on the day of birth. Such a foot has no fixed deformity and corresponds to the resolving pattern in previous discussion. Such feet have a high incidence of bilateral involvement and are more common in girls (Table 2.6). Conservative treatment results in a 90% good overall result.

2. *Moderate deformity*. Harrold has defined this group as having 20 of either fixed varus or equinus at the time of primary assessment. Conservative therapy results in between 40% and 50% good results. This type corresponds to the tendon contracture of the previous discussion.

3. *Severe deformity*. This includes all the severe club foot deformities and Harrold has defined them as having more than 20° of fixed varus or equinus at primary presentation. Deep creases are usually found posteriorly and medially and a successful outcome with conservative treatment only occurs in approximately 10% of cases. These correspond to the joint contracture of the previous discussion. If such feet are left untreated at birth the fixed deformities remain unchanged but the foot which is commonly stiff at the time of initial presentation gradually loosens up and this mobilization may be encouraged by gentle manipulation.

It would be a conclusion of the preceding discussion that conservative treatment would undoubtedly be indicated in the postural or resolving type of foot, where the outcome is likely to be extremely satisfactory. In the moderate deformity because there is approximately a 50% chance of success, treatment should be undertaken but reviewed very objectively after a period of 2–3 weeks when if no improvement is occurring in the fixed deformities or particularly if the foot is becoming swollen it should be abandoned in favour of operative treatment which should be delayed until the swelling has resolved and mobility has returned to the foot. This commonly takes approximately 4–6 weeks.

It would, however, be a principle of management that, if the foot without fixed deformity does well in the long term, the object of treatment is to convert a 'joint or tendon contracture' into the 'resolving pattern' by release of the fixed deformities. The risk of inadequate conservative or operative treatment is damage to the cartilage anlage, leading to inevitable deformity of the tarsal bones in the long term.

Form of primary management

Traditionally, there have been two types of primary conservative treatment, in both the foot is manipulated and then splinted. Splintage will either be by plaster of Paris or by strapping (Robert Jones). If the object of treatment is to restore mobility to the foot and overcome fixed deformities, manipulation should be performed as many times a day as possible and this would be an obvious advantage of the splintage by strapping. However, in the newborn foot in which there is a lot of fixed deformity, strapping is often ineffective in holding a position until such time as the forefoot element of the deformity is corrected. In such feet it is the author's practice to

Table 2.6

Group	No.	Fixed deformity	Boys:Girls	Unilateral/bilateral	Successful conservative treatment
I	49	0	18:21	36:13	89%
II	32	<20°	21:11	18:14	46%
III	48	>20°	34:14	32:16	10%

start correction with the foot in equinus with the use of serial plasters which are changed on a twice-a-week basis and then proceed to the use of strapping immobilization once the lateral border of the foot can be brought into the everted position. It is important when applying the serial plasters to be sure that the foot is locked in equinus so that a good stretch can be exerted on the tibialis posterior. As the foot is manipulated pressure is applied over the head of the talus to encourage reduction of the talo-navicular joint. This will have the effect of immobilizing the hindfoot and preventing a false correction from occurring as the result of a twist in the tibia.

Timing of surgical intervention

It is the author's practice to examine the feet on a weekly basis during the course of primary management but formally to assess them in relation to the observer independence signs at 3-weekly intervals. This allows an objective change in position to be noted. Failure of the foot to progress towards the resolving pattern is regarded as an indication for surgical treatment. Where the signs of a tendon contracture (Table 2.4) are observed a tendon release procedure with release of the posterior ankle capsule is indicated [17]. This operation should be regarded as an incident in continuing conservative treatment where a tendon contracture is converted to the resolving pattern. It is therefore undertaken during the course of primary management, and is best performed at approximately 6–8 weeks provided that adequate and competent anaesthesia is available for a child of this age. Where, however, the deformity is more marked and the signs of a joint contracture are present the timing of more radical surgery becomes difficult. There are many reports now in the literature of an early radical operation performed in the first few weeks of life [13,18,19].

The majority of these reports show good results but it is pertinent to ask whether the overall results deteriorate with time and are less likely to be successful if they are undertaken in a child who is perhaps 1 year of age. The reported literature is clear on this point; the results of radical procedure undertaken either in the first few weeks or at approximately 12 months of age are the same. An advantage of the later operation is that the foot is bigger and the operation is technically more simple. It is therefore the author's practice to wait until the child is crawling and showing evidence of wishing to stand before proceeding to a radical soft tissue procedure correcting both the hindfoot and forefoot deformities at one operation.

Siting of incisions for soft tissue procedure

Traditionally the club foot has been approached through a postero-medial incision starting well above the ankle and following the line of the vessels around the medial aspect of the ankle and along the medial side of the foot [20]. Access to the tight medial structures is satisfactory but there is commonly a deep scar tethering the skin to the underlying calcaneum and Achilles tendon. This factor may contribute to recurrent deformity. Healing of the wound is not usually a problem. More recently a number of surgeons, including the author, have been using two incisions, one placed on the postero-lateral aspect of the hindfoot and a second on the medial side of the foot reaching from the calcaneum to the medial malleolus and down the line of the first metatarsal. The advantages of this two-fold incision are that better access is gained to the lateral tissues behind the ankle, particularly the lateral malleolus and its ligaments; in addition, there is an important intact medial skin bridge on the inner side of the ankle. This produces a better cosmetic result. The medially placed incision allows good access to all the tissues which are tight, particularly the plantar fascia.

More recently the Cincinnati incision has been introduced [21]. This incision is currently popular and allows very good access to the subtaloid joint which some surgeons consider to be the most important part of the progressive release [22,23]. It heals well provided that no undue reflection of the distal flaps has occurred. It will, however, be realized that in the majority of late cases the plantar fascia is tight and requires release and it is not uncommon, if a radical release is required for the tissues on the medial side of the ankle, for it to be slow to heal and become necrotic. This incision, however, remains a very useful one provided that there is no undue cavus, and allows good access to the medial, posterior and lateral aspects of the ankle and foot.

Concept of a progressive release of tethers

It has been concluded in the sections on the anatomy of dorsiflexion and pathology that there are a number of tethers, both ligamentous and tendinous which may contribute to the maintenance of the club foot deformity (Fig. 2.6). It has also been suggested that one of the objectives of treatment is to convert the tendon or joint contracture to the 'resolving pattern'. When this later state has been achieved conservative therapy, mainly by manipulation, would finally correct the deformity. In considering surgical correction of these deformities it is suggested that these tethers should be progressively released until an adequate correction has been obtained. In contrast to manipulative therapy, surgical release should start posteriorly by releasing the ankle and lateral structures and by doing so unlock the rotatory element of dorsiflexion. When a joint contracture is present the medial side of the foot should then be approached to release progressively the plantar fascia, the distal attachment of tibialis posterior together with the short and long plantar ligaments, and the talo-navicular joint and the lateral tether between the navicular, cuboid and calcaneum. This last tether will also involve opening the calcaneo-cuboid joint to correct any fixed deformity. Such a protocol of progressive release will not result in over correction as the pivot of rotation between the talus and calcaneum has not been seriously disrupted. Division of the interosseous ligament between the talus and calcaneum with the necessary release of the medial side of the talo-calcaneo joints is liable to lead to progressive subluxation, valgus deformity and the complications of over-correction which have already been eluded to. This is not to say that in some extremely stiff feet, such as those associated with arthrogryposis, such a release may not be necessary but its indications are extremely rare.

A long term review by Green and Lloyd-Roberts [2] have confirmed the observation that in one third of cases coming to surgical treatment only a posterior release was necessary for satisfactory long term results.

In the older child over the age of 4 years where there has been considerable remodelling, both the talo-navicular and calcaneo-cuboid joints are abnormal and radiography shows a fixed medial subluxation of the calcaneo-cuboid joint. In these circumstances a progressive release will not be satisfactory unless the alignment of the calcaneo-cuboid joint is improved. This may be achieved, either by excising the calcaneo-cuboid joint (Dilwyn Evans procedure [11] or alternatively by realigning the joint by removing a wedge from the lateral aspect of the calcaneum. Many surgeons now currently feel that a medial release is not necessary in the Dilwyn Evans procedure but it cannot be stressed too much that the principle of the operation is a medial release coupled with a realignment of the calcaneo-cuboid joint by arthrodesis. The reported results of this operation show good satisfactory long term results, although radiologically the correction is seldom complete. The feet retain good mobility [25,26].

Problem of over-correction

With the more radical procedures that have recently been developed [13,22,23] lateral displacement of the calcaneum may result. Although the deformity is apparently well corrected as the result of these procedures it will be realized from study of the anatomy that the tethers have not necessarily been released, particularly those under the tarsus and metatarsal areas. While in the short term this may not be a problem, in the longer term the valgus in the heel becomes fixed and will result in a painful unstable ankle which is particularly difficult to treat. Over-correction, therefore, must be avoided in the long term and there is no doubt that a supple foot even with mild deformity will be very little trouble in the long term.

Later residual deformity

Following the posterior and postero-medial releases a number of cases will present with a mobile foot which is passively correctable but in which posturally the child walks in varus and supination. Although in many cases this will resolve without further treatment [27], in others the deformity seems to persist. Clinical experience has shown that a tibialis anterior transfer from the medial to the lateral side of the foot is often beneficial in these circumstances [28]. Care must be undertaken in carrying out this procedure that it is not put in tight and great attention must be paid to the joint laxity of the child, as it is not unknown for over-correction to occur in follow-up with the whole foot being pulled into eversion and valgus. Prompt return of the tendon transplant to the mid-line is indicated in these cases.

A number of children, particularly with arthrogryposis, and after repeated surgery remain with stiff deformed feet often with marked equinus. These children are too young for bony operations such as triple arthrodesis but too rigid for soft tissue procedures. Talectomy, in these circumstances, will result in a plantargrade foot of greatly improved shape. The reported results [2,29] are satisfactory. When this operation is performed, it is important to remove a segment from the Achilles tendon and to remove completely the talus without damage to the navicular.

There remain a few children who reach the age of early adolescence with persisting residual deformity in which the heel and forefoot are inside the line of weight bearing and who walk, therefore, in varus taking excessive weight on the lateral border of the foot and often complaining of recurrent ankle instability. These children are well treated by triple arthrodesis, but it is to be hoped that with the present improving understanding of the nature of the club foot, this procedure will become progressively less necessary in the course of time. It remains, however, a useful procedure for the stiff foot with a residual deformity.

References

1. Main, B. J., Crider, R. J., Lloyd-Roberts, G. C., Swann, M. and Kamdar, B. A. (1977) The results of early operation in talipes equino-varus. *J. Bone Joint Surg.*, **59B**, 337–341.
2. Green, A. D. L., Fixsen, J. A. and Lloyd-Roberts, G. C. (1986) Talectomy for arthrogryposis multiplex congenita. *J. Bone Joint Surg.*, **68B**, 697–699.
3. Scott, W. A., Hoskings, S. W. and Catterall, A. (1984) Club foot. Observations on the surgical anatomy of dorsiflexion. *J. Bone Joint Surg.*, **66B**, 71–76.
4. Swann, M., Lloyd-Roberts, G. C. and Catterall, A. (1969) The anatomy of the uncorrected club foot. A study of rotational deformity. *J. Bone Joint Surg.*, **51B**, 263–269.
5. Irani, R. M. and Sherman, M. S. (1963) The pathological anatomy of the club foot. *J. Bone Joint Surg.*, **45A**, 45–52.
6. Carroll, N. C., McMurtry, R. and Leete, S. F. (1978) The patho-anatomy of the congenital club foot. *Orthop. Clin. North Am.*, **9**, 225.
7. Bensahel, H., Hugueria, P. and Thermar-Noel, C. (1983) Functional anatomy of the club foot. *J. Pediatr. Orthop.*, **3**, 191–196.
8. Roberts, J. M. (1985) Personal communication.
9. Handelsman, J. H. E. and Badalamento, M. E. (1981) Neuro-muscular studies in club foot. *J. Pediatr. Orthop.*, **1**, 23–32.
10. Hutchins, P. M., Forster, B. K., Paterson, D. C. and Cole, E. A. (1985) The long-term results of early surgical release in club foot. *J. Bone Joint Surg.*, **67B**, 791–799.
11. Evans, D. (1961) Relapsed club foot. Operative techniques and results in thirty feet. *J. Bone Joint Surg.*, **43B**, 722.
12. Fahrenbach, G. J., Kuchn, D. N. and Tachdjian, M. O. (1983) Occult subluxation of the subtaloid joint in club foot. *J. Pediatr. Orthop.*, **3**, 334–340.
13. Ghali, N. N., Smith, R. B., Clayden, A. D. and Silk, P. F. (1983) The results of pantalar reduction in the management of congenital talipes equinovarus. *J. Bone Joint Surg.*, **65B**, 1–7.
14. Harrold, A. J. and Walker, C. J. (1983) Treatment and prognosis in congenital club foot. *J. Bone Joint Surg.*, **65B**, 8–11.
15. Laaveg, S. I. and Ponseti, N. (1980) Long term results of treatment of congenital club foot. *J. Bone Joint Surg.*, **62A**, 23–31.
16. Kite, J. H. (1964) *The Club Foot*. Grune and Stratton, New York.
17. Williams, D. H., Grant, C. E. P. and Catterall, A. (1987) Postero-lateral release for resistant club foot: early clinical results. *J. Bone Joint Surg.*, **69B**, 155.
18. Pous, J. G. and Dimeglio, A. (1978) Neonatal surgery in club foot. *Orthop. Clin. North Am.*, **9**, 233–240.
19. Ryoppy, S. and Sairanen, H. (1983) Neonatal operation, treatment of club foot. *J. Bone Joint Surg.*, **65**, 320–325.
20. Turco, V. J. (1981) *Club Foot: (Current Problems in Orthopaedics)*. Churchill-Livingstone, New York, Edinburgh, London, Melbourne.
21. Crawford, A. H., Marxen, J. L. and Osterfeld, D. L. (1982) The Cincinnati incision. A comprehensive approach for surgical procedures of the foot and ankle in childhood. *J. Bone Joint Surg.*, **64A**, 1355-1358.
22. McKay, D. W. (1983) New concept of and approach to club foot treatment (Section III). *J. Pediatr. Orthop.*, **3**, 141–148.
23. Simons, G. W. (1985) Complete subtalar release in club feet. *J. Bone Joint Surg.*, **67A**, 1044–1055.

24. Green, A. D. L. and Lloyd-Roberts, G. C. (1985) The results of early posterior release in the resistant club foot. A long term review. *J. Bone Joint Surg.*, **67B**, 588–593.

25. Tayton, K. J. J. and Thompson, P. (1979) Relapsing club foot. Late results of delayed operation. *J. Bone Joint Surg.*, **61B**, 474–480.

26. Addison, A., Fixsen, J. A. and Lloyd-Roberts, G. C. (1983) A review of the Dilwyn-Evans type of collateral operation in severe club feet. *J. Bone Joint Surg.*, **65B**, 12–14.

27. Wynne-Davies, R. (1964) Club foot? A review of eighty-four cases after completion of treatment. *J. Bone Joint Surg.*, **46B**, 53.

28. Kernohan, J. G., Kavanagh, T. G., Fixsen, J. A. and Lloyd-Roberts, G. C. (1985) A long term review of tibialis anterior transfer in congenital club foot. *J. Bone Joint Surg.*, **67B**, 490.

29. Hsu, L. C. S., Jaffrey, D. and Leong, J. C. Y. (1986) Talectomy for club foot in arthrogryposis. *J. Bone Joint Surg.*, **68B**, 694–696.

30. Catherall, A. (1991) A method of assessment of the club foot. *Clinical Orthopaedics and Related Research*, **264**, 225–232.

31. Catherall, A. (1994) Early assessment and management of the club foot. In *Children's Orthopaedics and Fractures* (M. D. K. Bewson, J. A. Fixsen and M. F. Macnicol, eds), Edinburgh: Churchill Livingston.

3

The surgical treatment of congenital displacement of the hip joint

J. A. Wilkinson

In a consecutive series of 201 infants between 10 months and 3 years of age, a two-stage surgical programme has evolved over the past 20 years. At the time of initial reduction, any soft tissue impediment is removed before the joint is splinted in flexion and abduction for 6 months to stimulate any growth potential for bony congruity and stability. Then the child is allowed to extend and medially rotate both legs and also take full weight for a further 6 months. Any muscle imbalance, articular incongruity or instability developing during this trial period is corrected by the realignment of the bony components, 1 year following the initial reduction.

The response to this surgery has been under constant review up to skeletal maturity. This assessment is confined to the first 117 patients with 140 displaced hip joints, who were treated between 1965 and 1980. Factors that have complicated and influenced the outcome of treatment have been investigated and assessed.

Introduction

The assessment of conservative treatment in a similar series of infants [1] reveal that the commonest cause of failure was due to re-displacement of the hip, either during the period of splintage or later. This failure resulted from eccentric reduction of the femoral head, often combined with fragmentation of the proximal femoral epiphysis. Those patients with a family history of congenital displacement of the hip

(CDH) were prone to do badly and infants with genetic acetabular dysplasia also failed to respond to conservative treatment.

Ludloff [2] was the first to record dissatisfaction concerning the results of conservative treatment, 'because even some early cases treated expertly failed to respond'. He found that many hips redislocated once the plaster cast or splints were removed and he claimed that his anatomical dissections of dislocated hip joints revealed variations from the normal structure which were responsible for the failure of conservative treatment. They included the infolding of the limbus and the interposition of the capsule, which were thought to be more frequent hindrances to closed reduction and retention than previously believed and were best eliminated by open operation. Ludloff also described the contracture of the anterior capsule and felt this to be another cause of reluxation, advocating its incision at the time of arthrotomy through an antero-inferior approach to the intra-articular structures.

Putti [3] first advised gentle stretching of such capsular contractures using a portable splint or divaricator which imposed a gradual degree of abduction on both legs. He claimed that his method reduced 95% of CDH in patients under the age of 12 months, and produced a perfect functional result. Later on, traction was added to abduction by various authorities [4,5]. The same concept of atraumatic reduction of the dislocated hip in an infant was developed by Scott [6] using a horizontal frame which he claimed reduced the prevalence of epiphysitis to less than 10%. The

Wingfield frame became a popular appliance, but it had to be tailored to fit each individual which restricted its use to orthopaedic centres with appliance workshops. The management called for specialized nursing care and many children had to be sedated in the earlier stages. They were kept on their frames up to 2 months and even then it was sometimes necessary to apply cross-traction to bring the femoral head down to the level of the acetabulum so as to attain a satisfactory reduction.

Somerville [7] found that the majority of patients thus reduced required surgery to gain concentric reduction and this prevented re-dislocation. He used a restricted anterior arthrotomy on the dislocatable hip, the laxity of the capsular ligaments allowing him to displace the femoral head downward to reveal the limbus at the back of the joint. Following its excision, stable reduction was best maintained by splinting the hip in extension, abduction and medial rotation, but this had to be followed by a lateral rotation femoral osteotomy 6–9 weeks later to maintain reduction and sometimes the osteotomy had to be repeated to prevent the femoral head resubluxing out of the acetabulum.

Fergusson [8] revived Ludloff's approach as a primary surgical reduction without preoperative traction, as he felt the latter was responsible for the enlargement and inversion of the limbus. He also found it necessary to splint the hip in abduction, extension and medial rotation, being led to believe that the Lorenz position produced pathological changes in the splinted hip joint. He did not find that the ligamentum teres or the limbus were obstacles to his surgical reduction. Others using his technique have encountered recurrent instability after the removal of the splint and have found it necessary to perform either pelvic or femoral osteotomies to prevent any residual subluxation [9–11].

So it appears that there are three primary requirements to attain atraumatic and concentric reduction and stabilization of an established congenitally displaced hip joint in the infant.

1. A release of the contracture of the anteromedial capsule, either by gentle stretching or by surgical incision.
2. A restricted arthrotomy to excise any soft tissue impediment causing eccentric reduction, so preventing undue pressure on the acetabulum and femoral head.
3. A period of postoperative splinting in flexion and abduction maintains concentric reduction and stimulates reciprocal bone growth of the femoral head and acetabulum, lowering the risk of residual subluxation and dislocation when the child is freed.

Bony realignment is usually necessary and is best performed during the second or third year of life in the majority of patients as the pelvis is thicker and more stable at that stage. A year after reduction, there is usually radiological evidence of persistent acetabular dysplasia on the side of dislocation. This is sometimes associated with varying degrees of subluxation but rarely with redislocation.

Selection of patients

There were 251 established dislocations in infants aged from 10 months to 3 years and 60% were girls. They formed a consecutive series, 30%

Table 3.1   Number of infants presenting with established CDH between 1965 and 1985

Group	Year treated	Length of follow-up	Number of patients treated	Number of CDH	Percentage		
					Right	Left	Bilateral
A	1965–70	15 yrs +	21	25	20	56	24
B	1970–75	10–15 yrs	42	51	17	49	34
C	1975–80	5–10 yrs	54	64	24	48	28
D	1980–85	< 5 yrs	84	111	29	23	49
	Totals		201	251			

being diagnosed in the first 2 months of life but failing to respond to early treatment; another 30% presented between 2 and 12 months, but 40% were not diagnosed until the second year of life [12] (see Table 3.1).

After the first 2 months, most displacements had become established or permanent. It was policy to delay treatment until the proximal femoral epiphysis had appeared radiologically, because this not only established the diagnosis, but also appeared to reduce the complications of epiphysitis in response to treatment. Similar observations have been made in other series [13].

In unilateral cases, the degree of acetabular development on the non-dislocated side, assessed by measuring the acetabular angle predicts the potential for spontaneous acetabular recovery on the side of dislocation [1].

On admission, careful examination was undertaken to exclude those infants with scars on the buttock caused by a previous septic arthritis [14], and also those with stigmata of spinal dysraphism including abnormal sacral hair distribution, local pigmentation and lipomata. Other signs of neuromuscular hypoplasia included calf wasting, calcaneo-valgus or cavus deformities of the foot and inequality of foot size. The presence and degree of familial joint laxity in both upper and lower limbs is significant especially in familial cases and may complicate treatment. It is important to question the parents repeatedly concerning any family history of CDH for when this is present, it gives a poor prognosis to the outcome of treatment and calls for greater vigilance at all stages of management.

Treatment

The child is first examined under general anaesthesia to assess whether the hip is reducible and also to detect any degree of adductor contracture. The latter can be released by tenotomy so that subsequent traction is applied directly to the capsular contracture without any hindrance. It is important to record the reducibility of the hip before and after tenotomy, and to assess the stability of reduction before and after the period of traction, when the hip is re-examined under anaesthesia. Most hips are found to be reducible but unstable at the beginning of treatment. Some may be irreducible, even after adductor teno-

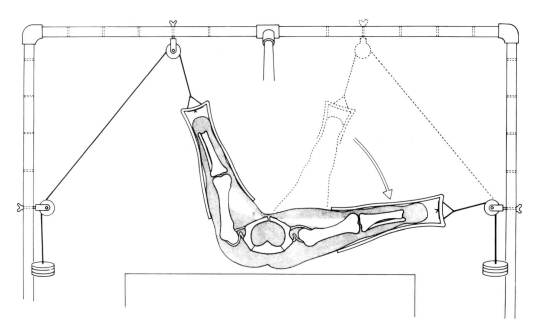

Fig. 3.1 Diagram of traction apparatus illustrating the two primary soft tissue impediments to reduction including infolding of the posterior capsule and a contracture of the anterior capsule. Correction of the latter allows eccentric reduction at the end of traction (previously published by Springer, [19]).

tomy, but this does not contraindicate traction as stretching of the capsular contracture often facilitates reduction (Fig. 3.1).

Traction

A simple form of balanced and vertical traction has been used over the past 20 years with a frame similar to the gallows frame [15], but wider to allow gradual abduction of both legs. The method is not unique as various forms of vertical traction have been used by others to reduce CDH [15–18]. The technique has been described [19] and has proved to be successful in the majority of infants providing a very low prevalence of femoral epiphysitis.

At the end of the 3- to 4-week traction period, the child is again examined under anaesthesia to assess the degree of initial reduction and the stability of the joint, the patients falling into three groups.

Group 1 comprised 15% of hips which reduced and proved to be non-dislocatable at the end of traction. If there was any doubt about the degree and stability of reduction, an arthrogram confirmed its concentricity (Fig. 3.2). If the hip was not dislocatable at the beginning of traction and remained stable at the end, the infants were allowed free without splinting but they were fol-

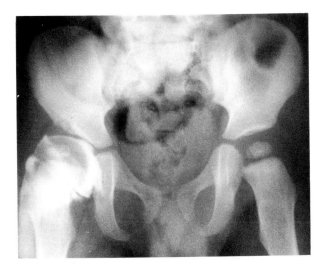

Fig. 3.2 Arthrogram of hip at the end of traction, stable reduction, the hip remaining non-dislocatable the arthrogram shows concentric reduction with no infolding of the limbus.

lowed up at regular intervals. Most recovered spontaneously, turning out to be cases of apparent displacement [20]. They have been excluded from the series.

If the hip was unstable at the beginning of traction, but stabilized during the treatment, the child was splinted in a Denis Browne harness for 6 months. The majority of these patients were found to have persistent radiological dysplasia a year after reduction and became candidates for pelvic osteotomy to stabilize the joint. At the time of surgery, the hip was explored and it was usual to find a small infolded limbus between the femoral head and the acetabulum. This impediment was extracted from the acetabulum and excised. These were genuine cases of CDH and have been included in the series.

Group 2 comprised 83% of hips that were unstable at the beginning of traction and remained so at the end, i.e. the hips were reducible but dislocatable. Arthrography showed that this was due to eccentric reduction and the impediment was a large infolded limbus between the femoral head and acetabulum. Pooling of the dye on the floor of the acetabulum confirmed the degree of eccentric reduction (Fig. 3.3). Posterior arthrotomy and excision of the limbus was preferred at this stage rather than providing a trial reduction; thus concentric reduction of the head was achieved and stabilized by the plication of the lax posterior capsule, before the hip was splinted in a Lorenz plaster with the thighs flexed above a right angle and abducted 70° (Fig. 3.4).

The child was sent home and 2 months later the plaster was replaced by a Denis Browne harness (Fig. 3.5) which was retained for a further 4 months, maintaining concentric reduction in flexion and neutral rotation. The child was allowed free at 6 months after reduction and quickly regained a normal standing posture and gait.

In bilateral hip displacement, when both hips remain dislocatable at the end of the traction, posterior arthrotomy was performed on each hip at the same time. The postoperative management was similar to that of unilateral cases.

Group 3 consisted of a very few cases that failed to reduce on vertical traction because of soft tissue impediment. In such cases, neither anterior nor posterior restricted arthrotomy should be attempted. It is better to undertake a formal surgical open reduction through an

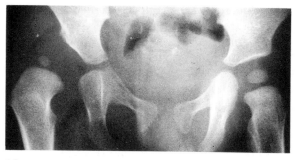

(a)

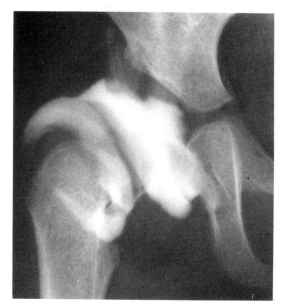
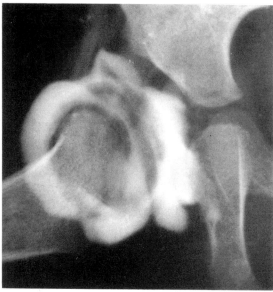

(b)

Fig. 3.3   (a) Right CDH presenting at 12 months with total displacement of femoral head into the upper and outer quadrant. (b) Arthrogram at the end of reduction revealing infolding of the limbus causing eccentric reduction of the femoral head. The hip was reducible but dislocatable and reduction was unstable due to the eccentricity of the femoral head.

anterolateral approach as described by Salter [21]. This allows an extensive incision of the capsule to provide unrestricted access to the acetabulum. It is usual to find a large circumferential limbus extending across the acetabulum, creating a total obstruction to the reduction of the femoral head. The ligamentum teres is usually intact and leads through a central hiatus in the limbus to the underlying bony acetabulum. Excision of the limbus reveals a bony acetabulum which is usually normal in size and depth, well able to accept a concentrically reduced femoral head. The hip is again splinted in a Lorenz plaster and the further care is as previously described.

Posterior arthrotomy

Should only be performed on hips that are dislocatable after the period of traction, as the aim is to reduce and stabilize the eccentrically reduced femoral head (group 2). It is unnecessary in patients whose hips are non-dislocatable at the end of traction, as the reduction is stable and it would also be difficult to displace the head out of the acetabulum to gain sufficient access to excise the limbus. It is important to proceed to posterior arthrotomy before any splints are applied to the child, as eccentric reduction can cause damage to both bony components. The posterior approach

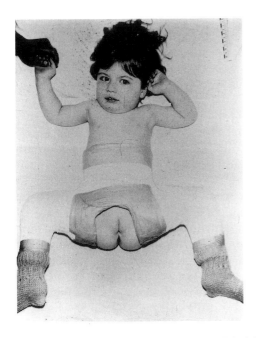

Fig. 3.4 Lorenz plaster (previously published by Springer, [19]).

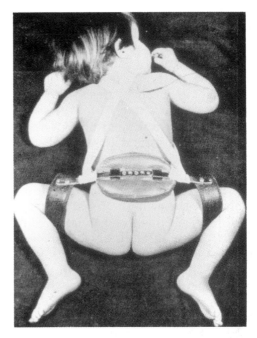

Fig. 3.5 Denis Browne harness (previously published by Springer, [19]).

has been developed to provide a direct access to the limbus which lies posteriorly. It provides an unimpeded view of the limbus allowing its complete excision, and also plication of the lax posterior capsule to stabilize the concentric reduction. It is not a major procedure and does not necessitate blood transfusion.

The child is placed in the lateral position with the affected hip upward and the affected leg is prepared and draped separately to allow free manipulation. The femoral head is reduced into the acetabulum and the hip is half flexed before making a 4-cm incision extending obliquely upward and backward above the tip of the greater trochanter. Splitting of the gluteus maximus reveals the posterior edge of the gluteus medius. This is retracted upward to reveal the gluteus minimus and piriformis tendon. These two structures are separated and stripped from the underlying capsule before being retracted superiorly and inferiorly, respectively. A blunt hook is placed under the tip of the greater trochanter to apply lateral traction and then the rim of the acetabulum can be felt deep to the posterior capsule.

An incision in the capsule, parallel, but 0.5 cm lateral to the rim of the acetabulum, releases any excess fluid in the joint. The incision is extended superiorly and inferiorly to allow the retractors to be placed within the joint. The blunt hook previously placed under the greater trochanter is replaced to retract the lateral edge of the capsule. The medial edge is incised at its mid-point at right angles to the previous incision to reveal the base of the limbus. Another blunt hook is introduced into the acetabulum around the free edge of the limbus to retract it out of the joint. It also defines the attachment of the limbus to the rim of the acetabulum, facilitating the complete excision along the limbus. The upper half is first detached and then the inferior part. Sometimes the limbus is adherent to the posterior articular surface of the acetabulum and has to be gently lifted off by blunt dissection. Occasionally, it is in two layers, the more superficial one lying free but the deeper one remaining adherent to the articular surface. Each layer has to be removed under direct vision. Never incise the capsule towards the base of the greater trochanter, as this will disrupt the arterial supply to the femoral head. Do not excise excess capsule, but reef the capsule by placing deep absorbable sutures well away from the edges; this reefing will take up the capsular hood and stabilize the reduction of the femoral head. It is not necessary to excise the ligamentum teres, as it never appears to obstruct reduction. Superficial sutures are placed in the fascia of the gluteus maximus, and the wound edges are closed with a subcuticular absorbable suture.

When both hips are dislocatable, one is explored and then the wound is sealed, before turning the child to perform the same procedure on the opposite side.

Postoperatively, the child is placed on the plaster frame in the supine position and both legs are flexed above a right angle and are allowed to abduct to their full extent. The lower legs are held in neutral rotation. It is necessary to test the reduction and stability of both hips before applying the wool and plaster and this must be done by the surgeon himself, as he is responsible for making sure that neither joint has redislocated. Failure to maintain reduction at this stage may have disastrous consequences, as the displaced femoral head becomes adherent to the capsular incision and makes further attempts at closed reduction impossible. Thus it is the most important step in the surgical management.

Postoperative radiographs confirm reduction (Fig. 3.6). The child is sent home and the plaster maintained for 8 weeks, allowing the capsular incision to heal and the joint to stabilize. It is then replaced with a Denis Browne abduction harness which will maintain reduction and also allow controlled movements to stimulate the develop-ment of the acetabulum and femoral head. It is retained for 4 months and then the child is allowed free to extend and medially rotate the thighs and weight bear on the leg. Within 4–6 weeks, the child is usually running around without a limp or any clinical evidence of previous displacement of the hip joint.

The initial response to gradual concentric reduction followed by 6 months of abduction splinting has to be assessed 1 year from the outset of treatment, as it is then decided whether to proceed to correct any residual incongruity of the bony components. At this stage, all but four of the 117 children in the series were walking normally and running without a limp. Two children redislocated one of their hips and two children developed abductor contractures producing apparent lengthening of the leg. The other children appeared quite normal and there was little evidence of stiffness of the affected joints.

Radiological assessment at 1 year from the onset of treatment was more critical. It confirmed the two redislocations which were due to extreme degrees of familial joint laxity, but there was evidence of residual subluxation or lateral drift in another 15 hips, i.e. 10% of the series. In five of these patients, the residual subluxation appeared to be due to a combination of genetic acetabular dysplasia and joint laxity, whereas 14 revealed no overt evidence to account for the instability.

In 10 of the hips, the femoral epiphysis lost some of its definition and appeared to undergo a mild degree of epiphysitis but there was no actual deformity or loss of epiphyseal height.

All the hips showed evidence of persistent acetabular dysplasia with increase of the acetabular angle above the normal standards of development (Fig, 3.7) [1]. Pelvic osteotomy was performed routinely 1 year following reduction as it was found that any delay tended to allow the

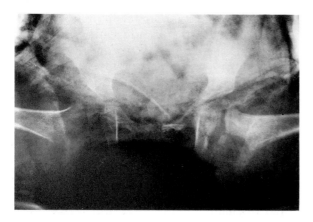

Fig. 3.6 Postoperative reduction, femoral head concentrically reduced following posterior arthrotomy. Patient in Lorenz plaster.

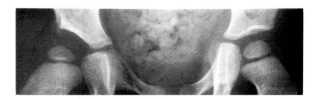

Fig. 3.7 Radiograph 1 year following posterior arthrotomy, right hip concentrically reduced but persistent acetabular dysplasia.

development of coxa magna and it was then difficult to obtain good acetabular cover following osteotomy.

Bony realignment (pelvic osteotomy)

In a previous assessment of the results of conservative treatment [1], 61% of the infants failed to respond adequately. Femoral head deformity, subluxation and in some cases redislocation, occurred because of severe degrees of epiphysitis secondary to traumatic manipulative reduction. Eccentric reduction also caused early subluxation and redislocation. In the 40% of patients whose hips were not damaged and were concentrically reduced, nearly half ended up with shallow hips (grade 2 and 3 results) which was thought at the time to be due to genetic acetabular dysplasia, especially in the unilateral cases.

In the present series, the above iatrogenic factors have almost been eliminated and concentricity of reduction has been attained by posterior arthrotomy and excision of the limbus. To improve on the 40% good results of conservative treatment, all the hip joints treated in this series have been subjected to routine pelvic osteotomy performed a year from reduction, i.e. after the child had been walking freely for 6 months. This period of freedom was found to be necessary, not only to ensure the normal development of femoral anteversion but also to observe the development of the femoral epiphysis following reduction.

As the child extended and medially rotated the hips following the removal of the abduction Denis Browne harness, taking full weight on the legs for the first time, the medial torsion placed on the proximal thirds of the femurs stimulated the development of the normal degree of femoral anteversion (approximately 30°). The postural torsion is normally transmitted to the acetabulum, but in previously dislocated hips the residual laxity of the capsular ligaments prevented this, resulting in a persistence of the primary acetabular retroversion. The combination of femoral anteversion and acetabular retroversion institutes the incongruity of the bony components with resulting instability (Fig. 3.8). Congruity of the bony components can be attained by either performing a lateral rotation femoral osteotomy or a pelvic osteotomy. The

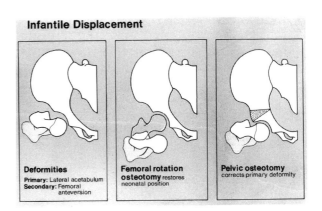

Fig. 3.8 Diagrams demonstrating bony incongruity, combination of acetabular retroversion and femoral anteversion with correction by femoral osteotomy and pelvic osteotomy (previously published by Springer, [19]).

former retroverts the femur and allows it to become congruous with the acetabular retroversion, while the latter anteverts the acetabulum to accommodate the normal degree of femoral anteversion.

Pelvic (innominate) osteotomy has been preferred in this series for a number of functional and cosmetic reasons. The technique previously described [19] not only reorientates the retroverted acetabulum outward and forward to improve the cover of the femoral head, but it also decompresses the bony components of the articulation. This prevents any postoperative stiffness and the development of avascular necrosis (Fig. 3.9).

If posterior arthrotomy had not been performed at the time of reduction, as in the non-dislocatable hip joints (group 1), the opportunity is taken to explore the hip at the time of pelvic osteotomy, as it does not add much to the operative procedure. It is usual to find a thin limbus infolded into the joint and it can be hooked out and excised. In cases of bilateral CDH, a second osteotomy is usually delayed for at least 4 months from the time of the initial pelvic osteotomy.

Postoperatively, a plaster spica is applied with both hips splinted in full extension with 20° of abduction and medial rotation. The latter is maintained on the side of dislocation by extending the plaster distal to the flexed knee joint. The cast is maintained for 6–8 weeks, a longer period being indicated if the capsule has been opened to explore the hip and plicate its lax capsule during which time the child can return home. At the end

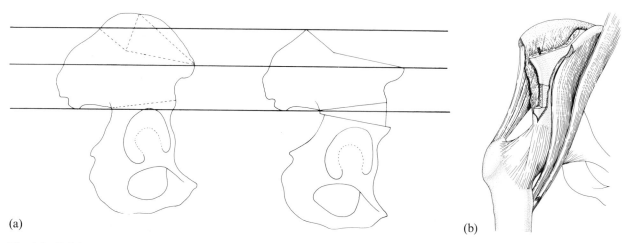

(a)   (b)

Fig. 3.9 Pelvic osteotomy. (a) Diagram showing excision of upper third of iliac crest. (b) drawing of pelvic osteotomy procedure (previously published by Springer, [19]).

of the 6–8 week period, the child is readmitted for removal of plaster, hydrotherapy and medial rotation exercises. The two fixation pins can be removed at that time.

Results

A yearly follow-up has been undertaken until the patients reach full skeletal maturity. When the families have moved away from the area,

arrangements are made for the children to be assessed either locally or return for review (Table 3.2).

Each parent is given a booklet of instruction on the management and assessment and they are warned that the 10–14 year period is the most testing time for the children's hip joints. During this period, the last spurt of skeletal growth occurs and this coincides with the pre-puberty secretion of hormones which produces hormonal joint laxity in the girls. At this age period, loss of

Table 3.2 **Results of surgery radiological results using modified Severin's classification**

Group	Year treated	Length of follow-up	Number of hips treated	Results				
				Successes			Failures	
				1	2	3	4	5
A	1965–70	15 yrs +	25	Perfect	Minimal stigmata	Slight stigmata and dysplasia	Moderate stigmata	Residual subluxation
				12	5	4	4	
				68%		16%	16%	
B	1970–75	10–15 yrs	51	26	11	8	3	3
				72%		16%	12%	
C	1975–80	5–10 yrs	64	27	26	6	1	4
				83%		9%	8%	
D	1980–85	<5 yrs	111	Not assessed for review				

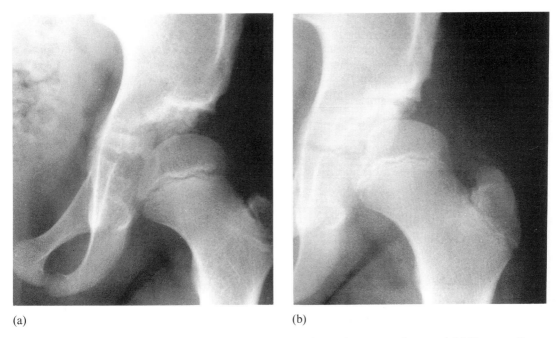

(a) (b)

Fig. 3.10 Late deformity and subluxation of the hip. Result at (a) 6 years of age and (b) 12 years of age. Although the early result was good, the late result showed recurrence of subluxation and loss of epiphyseal height.

epiphyseal height or premature fusion of the physis with or without late subluxation of the hip joint, can occur (Fig. 3.10). Any tendency to subluxate, i.e. those in group 3 (9%), is aggravated by these two factors and it may be necessary to repeat the pelvic osteotomy at this stage.

Yet the majority of patients need no further surgery and they mature with minimal stigmata and no residual instability (Fig. 3.11).

A retrospective review of groups 4 and 5 (8% failures) has revealed that half were due to iatrogenic epiphysitis, usually the result of splinting in

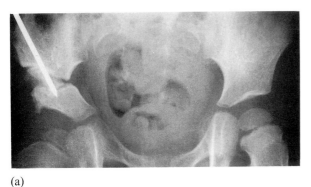

(a)

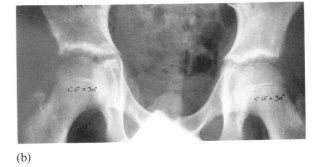

(b)

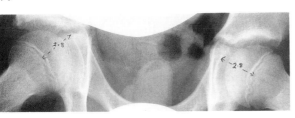

(c)

Fig. 3.11 Late good result from surgery.

the first 3 months of life, and sometimes to a combination of familial genetic factors. In the remaining half, there were no obvious causes for the failure to respond to treatment, but recent research has indicated that there may well be a muscle imbalance in these cases due to occult spinal dysraphism [22].

Discussion

From the very beginning of this surgical programme, it has been accepted that the persistence or establishment of congenital displacement of the hip beyond the first 10 months of life, is invariably due to the presence of an infolded limbus, or fold of posterior capsule, which has prevented spontaneous concentric reduction and recovery [7]. It has been confirmed that eccentric reduction of the femoral head is the commonest cause of redisplacement and epiphysitis following frame reduction, in a previous series treated conservatively. It is now accepted that a plaster cast or splints should never be applied to an infant before one is certain that the head is concentrically reduced in the acetabulum from the very outset of management [23]. It has been found from natural selection, that patients presenting for the first time in whom the radiographs reveal the presence of a femoral epiphysis within a displaced femoral head, respond much better to surgical management. This radiological sign not only confirms that diagnosis of total displacement of the hip joint, but it also indicates that a mature blood supply has developed in the proximal third of the femur. Experimental research has shown that the femoral head is more able to resist compression when the epiphysis occupies one third of the volume of the femoral head. This increases the resistance as compared to that offered by a purely cartilaginous head in the first 6 months of life [24].

It has been suggested previously that abduction on a vertical frame causes infolding of the limbus and its secondary hypertrophy [8], but this has been disproved in a small series of my patients who were simply placed on vertical traction and their legs were not abducted. In each case a limbus was found but the method was not continued, because the anterior capsular contracture was not stretched so effectively and limi-

tation of abduction of the hip persisted in these children.

Somerville [7] claimed to have few cases of epiphysitis in his series and the figures are comparable to the present series. In each the excision of the infolded limbus has been performed routinely on all dislocatable hips through a restricted surgical approach, before the application of splints and without any trial period of reduction. This low incidence of avascular necrosis common to both series (as compared to other series that have not included the routine excision of the limbus, i.e. the 15–30% prevalence reported by Salter, Kostuick and Dallas) is due to the concentricity of reduction and the stability of the hip joint. Truetta [25] pointed out that continuous severe pressure affects the growth by interference of the circulation adjacent to the growing cartilage. This could well explain the dire effect of an infolded limbus in the eccentrically reduced hip joint.

Posterior arthrotomy is preferred to the anterior approach described by Somerville, because it provides direct access to the limbus and allows adequate excision under direct vision and repair of the posterior capsule. It was once suggested that there was a risk to the capsular vessel which might cause an ischaemia of the femoral head, but Tucker [26] found this to be an erroneous view and this series has sustained his belief. Whenever anterior or anteromedial arthrotomy is performed, it is necessary to splint the legs in extension and medial rotation [2,7,8]. This position tends to wind up the capsule and so stabilize the reduction, whereas the Lorenz position relaxes the capsule. In this position, the stability of the femoral head is dependent upon the integrity of the anterior capsule which is intact if a posterior arthrotomy has been performed.

Summary

Thus, the first stage of surgical management is the concentric reduction of the hypoplastic femoral head into the primary acetabulum, involving minimal trauma and disturbance of its blood supply. The measure of the success of the manoeuvre is provided by the radiological appearance of the femoral head and the normal subsequent growth of both bony components.

Adductor tenotomy, controlled abduction with balanced traction on a vertical frame followed by posterior arthrotomy and excision of the limbus in 85% of the displaced hip joints, has proved to be an effective way of gaining concentricity of reduction. The Lorenz position has proved to be a very effective way of retaining concentric reduction over a period of 6 months. In view of the inherent tendency for persistent bony incongruity [27], osteotomy of the pelvis or femur is invariably necessary as a second stage procedure. Pelvic osteotomy has been preferred in this series as the incision leaves a lesser cosmetic blemish, whereas the osteotomy itself not only realigns the two bony components to produce a congrous articulation, but it can also be adjusted to decompress the hip joint and so prevent the late inhibition of epiphyseal growth which leads to permanent coxa plana in the adult hip.

References

1. Wilkinson, J. A. and Carter, C. O. (1960) Congenital dislocation of the hip. *J. Bone Joint Surg.*, **42B**, 652.
2. Ludloff, K. (1913) The open reduction of the congenital hip dislocation by an anterior incision. *Am. J. Surg.*, **10**, 438–454.
3. Putti, V. (1929) Early treatment of congenital dislocation of the hip. *J. Bone Joint Surg.*, **11**, 798–809.
4. Coonse, G. K. (1931) A simple modification of Perthes' splint for the early treatment of congenital dislocation of the hip. *J. Bone Joint Surg.*, **13**, 602.
5. Stewart, W. J. (1934) Further observations on the abduction-traction treatment of congenital dislocation of the hip. *J. Bone Joint Surg.*, **16**, 303.
6. Scott, J. C. (1953) Frame reduction in congenital dislocation of the hip. *J. Bone Joint Surg.*, **35B**, 372.
7. Somerville, E. W. (1953) Development of congenital dislocation of the hip. *J. Bone Joint Surg.*, **35B**, 363.
8. Fergusson, A. B. (1973) Primary open reduction of congenital dislocation of the hip using a median adductor approach. *J. Bone Joint Surg.*, **55A**, 671–689.
9. Tsuchiya, K. and Yamanda, K. (1978) Open reduction of congenital dislocation of the hip in infancy using Ludloff's approach. *Int. Orthop. (SICOT)*, **1**, 337.
10. Lehman, W. B. (1980) Early soft-tissue release in congenital dislocation of the hip. *Isr. J. Med. Sci.*, **16(4)**, 267.
11. Weinstein, S. L. (1980) The medical approach in congenital dislocation of the hip. *Isr. J. Med. Sci.*, **16(4)**, 272.
12. Catford, J. A., Bennet, G. C. and Wilkinson, J. A. (1982) Congenital dislocation: an increasing and still uncontrolled disability? *Br. Med. J.*, **285**, 1527.
13. Tonnis, D. (1982) *Congenital Hip Dislocation – Avascular Necrosis*. Thieme-Stratton, New York.
14. Fairbank, H. A. T. (1934) Congenital dislocation of the hip. *Cambridge University Medical Society Magazine*, **11**, 133.
15. Bryant, T. (1880) On the value of parallelism in the lower extremities in the treatment of hip disease and hip injuries with the best means of maintaining it. *Lancet*, **1**, 159.
16. Salter, R. B., Kostuick, J. and Dallas, S. (1969) Avascular necrosis of the femoral head as a complication of treatment for congenital dislocation of the hip in young children. *Can. J. Surg.*, **12**, 44.
17. Maw, H., Dorr, W. M., Henkel, L. and Lutsche, J. (1971) Open reduction of congenital dislocation of the hip by Ludloff's method. *J. Bone Joint Surg.*, **53A**, 1281–1288.
18. Lloyd-Roberts, G. C. (1971) *Orthopaedics in Infancy and Childhood*, 1st edn. Butterworths, London, p. 213.
19. Wilkinson, J. A. (1985) *Congenital Displacement of the Hip Joint*, Springer, Berlin.
20. Lloyd-Roberts, G. C. and Swann, M. (1966) Pitfalls in the management of congenital dislocation of the hip. *J. Bone Joint Surg.*, **48B(4)**, 666.
21. Salter, R. B. (1961) Innominate osteotomy in the treatment of congenital dislocation and subluxation of the hip. *J. Bone Joint Surg.*, **43B**, 518.
22. Wilkinson, J. A. and Sedgwick, E. M. (1988) Occult spinal dysraphism in established congenital dislocation of the hip. *J. Bone Joint Surg.*, **70B(5)**, 744.
23. Putti, V. (1933) Early treatment of congenital dislocation of the hip. *J. Bone Joint Surg.*, **15**, 16–21.
24. Hall, G. (1985) Personal communication.
25. Truetta, A. (1968) *Studies of the Development and Decay of the Human Frame*. Heinemann, London.
26. Tucker, F. R. (1949) Arterial supply to the femoral head and its clinical importance. *J. Bone Joint Surg.*, **31B**, 82.
27. Platt, H. (1953) Congenital dislocation of the hip. *J. Bone Joint Surg.*, **35B**, 339.

4

Orthopaedic management in spina bifida

E. A. Szalay

Introduction

The incidence of spina bifida is of the order of 1 in 2000 live births [1], making it one of the most common birth defects. Improved management has led to survival of most affected newborns, and a marked increase in adolescents and adults with spina bifida.

The first step in dealing with these children and their parents is realistic goal setting. Factors to be considered include level of neurological impairment, associated anomalies or other health problems, and intellectual and developmental achievements. Using these data, one seeks to maximize the individual potential of each child, without placing undue emphasis on unrealistic achievements. Mobility, activities of daily living, and cosmesis are important goals. Surgery should be prevented if possible; if surgery must be undertaken, hospitalization time and time out of school should be minimized by combining needed procedures into a single anaesthetic.

A myelodysplastic child should be enabled to achieve motor milestones at approximately the same age as does a neurologically normal child: sitting at approximately 6 months of age, standing at 10–12 months, and walking at 12–14 months. Limbs ideally should be free of deformity to allow shoeing and bracing, and appropriate assistive devices, such as corner chairs or standing frames, are provided when indicated.

Mobility

Ideal mobility is the ability to get from one place to another with minimum energy expenditure.

Most young children, regardless of level of neurological involvement, can be taught to 'walk' with braces and walker. Increasing body weight with age requires increased energy expenditure to 'walk' with braces. Many children with paralysis above the L4 level [2] cannot meet the long-term energy requirement for independent ambulation; for these children, ideal mobility is wheelchair ambulation. Our goal is to maximize function; a child in a wheelchair can keep pace with peers and may participate in sports, which cannot be done with braces and crutches.

None the less, ambulation, albeit short-term, is a goal for many children with spina bifida. Intellectual and motor development is encouraged if the child can be taught to stand and walk independently. The upright posture improves postural contractures such as equinus and knee flexion; weight-bearing encourages normal bone density and growth [3]. Most importantly, parents more readily accept the ambulatory limitation of their child if they feel that a reasonable attempt at ambulation has been made.

A number of factors influence ambulatory capability, and must be considered when setting long-range goals. Intelligence, balance, spatial orientation, and spasticity are partially determined by the status of the central neurological axis with respect to hydrocephalus and anomalies of the brain and spinal cord [4–10]; these problems may preclude ambulation even in children with excellent motor function. The level of neurological involvement is the next determining factor: long-term ambulation generally requires strong quadriceps and medial hamstring function, i.e. an L4 neurological level. Thirdly, fixed joint contractures must be addressed by stretching or by surgery to enable bracing; surgical risks must be weighed against long-term ambulatory potential. Last but not least, obesity is often a limiting factor, as many children with myelodysplasia become severely overweight.

Taking all these factors into consideration, emphasis must ultimately be placed on mobility rather than on ambulation *per se*. The concept of wheelchair mobility must be introduced early as a positive rather than a negative potential in those children who are likely to be unsuccessful at long-term community ambulation. Wheelchairs should be provided early for long-distance, independent mobility to those children capable of only household ambulation.

Role of the orthopaedic surgeon

In the perinatal period, the orthopaedic surgeon conducts a careful motor examination, preferably when the child is awake and vigorously active, to establish a baseline for voluntary muscular function. This allows early parental education regarding prognosis, ambulatory potential, and expected problems (Table 4.1) [11]. Stretching exercises and positioning suggestions may be offered. Radiographs of the spine are examined for congenital anomalies other than spina bifida. If congenital scoliosis or kyphosis is noted, its implications are explained to the parents, and plans for careful follow-up are made. The presence or absence of hip dislocations is noted and discussed with parents, along with whether or not treatment is contemplated. The care of anaesthetic skin, the need for long-term weight consciousness, and the importance of neurosurgical and urological care are communicated to the family.

As the child grows, examinations are repeated at appropriate intervals and are compared to the baseline examination, to update prognosis and to watch for neurological deterioration, development of scoliosis, or limb deformity.

Neurological deterioration may take the form of increasing spasticity, loss of motor levels, or change in bowel or bladder control. Shunt malfunction, hydromyelia, diastematomyelia and cord tethering are all potentially treatable causes of neurological deterioration; a high index of suspicion must be maintained to prevent functional loss in an already compromised individual [12].

Sixty to 100% of children with spina bifida develop scoliosis [13] and the orthopaedist must monitor the child carefully for its presence. Its diagnosis and management will be discussed in a later section.

Limb deformity such as congenital club foot and acquired postural or spastic contractures is

Table 4.1   Prediction of functional outcome based on neurological level

Highest functional level	Lower extremity function	Anticipated mobility	Expected problems
Thoracic	No voluntary L.E. motors	Childhood ambulation difficult with HKAFOS; wheelchair by adolescence	'Frog' contracture of hips; poor trunk control; scoliosis/kyphosis
High lumbar (L1–L3)	Functioning hip flexors and adductors	Ambulation in childhood with KAFOS; wheelchair by adolescence	Hip flexion/adduction contracture, knee extension contracture; hip dislocation; lordosis/scoliosis
Low lumbar (L4–L5)	Functioning quadriceps and medial hamstrings; may have tibialis anterior	May be long-term ambulators; require AFOS	Hip subluxation/dislocation; lower extremity torsional problems; calcaneus deformity of feet
Sacral	All muscles function except foot intrinsics	Independent ambulation, usually with no bracing	

noted, and decisions regarding management are made. Cosmetic considerations such as the ability to wear shoes, the desirability or practicality of bracing, and functional expectations are weighed against the physiological and psychological risks of surgical correction.

Lastly, the orthopaedist must coordinate physical and occupational therapy and prescribe and oversee orthotic and mobility aids.

Orthotics

Bracing can stabilize weak joints, help prevent postural contractures, and provide lower extremity and trunk stability to allow independent upper extremity activity. Bracing cannot correct fixed joint deformities nor increase the energy available for ambulation. Braces are hot and encumbering, and make dressing and toileting difficult. Ill-fitting braces may cause pressure sores in insensate skin. For these reasons, the decision to brace and the type of braces must be individualized for each patient.

Orthotics can be fabricated of plastic or of metal. Polypropylene braces can conform exactly to a deformed limb, and are useful in providing total contact to distribute weight and to decrease pressure concentration. They are cosmetically more acceptable because the child can vary shoe wear. However, the plastic braces are hot and often not sturdy enough for a very heavy child.

Metal braces are stronger, cooler, and more appropriate for a heavy child or adolescent. They may be attached to 'space shoes' if plantar ulcers are a problem. The metal uprights and attachment to unsightly 'orthopaedic' shoes make them less cosmetically desirable.

Principles of bracing in spina bifida

In children with neurological levels above L3, the parapodium [3], or standing frame, provides stable support to enable upright positioning of the child from 10 to 18 months old. This encourages head control, allows independent bimanual activity and helps the child develop confidence in the upright position. Some parapodia can be modified for swivel gait as the child gains confidence, or the child may then be fitted for ambulatory braces.

In all but the child with a very low neurological level, children most often benefit by a process of progressive brace weaning. They begin ambulation with a hip-knee-ankle-foot orthosis, i.e. a long leg brace with pelvic band, locked hips, and locked knees. The child then learns progressive control of joints, beginning with a toddler's walker and a swivel or swing-to gait with the hips locked. When this is mastered, the hips are unlocked and reciprocal gait is learned; the pelvic band may then be discarded. If quadriceps strength is sufficient, the child may then unlock the knee hinges, and the thigh pieces are removed when good knee control is achieved. This weaning process allows progressive learning of ambulation, and control of each joint is achieved independently. The type of final bracing is determined by the level of paralysis, with an upper lumbar level child requiring long leg braces, while a lower lumbar level child may wear short leg braces.

The hip

Myelodysplastic hip problems can result from positional contractures, muscle imbalance, or spasticity; establishing the aetiology of the deformity aids in treatment decision making.

Children with very high level or thoracic paralysis often develop a positional 'frog leg' deformity due to the tendency of the flail hip to fall into abduction when the child lies supine or prone. In children with neurological levels of L1 to L4, unopposed hip flexors and adductors commonly produce a flexion/adduction contracture which may progress to subluxation or dislocation. Hydrocephalus, central nervous system injury, or anomaly may cause spasticity; the spastic myelodysplastic hip may assume any of the deformities seen in a child with cerebral palsy.

Whether or not to treat the myelodysplastic posterior hip dislocation remains quite controversial. A dislocated hip in a child with spina bifida is usually not painful and does not prevent bracing or ambulation [14]. The surgical reconstruction of the dislocated hip is extensive, and redislocations have been noted postoperatively in as many as 45% [15]. For these reasons, treatment of the dislocated hip is not indicated in the child with a very high level of paralysis, or if other factors render the child a poor candidate for long-term ambulation.

In the child with excellent long-term ambulatory potential, such as a child with L4 function or below and no spasticity, surgical treatment of the dislocated hip may be considered.

A unilateral hip dislocation poses additional problems. In the ambulatory child, it produces an apparent limb length discrepancy. In the wheelchair-ambulatory child, the role of unilateral hip dislocation in the production of pelvic obliquity and scoliosis has not been clearly defined [16,17]. It has not been shown that treatment of a subluxating or dislocating hip will affect the development of scoliosis.

If, considering these factors, treatment is elected, early soft tissue releases (hip flexors and adductors) may be combined with prolonged night-time bracing in extension and abduction. The Sharrard iliopsoas transfer has been used to balance the hip musculature; some authors feel this procedure has a place in the treatment of the L4 level myelodysplastic. Others, however, feel that iliopsoas tenotomy achieves much the same end with significantly lower surgical morbidity [18].

In the older child with more significant subluxation or frank dislocation, bony procedures may be needed. The 'developmental' dislocation is often not marked by the severe acetabular dysplasia seen in congenital dislocation, and a varus femoral osteotomy may be sufficient to maintain reduction. If the acetabulum is deficient, the Chiari innominate osteotomy provides posterior as well as superior coverage.

Very rarely, spasticity may produce an extension contracture of the hip which results in loss of sitting ability and may progress to anterior hip dislocation. Treatment is indicated to prevent loss of sitting ability, and requires soft tissue release with occasional femoral shortening [19].

The knee

Knee deformities are also grouped as to aetiology as positional, due to muscle imbalance, or to spasticity.

A flexion contracture can result from prolonged sitting or crawling. In spastic children it may result from hamstring spasticity.

A knee flexion contracture may be an acceptable deformity in a wheelchair-ambulatory individual; in the ambulatory child, this contracture makes bracing difficult and decreases quadriceps efficiency. If treatment is elected, stretching and/or soft tissue release may address the mild contracture. Radical soft tissue release is needed for the severe deformity [20]. If the soft tissue release is limited by tightness of neurovascular structures or if bony derotation is desired, an extension/shortening/derotational osteotomy of the femur or tibia may significantly facilitate bracing and ambulation.

A rigid extension contracture of the knee may be seen in the child with an L3 neurological level due to strong quadriceps opposite flail hamstring muscles. The extended position of the knee is a braceable position – surgical release should only be considered if problems with wheelchair sitting or other positioning are encountered. A V-Y quadricepsplasty [20] may occasionally be indicated in the ambulatory child; quadriceps release and even patellectomy may be needed to achieve sufficient flexion for sitting in the non-ambulatory child.

Intoeing

A number of problems can cause intoeing in the myelodysplastic. Femoral anteversion, spasticity resulting in a gait similar to that seen in cerebral palsy, hamstring imbalance (functioning medial hamstrings while lateral hamstrings are flail), internal tibial torsion and foot deformities can all result in intoeing [21]. One must identify the aetiology of the intoeing so that orthotic or surgical correction can be appropriately directed. Adductor and/or hamstring release may be indicated; for bony deformities, femoral or tibial osteotomies may provide cosmetic or functional improvement that results in a more efficient gait.

Twister cables applied to braces have been used in the past and are seen to improve the gait in some children, at the expense of increased energy consumption and increased encumbrance. As energy limitation and encumbrance by braces are causes of ambulatory failure, twister cables are not advocated.

Out-toeing

The foot normally dorsiflexes during the swing phase to allow ground clearance; where dorsiflexion is limited, as in paralysis, or even when a fixed-ankle orthosis or cast is worn, a patient often externally rotates the limb to facilitate ground clearance. Other causes of externally rotated gait in myelodysplasia include external tibial torsion or a plano-valgus foot from heel-cord contracture or peroneal spasticity.

External tibial torsion is often seen with increased femoral anteversion, and may be associated in myelodysplasia with a valgus ankle joint [19]. Orthotic fitting becomes difficult, and pressure sores on the medial malleolus may occur. The torsion may be treated by supramalleolar osteotomy with simultaneous correction of the angular deformity of the ankle. Isolated ankle valgus is addressed in the ambulatory child by medial physeal stapling or hemiepiphysiodesis at an appropriate age to allow correction of the deformity by subsequent growth.

Limb length discrepancy

Limb length discrepancy is seen in the child with a unilateral hip dislocation, pelvic asymmetry, and especially in the child with an asymmetrical or unilateral paralysis. Careful attention is paid to this problem, with the goal being symmetry at skeletal maturity if the child is projected to be a long-term ambulator. It must be emphasized that limb length symmetry is only of importance if the child is projected to be a community ambulator at skeletal maturity.

Serial measurements of limb length are monitored, with epiphysiodesis or limb lengthening performed at an appropriate skeletal age. Shoe lifts in the face of an asymmetric pelvis or a subluxated hip may be seen to worsen the pelvic asymmetry while improving the gait only cosmetically.

Children with myelodysplasia often have advanced bone age and overall short stature; this must be considered when timing limb equalization procedures.

Foot deformity

Foot deformities are seen in almost two-thirds of children with myelodysplasia [22]. Feet must be plantigrade if bracing and ambulation are to be accomplished. Children whose ambulatory potential is poor often benefit psychologically and socially if foot deformities are corrected to allow normal footwear.

Deformities may be either congenital or acquired secondary to muscle imbalance or spasticity. The aetiology of the foot deformity must be defined if treatment is to be successful and recurrence avoided.

Congenital foot deformities include clubfoot and vertical talus. These are often severe in nature, resembling the arthrogrypotic foot. Serial casting is attempted by some to partially correct the deformity and minimize skin tightness at surgery. The author, however, does not employ serial casting in a rigid, insensate foot in which surgery is inevitable. Occasionally, a percutaneous heelcord tenotomy is performed, followed by several weeks of casting. In the minimally deformed foot, this may suffice to enable shoewear and significantly improve cosmesis.

If surgical correction is needed, a complete release is performed in the same manner as for a similar deformity in the nonparalytic foot. In contrast to the neurologically normal foot, however, unopposed tendons are not repaired. Talectomy may be required in the severely deformed foot or in the older child. One must beware of anomalous vascularity or sympathetic dysvascularity, and must be prepared for skin grafting if closure is difficult after correction of a severe deformity.

Deformities may result from muscle imbalance. Examples of these include the calcaneus deformity from a functioning tibialis anterior in a child who lacks triceps surae function, as seen in an L4 or L5 neurological level. The calcaneus gait can produce disastrous ulcerations as a result of weight-bearing on the point of the heel.

The treatment of foot deformities resulting from muscle imbalance is to balance the foot by removing or transferring the unopposed muscular influence. For the calcaneus deformity in the above example, treatment consists of tibialis anterior tenotomy with subsequent bracing, or transfer of the tibialis anterior to the heelcord [23].

The third cause of foot deformity in myelodysplasia and often the most difficult to treat is spasticity; deformities resulting from myelodysplastic spasticity resemble those found in cerebral palsy. Tenotomy may be performed, or muscle-balancing surgery may be cautiously attempted.

Increasing spasticity or development of foot deformity such as cavus may indicate a tethered cord or other central nervous system lesion. Before the foot deformity is addressed, the central nervous system must be assessed.

Spinal deformity

Patients with spina bifida develop scoliosis in from 60 to 100% of cases [13]. A distinction must be made between congenital and so-called 'developmental' or 'paralytic' curvatures.

Congenital curves result from malformations of the vertebrae aside from the dysraphism, and all newborns should be radiographically screened for such anomalies. If anomalies are noted, the spine is carefully observed for curve progression. As in congenital scoliosis without myelodysplasia, spinal fusion is performed as soon as curve progression is documented, even if that be at less than 1 year of age. Early posterior fusion alone may be performed in nondysraphic segments; in dysraphic areas anterior fusion or hemiepiphysiodesis is needed. A high index of suspicion is maintained for the existence of diastematomyelia and other cord anomalies in any patient with congenital anomalies [5], and myelographic computed tomography or magnetic resonance imaging should be undertaken to determine cord anatomy [12].

The 'developmental' or 'paralytic' scoliosis is an entirely different entity. The child is straight at birth and has no anomalies of the vertebral bodies, except the posterior bony dysraphism. The mechanisms for production of 'developmental' scoliosis are not well explained, as curves are often well above the level of the myelomeningocele. The literature suggests a strong correlation between this type of scoliosis and hydrocephalus or spinal cord anomalies such as syringomyelia and tethered spinal cord [8,24–28]; these lesions should be sought through diagnostic imaging.

The treatment for noncongenital scoliosis in spina bifida is generally surgical. Bracing may be used in the very young child as a temporizing measure, but the natural history of such curves is generally one of progression. When surgery is undertaken, better results are obtained with anterior spinal fusion with release and grafting or anterior instrumentation, followed by posterior fusion and segmental instrumentation [29–31]. When fusion to the pelvis is desired [31], the Galveston technique of intrailiac rod passage has proved useful. This is a major undertaking in these individuals, and carries a high complication rate [32], but these curves often become severe, and spinal stabilization provides prevention of further progression and pulmonary compromise while improving sitting balance and cosmesis.

A far more ominous problem is seen in the congenital kyphosis observed with very high level neurological lesions and high posterior defects. As neurosurgical care improves the survival rate of more severely involved infants, this problem occurs with greater frequency. Surgical correction in the young child is often unsuccessful and deformity recurs [33]; most successful results are obtained in the older child (8–12 years old) by resection of the apex and lordotic segment followed by rigid internal stabilization [31].

Fractures

Disuse and osteopenia in the nonambulatory or braced patient predisposes bone to fracture. Particularly vulnerable is the postoperative patient in whom cast immobilization has been used. Fractures in children with spina bifida often occur in insensate limbs, making diagnosis difficult. Children may present appearing slightly ill and mildly febrile, with a swollen, hot extremity. Significant sequelae from fracture may occur, such as fat embolism, pulmonary embolism, or hypovolemia from fracture bleeding.

Younger children may develop physeal changes from repeated microtrauma to the physis. This so-called 'Charcot physis' must be distinguished from neoplasm or other growth disturbance. Identification of the problem suggests protection of the physis to allow healing [34].

A high index of suspicion for fracture must be maintained for children with spina bifida. Postoperative casting should be minimized, with casts designed to permit early standing and weightbearing.

Conclusion

Myelodysplasia is a multi-system disease, and its orthopaedic care cannot be divorced from that of the pediatrician, neurosurgeon, urologist, and physical and occupational therapists. All must work together to maximize function and minimize deformity.

The orthopaedic care of myelodysplasia begins at birth by determination of neurological level and a search for congenital spinal anomalies or other congenital defects. Education of the parents begins by outlining expected ambulatory potential and predicting deformities that may be anticipated due to muscle imbalance.

As the child grows, developmental milestones are assisted by sitting or balance devices and bracing as indicated. Long-term mobility is achieved by bracing or by the use of a wheelchair. The child is not pressured to accomplish unrealistic goals, but is enabled to achieve his or her full individual functional capacity.

References

1. McLaughlin, J. *et al.* (1984) Management of the fetus and newborn with neural tube defects. *J. Perinatol.*, **4**, 3–11.
2. Waters, R. L. and Lunsford, B. R. (1985) Energy cost of paraplegic locomotion. *J. Bone Joint Surg.*, **67A**, 1245–1250.
3. Menelaus, M. B. (1980) *The Orthopaedic Management of Spina Bifida Cystica*, ed 2. Churchill Livingstone, Edinburgh.
4. Brown, H. P. (1978) Management of spinal deformity in myelomeningocele. *Orthop. Clin. North Am.*, **9**, 391–402.
5. Winter, R. B., Haven, J. J., Moe, J. H. and Lagaard, S. M. (1974) Diastematomyelia and congenital spine deformities. *J. Bone Joint Surg.*, **56A**, 27–39.
6. Mazur, J. A. *et al.* (1986) The significance of spasticity in the upper and lower extremities in myelomeningocele. *J. Bone Joint Surg.*, **68B**, 213–217.
7. McLone, D. G. and Naidich, T. (1985) Spinal dysraphism: experimental and clinical. In *The Tethered Spinal Cord* (ed. R. N. N. Holzman), Thieme-Stratton, New York, pp. 14–28.
8. Park, T. S., Cail, W. S., Maggio, W. M. and Mitchell, D. C. (1985) Progressive spasticity and scoliosis in children with myelomeningocele. *J. Neurosurg.*, **62**, 367–375.
9. Venes, J. L., Black, K. and Latack, J. T. (1986) Preoperative evaluation and surgical management of the Arnold–Chiari malformation. *J. Neurosurg.*, **64**, 363–370.
10. Williams, B. (1979) Orthopaedic features in the presentation of syringomyelia. *J. Bone Joint Surg.*, **61B**, 314–323.
11. Szalay, E. A. (1987) Orthopaedic management of the lower extremities in spina bifida, in Griffin, M. D., *Instructional Course Lectures XXXVI*, American Academy of Orthopedic Surgeons, Chicago.
12. Szalay, E. A., Roach, J. W., Smith, H. *et al.* (1987) Magnetic resonance imaging of the spinal cord in spinal dysraphisms. *J. Pediatr. Orthop.*, **7**, 541–545.
13. Mackel, J. L. and Lindseth, R. E. (1975) Scoliosis in myelodysplasia. *J. Bone Joint Surg.*, **57A**, 1031.
14. Barden, H. (1975) Myelodysplastics: fate of those followed for twenty years or more. *J. Bone Joint Surg.*, **57A**, 643–647.
15. Bazih, J. and Gross, R. H. (1981) Hip surgery in the lumbar level myelomeningocele patient. *J. Pediatr. Orthop.*, **1**, 405–411.
16. Kahanovitz, N. and Duncan, J. W. (1981) The role of scoliosis and pelvic obliquity in functional disability in myelomeningocele. *Spine*, **6**, 494–497.
17. Stillwell, A. and Menelaus, M. B. (1983) Walking ability in mature patients with spina bifida. *J. Pediatr.*, **3**, 184–190.
18. Breed, A. L. and Healy, P. M. (1982) The mid-lumber myelomeningocele hip: Mechanisms of dislocation and treatment. *J. Pediatr. Orthop.*, **2**, 15–24.
19. Szalay, E. A., Roach, J. W., Wenger, D. *et al.* (1986) Extension-abduction contracture of the spastic hip. *J. Pediatr. Orthop.*, **6**, 1–6.
20. Dias, L. S., Jasty, M. J. and Collins, P. (1984) Rotational deformities of the lower limb in myelomeningocele. *J. Bone Joint Surg.*, **66A**, 215–223.
21. Dias, L. S. (1985) Valgus deformity of the ankle joint: pathogenesis of fibular shortening. *J. Pediatr. Orthop.*, **5**, 176–180.
22. Duckworth, T. (1982) Management of the feet in spinal dysraphism and myelodysplasia. In *Disorders of the Foot* (ed. M. J. Jahss), Saunders, Philadelphia.
23. Banta, J. V. and Sutherland Wyatt, M. (1981) Anterior tibial transfer to the os calcis with achilles tenodesis for calcaneal deformity in myelomeningocele. *J. Pediatr. Orthop.*, **1**, 125–131.
24. Emery, J. L. (1986) The cervical cord of children with meningomyelocele. *Spine*, **11**, 318–321.
25. Hall, P. V., Campbell, R. L. and Kalsbeck, J. E. (1975) Meningomyelocele and progressive hydromyelia. *Neurosurgery*, **43**, 457–463.
26. Hall, P. V., Lindseth, R. E., Campbell, R. L. and Kalsbeck, J. E. (1976) Myelodysplasia and developmental scoliosis: a manifestation of syringomyelia. *Spine*, **1**, 48–56.

27. Hall, P. V., Lindseth, R. E., Campbell, R. L. *et al.* (1979) Scoliosis and hydrocephalus in myelocele patients. *J. Neurosurg.*, **50**, 174–178.
28. Sherk, H. H., Charney, E., Pasquariello, P. D. *et al.* (1986) Hydrocephalus, cervical cord lesions, and spinal deformity. *Spine*, **11**, 340–342.
29. Osebold, W. R., Mayfield, J. K., Winter, R. B. and Moe, J. H. (1982) Surgical treatment of paralytic scoliosis associated with myelomeningocele. *J. Bone Joint Surg.*, **64A**, 841–856.
30. Mayfield, J. K. (1981) Severe spine deformity in myelodysplasia and sacral agenesis. *Spine*, **6**, 498–509.
31. Allan, B. L. and Ferguson, R. L. (1979) The operative treatment of myelomeningocele spinal deformity. *Orthop. Clin. North Am.*, **10**, 845–862.
32. Sriram, K., Bobechko, W. E. and Hall, J. E. (1972) Surgical management of spinal deformities in spina bifida. *J. Bone Joint Surg.*, **54B**, 666–676.
33. Christoffersen, M. R. and Brooks, A. L. (1985) Excision and wire fixation of congenital rigid kyphosis in myelomeningocele children. *J. Pediatr. Orthop.*, **5**, 691–696.
34. Wenger, D. R., Jeffcoat, B. T. and Herring, J. A. (1980) The guarded prognosis of physeal injury in paraplegic children. *J. Bone Joint Surg.*, **62A**, 241–246.

5

Perthes' disease

G. Hall

We are at times painfully aware of the fact that there are many symptoms which we readily recognise in our clinical observations to which we can assign no cause, and it is also an undoubted fact that there are many conditions, even which exist today, of which we are ignorant, simply from our neglect to observe, or again, from faulty deduction even from good observation.

Alfred T. Legg [1]

Introduction

The statement made by Legg over half a century ago can equally apply today to the understanding of the condition which partly bears his eponym.

Although there has been a great deal of research and speculation, no significant advances in the understanding of Perthes' disease has occurred and the condition remains an enigma. The cause remains unknown; the prognosis is difficult to determine and the influence of treatment impossible to establish.

It now seems certain that Perthes' disease is the result of a series of vascular insults to the immature femoral head [2,3], and that these changes are most likely to occur in children with certain morphological changes first described by Burwell [4]. Once established, the outcome of the condition is variable and there are differing published views as to the natural history of the disease. Ratliff [5] has reviewed 34 cases of the condition and has suggested that in the long term only one in three cases obtain a good end result. Using a different method of assessment Eaton [6]

claims 61% of his cases achieved good results in adult life. This suggests that the prognosis of Perthes' disease is usually benign.

Similarly, when trying to establish the influence of treatment on the outcome of the disease, differing reports are obtained from the literature. Brotherton and McKibben [7] have suggested that traction in abduction can improve the prognosis, while Lloyd-Roberts [8] maintains that an osteotomy below the hip has a similar effect.

It is therefore very difficult for clinicians dealing with this condition to have a clear understanding of the natural history of the disease, and the possible influence of treatment on the outcome.

An attempt has been made to resolve this dilemma by reviewing a large series of children with Perthes' disease treated in Wessex over the last 50 years.

Patients and methods

One hundred and nine cases of Perthes' disease have been reviewed in an attempt to establish the natural history of the condition as well as the possible value of various prognostic features. All of the children in this review were treated in Wessex, either at the Bath and Wessex Orthopaedic Hospital or the Lord Mayor Orthopaedic Hospital, Alton, Hampshire. The original hospital records and radiographs were studied and a clinical and radiographic review performed on the patient in adult life. The average length of review from onset of the disease is 34 years (range 8–57).

End result

It is vital when comparing two differing forms of treatment that the outcome of the treatment is expressed in the same way. Many papers have been written where the outcome of the disease has been assessed before skeletal maturity, and obviously as children have such a growth potential it is foolhardy to be dogmatic about the outcome. The later in life that the review is performed the greater its value, and Ratliff [5] has suggested a method of assessing the outcome of Perthes' disease which is both clinical and radiographic, and is weighted heavily towards the clinical picture.

Assessment in adult life

The results obtained using the Ratliff method of assessment showed that the majority of hips (71.3%) had good results, being totally free of pain and functionally without impairment with a concentric hip free of degeneration on the radiograph. The average age of the patient when reviewed was 42 years. Only 10.6% of cases had poor end results in adult life assessed by this method, and four of the 109 hips reviewed had required surgery for pain relief.

At healing of the disease

A good result from Perthes' disease is obviously a hip that functions well throughout life without premature degeneration. It is of course helpful when attempting to evaluate the effect of treatment on the outcome of the disease to make an assessment of the result at an earlier stage.

In this review a radiographic assessment of the result was also made when the disease had healed, but before skeletal maturity. The shape of the healed femoral head was determined using the concentricity of Mose and also a visual assessment of the result was made using the method described by Catterall [9]. The cases were

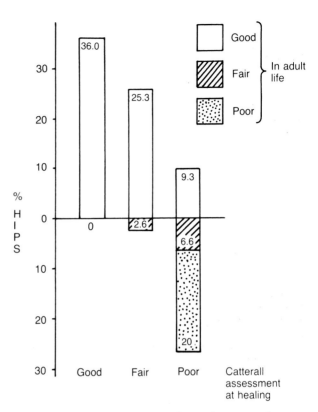

Catterall visual assessment/end result

Fig. 5.1 Comparison between the result measured at healing of the disease with the actual result in adult life.

then assessed in adult life using the methods described by Ratliff, and also using the concentricity of Mose [10] on the adult radiograph. Comparison of these results suggests that a considerable improvement occurs in adult life (Fig. 5.1).

This improvement can also be seen by measuring the concentricity of Mose both at healing and on the adult radiograph. When the concentricity of Mose was measured at healing of the disease, 24.4% of hips had less than 2 mm of flattening and yet in adult life 54.2% of hips showed good concentricity with less than 2 mm of flattening.

The epiphyseal quotient is the ratio of epiphyseal height and width expressed as a percentage of the normal hip and gives an indication of the degree of flattening of the femoral head. This quotient has been used as an assessment of the result of Perthes' disease at healing of the disease and is thought to give a reasonable indication of the likely end result in adult life. In fact, only one

The 'head height'

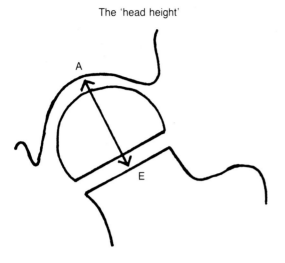

Fig. 5.2 The head height was measured from the acetabular roof to the epiphyseal plate.

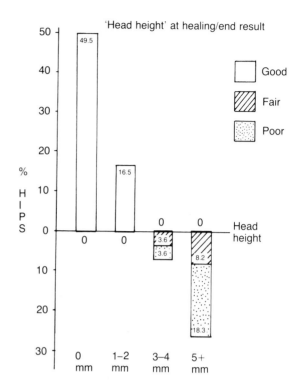

Fig. 5.3 The measurement of the head height on the initial radiograph is of great importance in determining the end result. A difference of more than 2 mm in head height always has a poor result.

hip in this review, with a quotient above 60%, had a poor result in adult life. However, 8.6% of hips with a severely flattened epiphysis with a quotient of 60% or less achieved a good result in adult life. The degree of distortion of the femoral head therefore does seem to be a fairly good indicator of the likely long term result of the disease.

A more accurate assessment of the outcome can, however, be gained by measuring the 'head height' (Fig. 5.2). This height probably represents the cartilaginous anlage of the hip and can be determined by measuring the distance between the acetabulum and the epiphyseal plate on both the affected and normal sides. When this height is related to the end result, it is seen quite clearly (Fig. 5.3) that those cases in which collapse of the cartilaginous anlage did not occur all achieved a good result. It is therefore apparent that any assessment of the likely end result which is not based upon the overall shape and position of the cartilaginous anlage of the hip will give a misleading impression of the prognosis.

Prognostic factors of Perthes' disease

Since the first descriptions of Perthes', attempts have been made to establish at an early stage the likely outcome. Legg described a 'cocked hat' appearance of the epiphysis and tried to relate it

to the end result. The features which may influence the possible outcome of the disease can be divided into radiographic and non-radiographic.

Non-radiographic features

In this review it would seem that the mode of onset, severity and duration of symptoms do not influence the end result. It has been suggested that girls have a worse prognosis than boys. In this review the ratio of girls to boys was as expected, approximately 1:4, and in fact there was no appreciable difference in the end result between girls and boys. It has been recognized that the child's age at the onset of the condition has a profound influence on the outcome, and that after the age of 8 years the outlook worsens. In this review a similar pattern emerges and children presenting after the age of 8 years have a relatively high proportion (88%) of unsatisfactory results (Fig. 5.4).

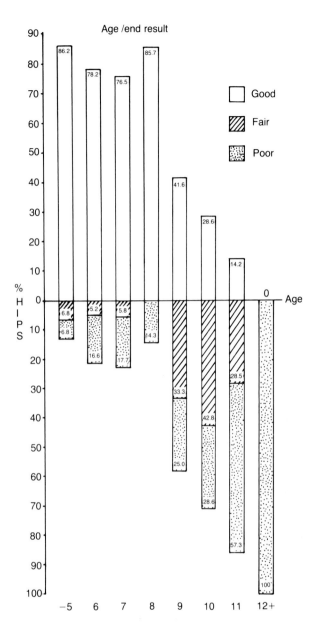

Fig. 5.4 The influence of age on the outcome of the disease.

Radiographic features

The diagnosis of Perthes' disease is entirely radiographic. Fragmentation, alteration in the density and shape of the hips' ossific nucleus as well as other specific radiographic changes characterize the disease. There have been several attempts in the past to establish from the initial radiograph various features which may guide the clinician to the likely outcome. The degree of involvement of

the ossific nucleus would seem to vary from case to case and it has been shown by Katz [11] and also by Catterall that the outcome is partly related to this. Not surprisingly, the children with more involvement of the femoral head tend to have a worse end result than those with a lesser degree of involvement. In this review there was a

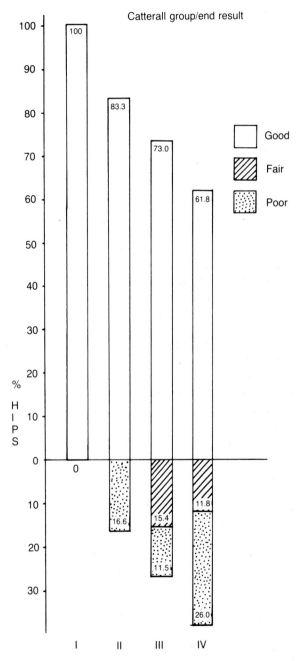

Fig. 5.5 The amount of ossific nucleus affected by the disease as defined by the Catterall group has a slight influence on the outcome.

progressive decline in the proportion of good results occurring in adult life with increasing involvement of the ossific nucleus (Fig. 5.5). Children with minor involvement of the ossific nucleus (Catterall groups 1 and 2) tended to fare better than those with whole head involvement, but even in the group of children with whole head involvement nearly half had satisfactory results in adult life.

The discrepancy between the results in this review and those of Catterall must be partially attributable to the difference in assessing the result. Catterall's group of children was assessed at healing of the disease, and as shown earlier, a considerable improvement can occur as the child matures.

'Head at risk' signs

Catterall has also described five features seen on the radiograph which are thought to help judge the outcome. He has termed these the 'Head at risk' sign, and suggested that when seen on the initial radiograph, the prognosis was poor.

Subluxation of the hip is one of the 'at risk' signs, and is described by Catterall in this context as an increase of medial joint space of more than 2 mm when compared to the normal side. Sixty-seven per cent of hips exhibited an increase of medial joint space of more than 2 mm on the initial radiograph, and of these 70% achieved good results in adult life. An increased medial joint space, therefore, is not a very accurate way of determining the likely end result and other ways of assessing subluxation of the hip should be considered.

A joint is subluxed when there is lack of apposition of the joint surfaces. In the hip this can be determined either by measuring directly the percentage of head uncovered by the acetabulum, or the centre edge angle of Wiberg. A reasonable estimate of the degree of subluxation can also be obtained by observing Shenton's line. These methods of assessment of subluxation give a more accurate means of determining the end result, and certainly the more profound the subluxation the worse was the outcome in adult life. The hips with an obvious break in Shenton's line on the initial radiograph generally tended to have poor end results, with only 25% achieving a good result. Similarly, in those hips which exhibited

more than 20% uncovering of the hip, only 25% achieved a good end result.

The other 'at risk' signs are calcification seen laterally to the growth plate, a reaction in the metaphyseal region of the hip, a horizontally placed growth plate and the presence of a Gage sign.

Although Gage [12] first described his sign as a prominence of the contour of the superior aspect of the femoral neck, it has widely become used to denote an angular type defect in the lateral epiphyses which is not seen on the unaffected side. The individual merits of the 'at risk' signs are of doubtful significance and only the Gage sign is of any statistical significance as a prognostic indicator. Of the 109 hips reviewed, however, all but five however, showed one or more of the 'at risk' signs. Nine hips exhibited all five 'at risk' signs and of these four achieved a good end result in adult life. These results would tend to suggest that if treatment is based on the 'at risk' concept alone, half or more of the affected hips would be treated unnecessarily as they will probably achieve a good end result without intervention.

Femoral head shape

As a poor end result of Perthes' disease is usually associated with a mis-shapen femoral head, it would seem reasonable to attempt to predict this deformation in shape at an early stage.

A direct measurement of the affected ossific nucleus can be made and related to the unaffected side. This ratio can be expressed as a percentage (the epiphyseal quotient) and related to the end result. This measurement of the deformation of the ossific nucleus gives a more accurate indication of the outcome than the other prognostic features noted (Fig. 5.6). It is curious to note, however, that a number of hips show quite severe flattening of the ossific nucleus and still achieve a satisfactory outcome in adult life.

The structure of the developing hip in a child is, of course, not entirely bony in origin. Presumably deformation of the cartilaginous anlage can also occur in Perthes' disease. The shape, size and position of this cartilaginous anlage can be outlined by arthrography of the joint and, this can on occasion demonstrate that the ossific nucleus has collapsed leaving a relatively intact cartilaginous anlage. A reasonable estimate of the

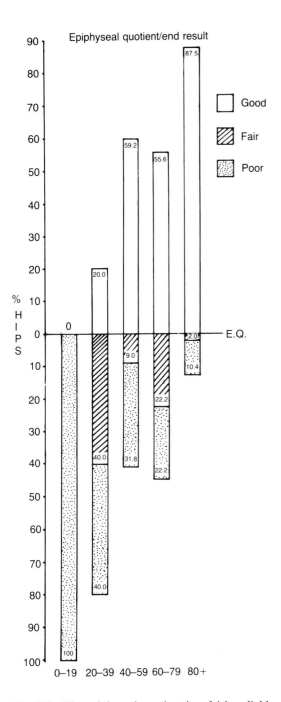

Epiphyseal quotient/end result

☐ Good

▨ Fair

⬚ Poor

E.Q.

0–19 20–39 40–59 60–79 80+

Fig. 5.6 The epiphyseal quotient is a fairly reliable indicator of the outcome.

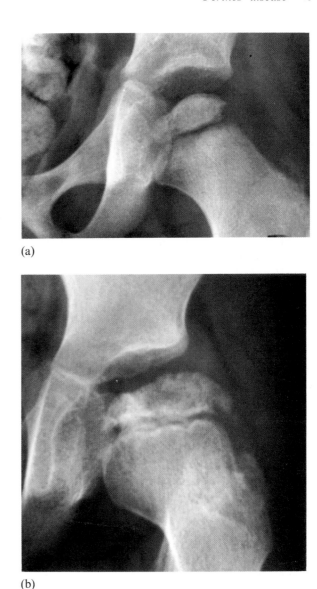

(a)

(b)

Fig. 5.7 Apparent increase in superior joint surface produced by collapse of the ossific nucleus without cartilagenous collapse.

shape of the anlage can be obtained by measurement of the distance between the acetabulum and the femoral epiphysis. In some cases of Perthes' disease it appears that there is an apparent increase in the superior joint space after collapse of the ossific nucleus and yet in other cases there is

no such increase (Fig. 5.7) When the distance between the acetabulum and epiphyseal line is compared to the unaffected side and related to the end result it would appear that this is a very effective means of judging the outcome. Ninety-three per cent of cases exhibited loss of head height on the original radiographs, and all of the cases had an unsatisfactory result. Of the 84 cases who exhibited no loss of head height on the original radiograph, 93% achieved a good result in adult life. The group of children who showed

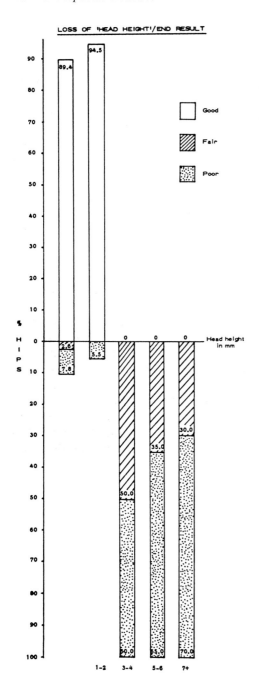

Fig. 5.8 The measurement of the head height on the initial radiograph is of great importance in determining the end result. A difference of more than 2 mm in head height always has a poor result.

no collapse on the original radiograph and yet did not achieve a satisfactory result all developed loss of head height on subsequent radiographs. It would therefore seem that the measurement of the shape of the cartilaginous anlage is the best

indicator of the likely outcome of the disease. Unsatisfactory results only occurred in this review in the children whose hips exhibited distortion of the cartilaginous anlage. When the shape of the hip anlage was maintained throughout the disease process, the outcome was always good (Fig. 5.8).

Effect of treatment

The children in this review were all treated after the diagnosis of Perthes' disease was made by a period of recumbency and straight Pugh type traction until signs of healing of the femoral head occurred. None of the patients in this review appeared to have suffered from the irritable hip syndrome prior to their admission for Perthes' disease.

To assess the possible effect of treatment on the outcome of the disease it is interesting to compare the results of this series of patients with other groups treated in differing ways. This of course has obvious pitfalls. It is important that the results are assessed in a similar way and at a similar stage of the condition, and that the severity and age at onset of the disease are taken into account.

Catterall has reported a group of 54 children who were untreated and found that 31% had good results, 28% fair and 41% poor results. These results are directly comparable with the results in this review where 36% had good results when assessed at healing of the disease. This would suggest that simple traction without containment has very little effect on the outcome. Some further evidence that traction alone has little benefit on the outcome of the disease can be gained by studying whether those patients in whom treatment was delayed by a significant time tended to have a worse outcome than those in whom treatment was started at the onset of symptoms. Although this is a crude assessment in that patients had symptoms for at least 6 months before treatment started, this delay in instituting treatment did not seem adversely to affect the outcome of the condition.

The possible effect of containment can be judged by comparing the results of this review with those of Brotherton and McKibben [6]. In their series, children were treated by abduction traction, and therefore any benefit to be derived from abduction should be apparent. The assessment of the Brotherton and McKibben review is the same as this review, and therefore a fair comparison can be made. It would seem that there is little if any benefit to be derived from the addition of abduction to traction.

This review would suggest that by and large Perthes' is a fairly benign condition and simple traction would not seem to influence the outcome.

Pathogenesis of head collapse

Quite clearly, the outcome of Perthes' disease is determined by the degree of deformation of the cartilaginous anlage which occurs during the course of the disease. The two factors which have been shown to influence the degree of distortion of the femoral head are: the age of the child at onset of the disease and the degree of involvement of the ossific nucleus. There is no evidence to suggest that the older child suffers from a more severe form of the condition and it is therefore likely that the deformity of the femoral head is related directly to the maturity of the child.

As the child's hip develops, there is alteration in the relative proportion of cartilage to bone. At birth the femoral anlage is totally cartilaginous, the ossific nucleus develops in the centre of this anlage and grows at a proportionally higher rate than the cartilaginous hip. By the age of 6 years the ossific nucleus occupies 30% of the femoral head and by 12 years of age the proportion of bone in the developing hip is 80%. As Perthes' disease appears to be entirely a condition affecting the developing nucleus, it is not surprising that the relative proportion of the hip occupied by ossific nucleus influences the mechanical strength of that developing hip.

In the younger child the majority of the affected hip is in fact cartilaginous: it therefore can withstand the mechanical deforming factors and deformation does not occur. At a later stage in development when the ossific nucleus occupies more of the hip, avascularity of that nucleus will produce a more pronounced effect on the ability of that hip to withstand deformation and subsequently collapse of that hip will occur (Fig. 5.9). It would appear that the critical level of development of the hip is when approximately 50% of the hip is ossific, which occurs at approximately 8 years of age. It is easy to understand why an ossific nucleus only partially affected by the disease can withstand deformation more than one with whole head involvement.

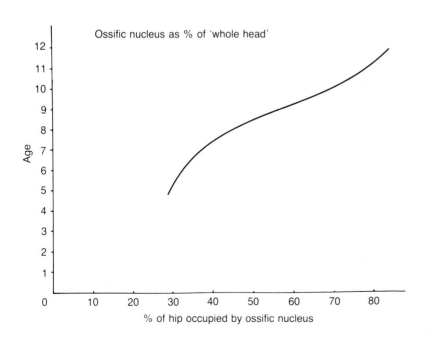

Fig. 5.9   Diagram shows how the proportion of bone in the hip increases with age.

Load testing of immature pig hips

To test this hypothesis, load testing experiments were performed on the hips of freshly killed piglets. Like the human hip, the hip of the piglet develops from a cartilaginous anlage with an increasing proportion of ossific nucleus as the pig matures.

Compression loading was performed on hips of varying maturity, and the degree of deformation produced by a given load noted. The experiments were repeated on hips of differing degrees of maturity after their ossific nuclei had been removed.

The results of these simple load testing experiments showed that the immature totally cartilaginous hip deforms quite readily under load. Once the ossific nucleus develops, however, the strength of the hip increases dramatically. When the ossific nucleus is removed from the developing hip the load/deformation characteristics change considerably. A hip which is mainly cartilaginous can withstand removal of its ossific nucleus without unduly affecting its load characteristics. However, when the hip's ossific nucleus is larger, removal of that ossific nucleus has a profound effect on the load bearing capacity of that hip. The load bearing characteristics of the developing hip appear to alter dramatically at the critical level when 50% of the hip is ossific nucleus.

It is interesting to relate the experimental findings with the clinical review. At the age of 8 years, approximately 50% of the child's hip is composed of the ossific nucleus. This relates well with the experimental evidence found in the piglets' hips.

When the end result is equated to the relative size of the ossific nucleus rather than the child's age it becomes apparent that the size of the ossific nucleus determines the outcome.

It would therefore seem that the outcome of Perthes' disease is directly related to the size and proportion of the ossific nucleus affected by the disease, and that the size of the ossific nucleus is determined by the skeletal maturity of the child.

Conclusions

For more than 70 years clinicians have advocated treatment of children suffering from Perthes' disease. A review of the literature has failed to substantiate that treatment either by weight relief or containment has any effect on the outcome of the condition. Therefore the basic question must be asked: should Perthes' disease be treated?

This review has confirmed that the overall outcome of Perthes' disease is generally satisfactory. Only four hips in this review have required surgery in adult life for pain relief. The average age of the patient when this surgical intervention took place was 38 years. With the success of modern treatment of osteoarthrosis of the hip again it is difficult to justify the treatment of children with Perthes' disease, and it would therefore seem reasonable to restrict any attempts at treatment to those cases in which a poor outcome can be predicted with certainty.

References

1. Legg, A. T. (1910) *Boston Medical Journal*, **162**, 202–204.
2. McKibben, B. and Ralis, Z. (1974) Pathological changes in a case of Perthes' disease. *J. Bone Joint Surg.*, **56B**, 438.
3. Kemp, H. B. S. (1973) Perthes' disease with an experimental and clinical study. *Ann. R. Coll. Surg.*, **52**, 18.
4. Burwell, G. *et al.* (1978) Perthes' disease. An anthropometric study. *J. Bone Joint Surg.*, **60B**, 461.
5. Ratliff, A. H. C. (1977) Perthes' disease – study of sixteen patients followed up for 40 years. *J. Bone Joint Surg.*, **59B**, 248.
6. Eaton, G. O. (1967) Long term results of treatment of coxa-plana. *J. Bone Joint Surg.*, **49**, 1031.
7. Brotherton, B. J. and McKibben, B. (1978) Perthes' disease treated by prolonged recumbency and head containment. *J. Bone Joint Surg.*, **59B**, 8.
8. Lloyd-Roberts, G. C. *et al.* (1978) A controlled study of the indication for and the results of femoral osteotomy in Perthes' disease. *J. Bone Joint Surg.*, **58B**, 31.
9. Catterall, A. (1971) The natural history of Perthes' disease. *J. Bone Joint Surg.*, **53B**, 37.
10. Mose, K. (1964) *Legg–Calvé–Perthes' Disease.* Universitets for Laget, Arthus.
11. Katz, J. F. (1967) Conservative treatment of Legg–Calvé–Perthes' disease. *J. Bone Joint Surg.*, **49A 6**, 1043.
12. Gage, H. C. (1933) A possible early sign of Perthes' disease. *Br. J. Radiol.*, **6**, 295.

6

Slipped upper femoral epiphysis

W. E. G. Griffiths

The condition of slipped upper femoral epiphysis (SUFE) was first described by Ambroise Paré in 1572. Also known as epiphysiolysis or adolescent coxa vara, it may be defined as posterior displacement of the femoral capital epiphysis in otherwise normal adolescents.

In the Portsmouth Health District, UK, a population of approximately 530 000 produced 65 new cases of SUFE in the 13 years from July 1973 to July 1986, that is, an average of approximately one case per 106 000 population per year. Of these cases 48 were male (75%) and 14 were bilateral at presentation (21.5%). The males ranged from 8 years 2 months to 17 years 8 months in age, an average of 14 years 4 months. The females ranged from 8 years 6 months to 17 years 9 months, an average of 12 years 7 months.

Of the 79 hips 45 were mild or early slips (58%) and the remainder were sufficiently severe to merit surgical reconstruction of the relationship between head and neck of femur, in order to eliminate deformity and reduce the risk of osteoarthritis in later life.

The management of mild degrees of slippage is now generally agreed by most authorities to consist of internal fixation *in situ* with slender steel pins. Conservative treatment alone has been abandoned as a result of complications such as chondrolysis after immobilization in plaster spica, or increasing slippage while on traction. A bone graft may be used instead of steel pins, but this guarantees the fusion of the growth plate prematurely.

The management of cases of severe degrees of slippage has, throughout several decades of spectacular advance in most other problem areas of orthopaedics, continued to present a challenge almost unique in its ability to stimulate controversy. Insidious in onset, often with minimal symptoms and signs, the average interval between onset and diagnosis is approximately 5 months, by which time the radiological changes may be far advanced, and *in situ* pinning no longer acceptable. Different schools advocate different methods of management, including manipulative reduction with or without traction, hip spica, or surgery, while surgical reconstruction can be achieved in different ways, including correction at the site of slippage through the physis, or at the base of the neck of the femur, or through the trochanteric region. A cortico-cancellous bone graft may be used to stabilize and fuse the growth plate in the slipped position without attempting reduction; and there are advocates of pinning *in situ* even for the more severe slips in the hope of remodelling taking place, though the evidence for this lacks substance. Aggressive surgical treatment carries an increased risk of the dreaded complication of avascular necrosis of the capital epiphysis, while chondrolysis may follow any treatment, or no treatment at all.

Blood supply to the capital epiphysis

A rational appraisal of this controversial subject must begin with a study of the blood supply to the adolescent capital epiphysis. Trueta [1] traced the developing stages through which the blood supply passes, from embryo to adult: in the adolescent phase the blood supply is mainly from the lateral epiphyseal vessels, themselves derived from the medial circumflex artery, with some variable anastomosis from the ligamentum teres. No vessels cross the growth plate itself at this stage. Green [2] emphasized the importance of the vessels carried up the postero-inferior aspect of the neck of the femur in the retinacula of Weitbrecht. Blood from these vessels enters the periphery of the capital epiphysis, bypassing the epiphyseal plate.

Direction of slippage

From radiographic observation, the direction of slippage appears to have three elements, the caput moving posteriorly, medially, and into internal rotation with respect to the neck of femur, and for many years this tri-plane concept governed the principle of surgical reconstruction. However, M. J. Griffith [3] argued that the triplane idea is unnecessarily complicated, and from morphological studies on cadaveric specimens he showed quite clearly that the epiphyseal plate can be represented by part of the surface of an imaginary cylinder, whose axis exists at an angle of 65° to the femoral shaft, in the trochanteric region, in the plane of anteversion (Fig. 6.1a). As

the epiphysis slips, it moves in a purely posterior direction about this curved surface. On the AP radiograph the head of the femur sinks over the horizon like the setting sun, and the loss of height of the capital epiphysis compared to the normal side may be the only early radiological sign. The appearance of medial or even lateral displacement can then be produced simply by taking further radiographs in positions of internal and external rotation; lack of understanding of this simple principle has in the past led to confusion in presenting and interpreting results of manipulative 'reduction'. In practice, three methods are commonly used to take lateral radiographs of the upper end of femur.

(i) Frog lateral: an AP projection of the pelvis, with both thighs semiflexed, 45° abducted, and externally rotated to the maximum.
(ii) 'Shoot through' lateral of the affected hip is taken with the patient supine and the other hip flexed up out of the way: the plate is tucked above the iliac crest.
(iii) The 'turn over' view, with the patient supine and the pelvis tilted up on the unaffected side, the affected leg is partly flexed and externally rotated.

One or more of these views may be unobtainable if the patient is in severe discomfort, or if both hips are severely affected. The last method is probably the most reliable for routine use.

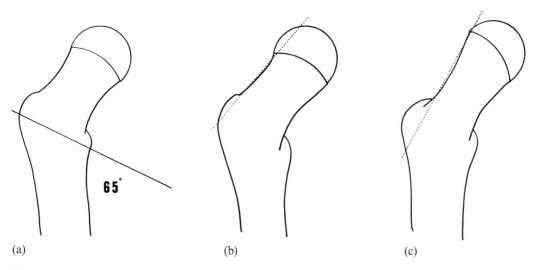

(a)   (b)   (c)

Fig. 6.1 (a) Showing the axis about which the epiphysis slips, posteriorly away from the observer. (b) Trethowan's line negative. (c) Trethowan's line positive.

Pathological changes

As the caput advances posteriorly it strips up the periosteum on the posterior aspect of the femoral neck, laying down a curving beak of new bone formation (Fig. 6.2a, b). The exposed anterior margin of the neck (Fig. 6.2b, c) will tend to remodel away after an interval, although a nubbin of bone can lead to a mechanical blockage in flexion and abduction. If slippage accelerates, tearing will occur at the junction of the anterior periosteum of the neck with the hyaline cartilage of the receding caput, leading to haemarthrosis and increased pain. Acute separation of head and neck may follow a minor force such as stepping off the kerb (Fig. 6.2d) presenting clinically in the same way as a subcapital fracture, with severe pain and complete loss of function. More commonly, slow chronic slippage continues over many months resulting in severe remodelling of the femoral neck.

Slippage of any appreciable severity tends to be followed by premature fusion (Fig. 6.2e), though this is unpredictable and does not always happen. In cases of unilateral disease the normal hip continues to grow, but in most cases the resulting discrepancy in leg length is very small because little growth potential is left, the capital epiphysis contributes much less than the lower epiphysis of the femur, and the neck of the femur is at an angle to the vertical.

Microscopically, the epiphyseal plate consists of four layers of cells: the resting layer of cartilage cells adjacent to the epiphysis, the proliferating layer, the hypertrophied layer, and the zone of provisional calcification adjacent to metaphyseal bone. During slippage, cleavage occurs through the hypertrophied layer.

Aetiology

Harris [4] observed that there was a tendency for SUFE to occur in adolescents of heavy build and immature secondary sexual characteristics, the 'adiposo-genital' syndrome, and also in a second, smaller group of rapidly growing, tall thin individuals. It was known that anterior pituitary growth hormone stimulated the proliferative layer, leading to a thicker growth plate, less resistant to shearing force, while oestrogen, and to a lesser extent testosterone, inhibited the an-

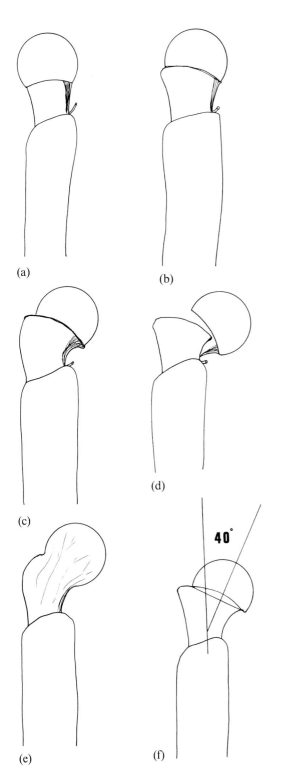

Fig. 6.2 (a) Normal lateral aspect of upper end of femur. (b) Early chronic slip, epiphyseal plate open: type 1. (c) Severe chronic slip, epiphyseal plate open: type 3. (d) Acute on chronic slip: type 2. (e) Severe chronic slip, epiphyseal plate closed: type 4. (f) To show the angle of slippage.

terior pituitary production of growth hormone. He suggested that an imbalance in the ratio between these two sets of hormones in adolescence would therefore predispose to SUFE. In the adiposo-genital syndrome there is a deficiency of sex hormone and in the tall thin cases an excess of growth hormone. He supported this experimentally by measuring the resistance to shear force in the upper tibial epiphysis of the rat, showing that it could be increased by oestrogen, and reduced by growth hormone. Further evidence from clinical assessment of hormone levels in patients with SUFE is, however, lacking, and this would appear to be a ripe field for future investigation.

We have already defined SUFE as occurring in otherwise normal children, but it is worth recording that it may also occur as part of the manifestation of a variety of disorders, including hypopituitarism, hypothyroidism, also treated hypothyroidism resulting in a growth spurt, hyperparathyroidism, renal osteodystrophy, rickets, Morquio's disease, multiple epiphyseal dysplasia, achondroplasia, or after sepsis or radiotherapy.

Clinical features

SUFE presents mainly between the ages of 10 and 16, females younger than males, as a problem of pain in the groin or knee, and limp. Pain may be non-existent, or slight, or vary in intensity over a period of many months. It cannot be said too often that obscure knee pain in an adolescent should alert the clinician to the possibility of hip disease, but in practice the diagnosis is frequently delayed, and there is nearly always a radiograph of the knee in the envelope. Pain is only severe when acute separation supervenes.

Only about half the cases exhibit the typical overweight, sexually immature physique or are very tall and thin; the remainder vary as normal children do.

Trendelenburg test is positive except in early chronic slippage. The gait is striking, with the foot on the affected side held in external rotation, and even in early cases, fixed external rotation of the hip shows up in flexion, as the posteriorly displaced epiphysis sits more comfortable in the obliquely facing acetabulum in external rotation when the hip is flexed. Wasting of the buttock

and thigh will occur in time. The incidence of bilateral disease is in general thought to be about 35%, though figures vary in many different reports. There will be less than this at initial presentation, as the second side may slip later. This figure will also clearly be reduced if prophylactic pinning is done.

Radiographic diagnosis of the early chronic slip may be easily overlooked on AP projection only, as the only definite sign is loss of height of the capital epiphysis compared to the other side (if that is normal), as the caput recedes over the horizon of the neck. The epiphyseal plate may appear broader because of its geometric tilt. Trethowan's line is useful but not absolutely reliable as a few degrees of retroversion will negate it (Fig. 6.1b, c).

Classification

Dunn and Angel [5] emphasized that a clear and practical classification is essential if reliable comparisons between different methods of treatment are to be used, and suggested the following.

(i) Acute traumatic. These cases are rare, involving violent trauma to mainly younger children with previously normal hips; there is no pre-existing break. These are really separate from the syndrome of SUFE.

(ii) Type 1. Chronic slip, early (Fig. 6.2b). There is no universally accepted method of differentiating between mild (early) slippage and severe slippage, the threshold being variously taken as 1 cm or 1/3 diameter, or 40° backwards angulation using the head/shaft angle or head/neck angle (Fig. 6.2f).

(iii) Type 2. Acute on chronic slip (Fig. 6.2d). In this situation an epiphysis which has already slipped sufficiently to create an identifiable beak on lateral radiograph, undergoes a further sudden movement, losing its adhesion to the metaphysis. The tone of the hip flexors and abductors and short external rotators produces proximal displacement of the femur, with external rotation and shortening clinically, accompanied by acute pain. On lateral radiograph the caput lies on the side of the femoral neck, with point contact between the beak and the concave aspect of the head. The periosteum is torn anteriorly, and stripped posteriorly from the femoral neck. Adaptive shortening of the retinacular vessels takes place within hours rather than days.

(iv) Type 3. Severe chronic slip, growth plate open (Fig. 6.2c). As this develops over a period of months, the epiphysis slips backwards and downwards, slowly stripping up the posterior periosteum which lays down a gradually increasing beak of new bone, thereby remodelling the shape of the metaphysis. The uncovered anterior margin will eventually remodel away, though this process lags behind and often leaves a protuberant bony nubbin. Severe deformity of the femoral neck will eventually result, again with shortening, fixed external rotation and limited flexion and limp, though not necessarily pain.

(v) Type 4. Severe chronic slip, growth plate closed (Fig. 6.2e). Metaphyseal vessels now cross the growth plate remnant to anastomose with capital vessels, and on no account must these anastomoses be disrupted. Any surgical reconstruction *must* now take place away from the head/neck junction.

Management

Acute traumatic slip demands emergency treatment for severe pain. Manipulative reduction (open if necessary) and internal fixation must be done as soon as anaesthesia is safe, as in the normal trauma situation. The risk of damage to the capital blood supply at the time of injury is

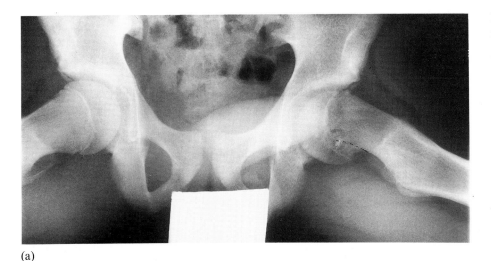

(a)

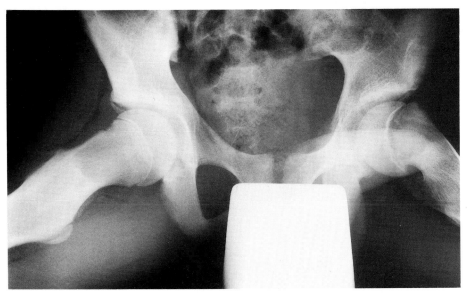

(b)

Fig. 6.3 (a) This male patient aged 16 years 8 months was admitted with moderately severe chronic slip of the left upper femoral epiphysis measuring 34° on January 4th 1982, but suffered increased pain, deformity and limitation of movement over the next 4 days while in bed on skin traction awaiting surgery. (b) The same patient on January 8th: a previously borderline case had now become unquestionably severe, with slippage measuring 52°. Open replacement was necessary.

great, delay will only increase it, and the best chance for a viable head lies in swift reduction and secure fixation.

Type 1. Early chronic slip. Conservative treatment is dangerous: traction in bed does not truly relieve the hip joint from compressive forces, so increased slippage is still possible (Fig. 6.3). Immobilization in a plaster spica leads to a high incidence of chondrolysis.

Internal fixation *in situ*, that is to say without reduction, using slender steel pins, is now generally agreed to be the treatment of choice, except by those who prefer epiphysiodesis (see type 3). A large bore nail such as Smith–Peterson should not be used as the dense cancellous bone of the caput will not accept it readily, and displacement or vascular damage may occur.

Of the various designs of slender pins, the Crawford Adams (Fig. 6.4a) is the most suitable for this purpose, with a 2 mm steel shank, and a built-up threaded section to grip the outer cortex. Beyond the thread the pin ends in a triangular section for ease of insertion and removal using a long slender triangular chuck in an ordinary hand drill. Four pins introduced under image intensifier control are sufficient to stabilize an early chronic slip. For moderately severe slips not bad enough for reconstruction, it is wise to begin drilling the outer cortex of the femur well anterior to the mid-lateral line and aim posteriorly so as to penetrate the middle of the epiphysis.

There is some controversy regarding the question of prophylactic pinning of the unslipped hip on the other side. As the risk of bilateral disease is

of the order of 35%, the author prefers to pin the unslipped side in all cases except those close to maturity. From past personal experience, patients cannot be relied upon to report early symptoms which may in any case be minimal. The morbidity of prophylactic pinning carefully done is extremely small. Radiography of the good hip every 4 months has its advocates but that too is not free from morbidity. The risk of bilateral disease is increased in patients of Negro or Polynesian race, or heavy build, or if the tri-radiate cartilage is still open. Pins should be removed 6 months after radiological evidence of closure of epiphysis. Occasionally pins require replacing with larger ones as the epiphysis grows off the proximal ends of the pins.

Type 2 acute on chronic. Debate continues whether manipulation to reduce severe displacement should be done in every case, or sometimes, or never.

Many reports fail to differentiate between severe chronic and acute on chronic slips, but from the experience of operating upon both types it is plain that manipulation of a purely chronic slip must never be done. Anything short of brute force will not shift a chronic slip (at operation a broad curved gouge is necessary to lever the head and neck apart), and if the head did shift, the effect on its blood supply would be disastrous.

In cases of acute on chronic slip, on the other hand, by definition there is loss of cohesion between head and neck, and a gentle manipulation has at least a chance of improving the relationship, exactly as in a subcapital fracture in

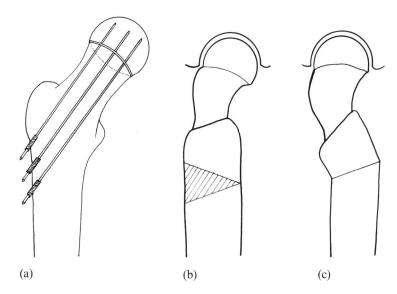

Fig. 6.4 (a) Crawford Adams pins internally fixing an early slip *in situ*: only three pins shown. (b) Trochanteric osteotomy: removal of an anteriorly based wedge from the trochanteric region, with closure of the wedge leading to (c) restoration of the capital epiphysis comfortably into the acetabulum.

(a)   (b)   (c)

an elderly patient. Certainly early closed reduction followed by pinning in anatomical position can lead to perfect restoration of hip function and development. In the ideal situation, reduction within hours of the acute episode, and only in the presence of minimal beak formation, would appear to carry only a small risk of damage to the retinacular vessels.

This risk would clearly increase:

(i) in the presence of a large beak;
(ii) after the passage of enough time following the acute episode to allow adaptive shortening of the soft tissues carrying the retinacular vessels, say 24 hours (N.B. some authorities define 'acute' slip so as to include any case within 3 weeks of an acute episode).
(iii) if over-reduction takes place, even momentarily.

It has been stated that there is no such thing as gentle manipulation of the retinacular vessels, and great care must be taken to avoid the trap of misreading radiographs taken in different degrees of rotation which, as have been clearly shown, can mimic reduction.

In practice it is rare to be presented with the ideal combination of circumstances favourable to closed reduction, the usual problem being delay between the moment of acute slippage, and either diagnosis, or availability of operating facilities. Probably after 24 hours, and certainly after 48 hours manipulation should not be done.

Acute on chronic slippage implies a degree of slipping already too great for pinning *in situ*, so if manipulation fails or only partly succeeds, surgical restoration of anatomy must now be contemplated, with the following options available.

(i) Allow the acute slip to stabilize in its presenting position, or partly reduced, either by immobilization or temporary internal fixation with pins. Prolonged immobilization would lead to a risk of chondrolysis, but the epiphysis will stabilize in quite a short time, say 3 weeks. This can then be followed by (ii).
(ii) elective trochanteric osteotomy, which carries little if any risk to the capital vascular supply. (Basal cervical osteotomy is also done, for the same reason but this is much less popular.) The object is to restore the caput neatly into the acetabulum by removing a wedge based anteriorly (Griffith [3]) or antero-laterally (Southwick [6]). No further growth or remodelling will take place but some length will be gained by

geometrical realignment. Viewed from the lateral aspect a somewhat Z-shaped upper end of femur results, and the critics of this line of treatment would say that perfect restoration of anatomy is never achieved, the abduction mechanism is permanently misaligned and progression to early osteoarthritis, say by the 4th decade, is a common sequel. The misshapen upper end of femur then leads to technical problems with total hip replacement. Avascular necrosis, however, is practically eliminated: the surgeon will not have to face early failures (Fig. 6.4b, c).

(iii) Open replacement; an intracapsular procedure variously referred to as cuneiform osteotomy, trapezoid osteotomy or cervical osteotomy has the attraction of restoring as accurately as possible the head/neck relationship at the site of the lesion itself, and is done immediately after diagnosis, without preliminary traction or spica. The anterior approach to the joint can be used [7] but a lateral approach detaching the greater trochanter is better, allowing visualization of the anterior, lateral, and posterior aspects of the femoral neck. The greater trochanter is detached extracapsularly, and after the capsule is opened, great care is taken not to disrupt the continuity of the retinacular vessels running up the back of the femoral neck from the capsular reflection at its base.

The head of the femur is levered gently off the neck (Fig. 6.5a) and the exposed end of the metaphysis trimmed carefully so as to remove a wedge or trapezium (viewed from lateral aspect) of bone, plus the beak of new bone. Bleeding back should be demonstrated by curetting the concave inner aspect of the epiphysis at this stage, showing that it is still viable.

The minimum amount of trimming of bone is done to allow easy reduction of the neck against the head without tension in the retinacular vessels. Dunn [5] recommends 20° valgus alignment rather than square reduction. Five Crawford Adams pins are used to fix the reduction (Figs 6.5b, c, 6.6a, b, c) and one or two screws to replace the greater trochanter. Postoperatively, the leg is maintained on light skin traction allowing supervised movements for 4 weeks, followed by partial weight bearing for a further 8 weeks. If avascular necrosis supervenes, the changes will be apparent, clinically and on radiography, within 6 months. In Dunn's series of 73 open replacements, nine out of 24 cases of acute on chronic slip went on to avascular necrosis, but only two of these were complete, and seven partial (segmental or mottling only).

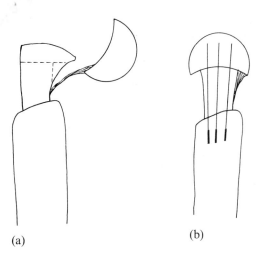

(a)

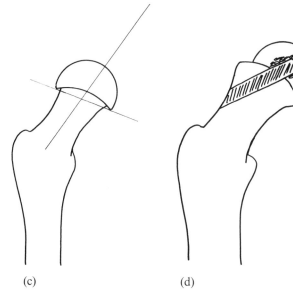

(b)

(c)   (d)

Fig. 6.5   (a) Open replacement: to show the amount of bone requiring removal at open replacement, including the beak, so as to allow reduction of head and neck without tension in the retinacular vessels. (b) Reduction and fixation achieved, square on the lateral view. (c) Up to 20° valgus is preferred on AP projection. (d) Epiphysiodesis.

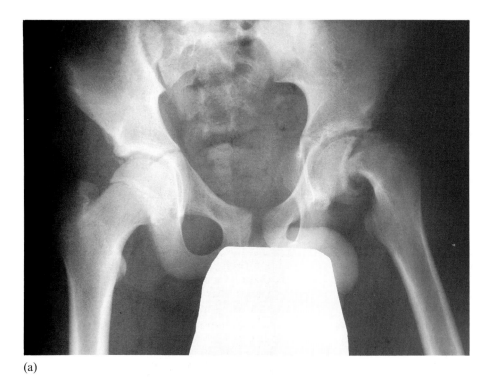

(a)

Fig. 6.6   (a) A severe case of acute on chronic left SUFE in a male aged 14 years 1 month: preoperative radiograph. (b) After open replacement. The greater trochanter has been refixed distally in order to tense the abductors. (c) Twelve months postoperatively, an excellent result, clinically and radiologically. The other side has been pinned prophylactically.

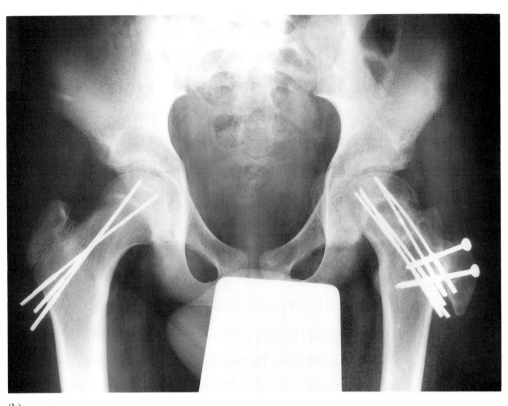

(b)

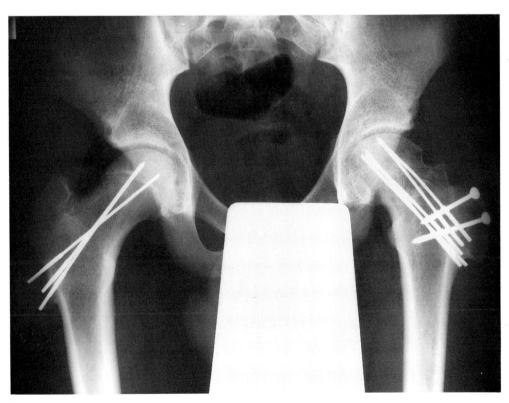

(c)

Type 3. Severe chronic slip, growth plate open. The author prefers a simple and reliable method of measuring backward angulation on the lateral radiograph, taking the axis of the femoral neck from the line of the original anterior cortex, ignoring the beak (Fig. 6.2f). The angle is measured between this line and the line bisecting the epiphysis. Severe chronic slip is defined as being over 40° of backward angulation.

Manipulation of a pure chronic slip without an

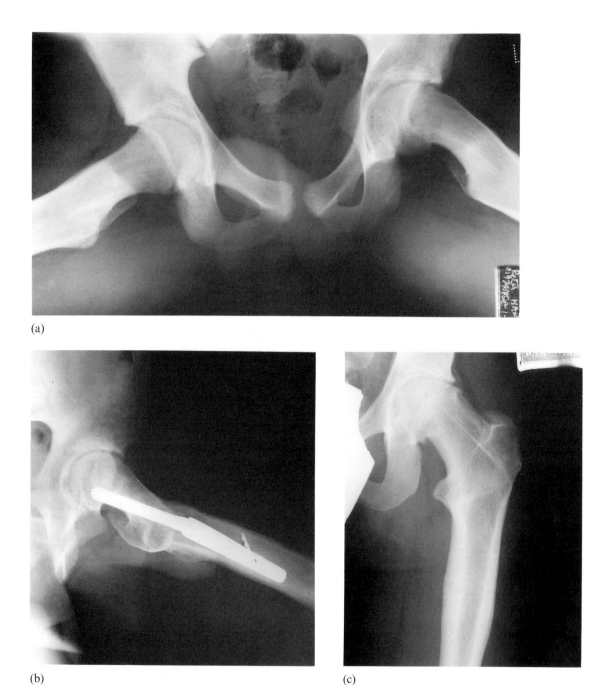

(a)

(b)　　　　　　　　　　　　　　　　　　　　(c)

Fig. 6.7 (a) Severe chronic slip, growth plate closed, left hip only, in a male patient aged 15 years 5 months. (b) After trochanteric osteotomy, closing an anteriorly based wedge. (c) The appearance 3 years later. There is some flattening of the superior surface of the head of femur, and early osteophyte formation.

acute episode has no place, and the options now are as follows:

(i) Stabilization by pins *in situ*, with no attempt to restore the anatomical relationship, allowing remodelling to take place with further growth. This course has been advocated, but it is difficult to see how this can work for very severe slips which will remain very limited by fixed external rotation and surely progress to early osteoarthritis. The younger child should however have greater remodelling powers.

Simple stabilization in this way carries practically no risk of avascular necrosis, though chondrolysis has been reported.

(ii) Trochanteric osteotomy as above. Preliminary stabilization by pins, or traction etc., is not necessary.

(iii) Basal cervical osteotomy.

(iv) Open replacement, as above. In the absence of acute separation the capital epiphysis will need to be levered off the metaphyseal surface of the neck using a broad curved gouge.

(v) Epiphysiodesis (Heyman–Herndon procedure [8], Fig. 6.5d). This consists of stabilizing the slipped epiphysis with a cortico-cancellous bone peg and chips which act as internal fixation plus graft, rapidly uniting the femoral head and neck. This is accompanied where necessary by a 'nubbinectomy' to reduce mechanical blockage to abduction and flexion. The risk of avascular necrosis is practically non-existent, but no attempt is made to restore normal anatomy [9].

Dunn [5] (1/40) and Fish [7] (0/36) separately reported a very low incidence of avascular necrosis after open replacement for severe chronic (type 3) slip, and therefore this would seem the operation of choice as normal anatomy is most nearly restored.

Type 4. Severe slip, growth plate closed. The metaphyseal vessels now contribute the main source of blood supply to the head, crossing the growth plate remnant, and if surgical reconstruction is felt to be necessary on grounds of deformity, limited movement or exceptionally pain, or to improve the prognosis for the longevity of the joint, it must now be done at a level away from the head/neck junction, to avoid jeopardizing these vessels. Osteotomy in the trochanteric region is usually done with the aim of restoring the head of femur comfortably into the acetabulum (Figs 6.4b, c, 6.7a, b, c).

In summary, the surgeon faced with a case of severe SUFE must first decide which type of slip he is dealing with, and then has a choice of options. Each option has its potential penalties; of the surgical procedures described only pinning *in situ* is straightforward; the others are all difficult technical procedures requiring attention to detail and special training.

Major complications

Avascular necrosis

Severe radiological collapse of the femoral head results in shortening, limited movement, limp, and wasting of thigh and buttock with a positive Trendelenburg test. Pain however, is conspicuous by its absence in the majority of cases, and if the temptation to perform arthrodesis can be resisted, a pseudarthrosis gradually appears with a wide and very useful joint space (Fig. 6.8). Walking without a stick is eventually possible, limp is reduced by a heel raise, and reasonable function for many years may ensue. There is no contraindication to total joint replacement later in life.

Chondrolysis

Also known as acute necrosis of cartilage.

This complication is uncommon, except in Negroes and Polynesians. It may follow any mode of treatment, or no treatment at all, and may be uni- or bilateral. It is manifested by a uniform loss of joint space radiologically, and progressive stiffness clinically, sometimes leading to severe deformity in flexion and adduction.

The aetiology is obscure: cartilage nutrition through synovial fluid is probably interfered with by immobilization in some way.

Microscopically, hyaline cartilage is replaced by fibrocartilage in a thin irregular layer, with normal bone beneath, at least to begin with: atrophy may follow. Dense intracapsular adhesions are formed and the capsule itself becomes inflamed and thickened up to 2.5 cm. Synovium practically disappears. In some less severe cases, gradual recovery takes place. There is no known effective treatment leading to recovery of normal hyaline cartilage. Manipulation under anaesthesia can improve the range of motion: sometimes osteotomy is necessary to reduce fixed deformity.

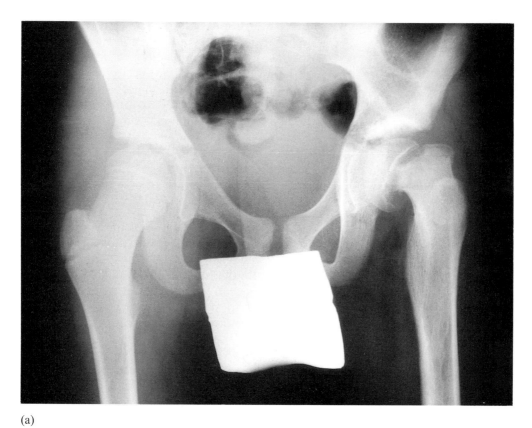

(a)

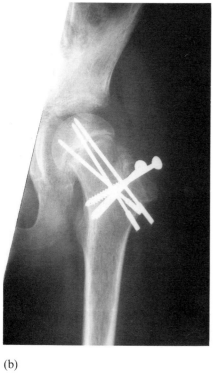

(b)

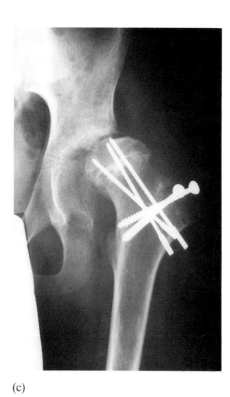

(c)

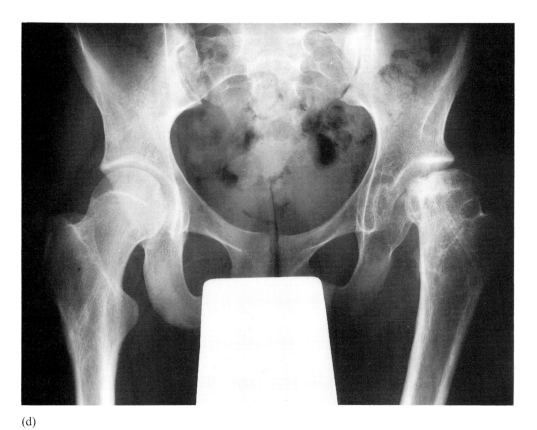

(d)

Fig. 6.8 (a) A case of acute on chronic displacement in a male aged 11 years 2 months, treated by open replacement. (b) Excellent reduction was achieved, but, (c) within 6 months, avascular necrosis of the capital epiphysis was obvious; subluxation is also occurring. (d) The eventual result, with 4 cm shortening, flexion to 90°, no pain, positive Trendelenburg (6 years later).

Osteoarthritis

Murray and Duncan [10] pointed out that many cases of 'idiopathic' osteoarthritis presenting in middle life on closer scrutiny can be seen to exhibit a minor degree of old slipped epiphysis, deduced from the shape of the head and neck of femur on radiography. They felt that athletic activity in adolescence might be a factor in the aetiology of such cases. Less commonly, the aetiology is obvious and the osteoarthritis severe (Fig. 6.9).

Jerre [11] in reviewing a large series, found that in addition to the cases of bilateral slip already diagnosed in adolescence, there were many undisclosed cases of minor slippage which came to light at review many years later: of 30 such cases, 18 had evidence of degenerative change on radiography at an average age of 37 years, though without symptoms at that time.

Dunn and Angel [5] described the articular cartilage of the femoral head as being thicker at its zenith than at its periphery, and suggested this might account for early degeneration if anatomy is not accurately restored, as weight is then borne on the thinner peripheral cartilage.

Osteoarthritis may follow, sooner or later, any of the surgical procedures described above, which all aim to minimize the deviation from the normal head/neck anatomical relationship, and it is reasonable to suppose that the greater the deviation, the worse the prognosis. Severe cases usually culminate in total hip replacement.

At the present time, the following questions remain open to debate.

1. Exactly where should one pitch the threshold of

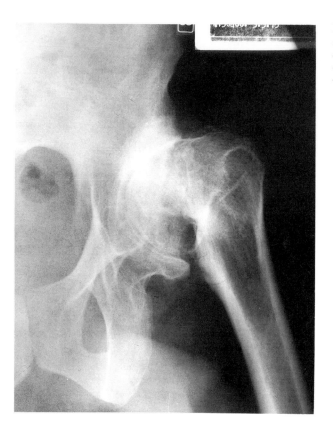

Fig. 6.9   This man presented at the age of 37 years with a history of slowly increasing limp, pain, stiffness and deformity of the left hip dating back to his teens. Osteoarthritis was severe, and the aetiology in this case was obvious. Total hip replacement was necessary.

severity, between cases suitable for pinning *in situ*, and those in which surgical reconstruction should be done.

2. In acute slippage, when, if ever, should manipulation be attempted.
3. Should surgical reconstruction be carried out at the level of the physis or base of the neck or trochanteric region?
4. Which method carries the greatest risk to the greater number?
5. What should be done for acute on chronic slip with severe displacement?

Open replacement most nearly restores anatomy at the level of the lesion, and has been shown to be safe in cases of severe chronic slip. In acute on chronic slips, especially those with severe displacement of up to 90° backward angulation, clearly something must be done to effect at least partial reduction before fixation is achieved. Open replacement carries a risk of avascular necrosis of the order of 20–25%. It has been suggested that the blood supply to the capital epiphysis may already be irreversibly damaged in the process of acute slippage in some cases. A pre-operative bone scan might clarify this point,

but reduced uptake in the capital epiphysis can be obscured by increased activity in the beak of new bone.

Trochanteric osteotomy carries virtually no risk of avascular necrosis, but the proponents of open replacement through the physis would argue that it is better to produce a near normal head/neck relationship with an excellent long term prognosis for the great majority, accepting a small number of early failures some of which will require further surgery, than to do a procedure which is relatively safer in the short term, but which condemns many of its recipients to osteoarthritis at an early age, with the prospect of difficult revision surgery in view of the deformity of the upper femur.

There is a lack of long term prospective reviews of properly classified series which might eventually give answers to these questions.

Acknowledgement

I should like to thank Mr R. J. McLean ABIPP of the Department of Medical Photography,

Queen Alexandra Hospital, Portsmouth, for his help in producing the illustration and photographs.

References

1. Trueta, J. (1957) The normal vascular anatomy of the human femoral head during growth. *J. Bone Joint Surg.*, **39B (2)**, 358–394.
2. Green, W. T. (1945) Slipping of the upper femoral epiphysis. Diagnostic and therapeutic considerations. *Arch. Surg.*, **50**, 19–33.
3. Griffith, M. J. (1976) Slipping of the capital femoral epiphysis. *A. R. Coll. Surg. Engl.*, **58**, 34–42.
4. Harris, W. R. (1950) The endocrine basis for slipping of the upper femoral epiphysis. *J. Bone Joint Surg.*, **32B**, 5–11.
5. Dunn, D. M., and Angel, J. C. (1978) Replacement of the femoral head by open operation in severe adolescent slipping of the upper femoral epiphysis. *J. Bone Joint Surg.*, **60B (3)**, 394–403.
6. Southwick, W. O. (1967) Osteotomy through the lesser trochanter for slipped capital femoral epiphysis. *J. Bone Joint Surg.*, **49A**, 807–835.
7. Fish, J. B. (1984) Cuneiform osteotomy of the femoral neck in the treatment of slipped capital femoral epiphysis. *J. Bone Joint Surg.*, **66A**, 1153–1168.
8. Herndon, C. H., Heyman, C. H. *et al.* (1963) Treatment of slipped capital femoral epiphysis by epiphysiodesis and osteoplasty of the femoral neck. *J. Bone Joint Surg.*, **45A**, 999–1012.
9. Melby, A., Hoyt, W. A. and Weiner, D. S. (1980) Treatment of chronic slipped capital femoral epiphysis by bone graft epiphyseodesis. *J. Bone Joint Surg.*, **62A**, 119–125.
10. Murray, R. O. and Duncan, C. (1971) Athletic activity in adolescence as an aetiological factor in degenerative hip disease. *J. Bone Joint Surg.*, **53B (3)**, 406–409.
11. Jerre, T. (1950) A study in slipped femoral epiphysis. *Acta Orthop. Scand.* **Suppl.**, **6**.

7

Spinal deformities

R. A. Dickson

Basic principles

In order to understand the treatment of spinal deformities it is important to have a clear appreciation of basic principles. 'Spinal deformities' has its own language as regards terminology and classification and much of the vocabulary is confusing if not meaningless. The aetiology of spinal deformities is perhaps the most important basic principle to grasp, as knowledge of this explains much about the natural history of spinal deformities. Then, before considering individual types of spinal deformity an overall management strategy is a necessity.

Terminology

Scoliosis is defined as a lateral curvature of the spine, a curvature in the coronal plane. This is an unsatisfactory definition as few, if any, scolioses exist solely in the coronal plane. The great majority are associated with axial rotation and thus the deformity also involves the sagittal plane. Moreover, vertebral shape in the transverse plane is also asymmetrical.

Kyphosis and lordosis are terms describing spinal shape in the sagittal plane only. Kyphosis refers to a curvature of the spine convex backwards (the posterior elements form the curve convexity), while lordosis describes a spinal curvature convex anteriorly (the vertebral bodies form the curve convexity). The terms 'structural' and 'non-structural' are applied to spinal deformities in an effort to distinguish those that are important from those that are not [1]. Unfortunately, the terms 'structural' and 'non-structural' do not describe any of the important distinguishing features (Fig. 7.1). A structural scoliosis, for example, is defined as a lateral curvature of the spine with rotation [1] and even this definition does not provide the information required. A structural scoliosis is important because it involves the spine primarily and has progression potential with spinal growth. It would be better termed 'primary' or 'progressive'. In contradistinction, a non-structural scoliosis is defined as a lateral curvature only, i.e. without rotation [1], but this again does not describe its important features. A non-structural scoliosis is not an intrinsic problem of the spine or its supporting mechanisms but occurs for some other reason, e.g. leg length inequality tilting the pelvis, or painful paraspinal muscle spasm accompanying a disc derangement. Moreover, these non-structural curves have no progression potential of their own and thus the term 'secondary' or 'non-progressive' would be infinitely preferable.

Scolioses are described according to the side of the convexity of the curve and where the apex of the curve is located. Thus right thoracic or left lumbar conveniently and quickly assigns a curve to a particular pattern. If the apex of the curve is T12 or L1 then it is referred to as thoraco-lumbar. If there is more than one curve in the spine, e.g. a combination of right thoracic and left lumbar curves, then this is called a double curve. If there

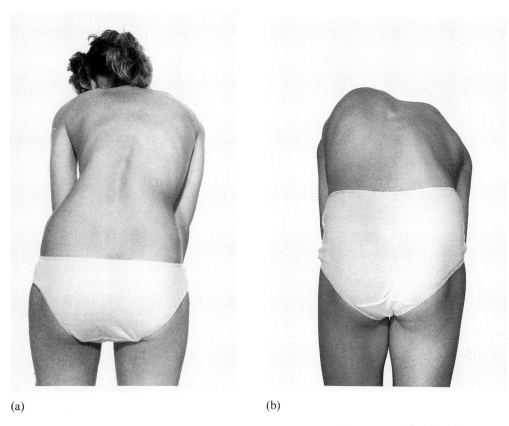

(a)   (b)

Fig. 7.1   (a) Non-structural scoliosis in a girl with an adolescent disc protrusion. There is a lateral curvature without rotation. (b) Structural scoliosis in a girl with idiopathic scoliosis. There is a marked rotational prominence.

are more than two curves then the expression 'multiple curve pattern' is applied.

The Cobb method of measurement is universally used to register radiographically the size of the deformity [2]. On an AP film lines are drawn parallel with the upper border of the upper end vertebra (the vertebra above the apex which is maximally tilted into the curve concavity) and along the lower border of the lower end-vertebra (the vertebra below the apex which is maximally tilted into the curve concavity) and these two lines are produced until they intersect. The angle subtended is referred to as the Cobb angle of the curve. While this may be a quick and easy method of estimating curve size, it is notoriously misleading. The bigger a curve becomes the more it is rotated away from the coronal plane of the patient such that the AP view progressively underestimates the true size of the deformity. Therefore a curve of 60° is much more than twice as bad as a curve of 30° and, similarly, a curve

that has been corrected surgically from 60° to 30° has achieved a much greater than 50% correction. Thus Cobb angle data cannot be handled in an arithmetic way by deriving percentage changes or means. Yet every article published about scoliosis with reference to curve size derives a mean Cobb angle which is quite inadmissible.

If the deformity is a kyphosis, existing solely in the sagittal plane, then the Cobb angle is a very reasonable method of measurement. Because of the rotation accompanying structural scoliosis, other measurements of deformity size are more relevant. From the AP radiograph the amount of apical rotation can be measured by the method of Pedriolle [3] and this is accurate for curves with a Cobb angle not much in excess of 60°. Because of the difficulty in obtaining a satisfactory radiographic measure of the size of the overall deformity, much attention has recently been focused on measurement of surface shape and there are a number of methods available including the sophisticated integrated shape imaging system (ISIS). In practice, the angle of trunk inclination (ATI) can be easily measured with a simple inclinometer [4]. Because it is body shape that requires correction in the great majority of cases coming to surgery, then it is important that some measure of surface shape be routinely used.

Classification

The basic classification proposed by the Scoliosis Research Society is simple and short [1]. The classification comprises idiopathic deformities, congenital deformities, neuromuscular deformities, deformities in association with neurofibromatosis, mesenchymal disorders (heritable disorders of connective tissue, mucopolysaccharidoses and skeletal dysplasias), trauma, infection and tumours. The classification is not strictly of spinal deformities, except idiopathic, but of the associated conditions. Table 7.1 shows the classification in more detail. While of descriptive use, it misleads into believing that there is something different about the deformities of, say, neurofibromatosis and osteogenesis imperfecta. This of course is not so, the deformities are the same, it is the conditions which differ.

Pathogenesis

Once the pathogenesis of idiopathic scoliosis is appreciated [5] it is not difficult to understand why spinal deformities are particularly prevalent when there is some associated condition as listed above in the classification. Indeed the aetiology of idiopathic scoliosis has been known for more than a century [6], but these published works have received scant attention and a seemingly enormous advantage of the development of X-rays has done more to confuse than to assist this issue by highlighting the lateral curvature component of the deformity. Thus X-rays have reduced down to two dimensions a deformity which is clearly happening in three. Accordingly, although for no obvious reason, most workers have sought to try and find something different between the convex and concave sides of a scoliosis without thinking about rotation. In the

belief, and belief only, that our normal healthy, and usually pretty, teenage girls with idiopathic scoliosis have subclinical muscular dystrophy, poliomyelitis, or other as yet unnamed neuro-

Table 7.1   Aetiological classification of spinal deformities: primary, progressive or structural deformities

A.   Idiopathic deformities
   1. Idiopathic scoliosis
     a. Early onset
     b. Late onset
   2. Idiopathic kyphosis
     a. Type I – classical Sheuermann's disease
     b. Type II – 'apprentice's spine'

B.   Congenital deformities
   1. Bone deformities
     a. Scoliosis   (1) Failure of formation
     b. Kyphosis   (2) Failure of segmentation
     c. Lordosis   (3) Mixed
   2. Cord deformities
     a. Myelodysplasia scoliosis
     b. Myelodysplasia kyphosis
     c. Myelodysplasia lordosis

C.   Neuromuscular deformities
   1. Cerebral palsy
   2. Poliomyelitis
   3. True 'neuromuscular disorders'

D.   Deformities in association with neurofibromatosis
   1. Dystrophic deformities
   2. Idiopathic-type deformities

E.   Mesenchymal deformities
   1. Heritable disorders of connective tissue
   2. Mucopolysaccharidoses
   3. Bone dysplasias
   4. Metabolic bone disease
   5. Endocrine disorders

F.   Traumatic deformities
   1. Vertebral
   2. Extravertebral

G.   Deformity due to infection
   1. Pyogenic infection
   2. Tuberculosis

H.   Deformity due to tumours
   1. Intradural tumours
   2. Syringomyelia
   3. Paravertebral childhood tumours
   4. Primary extradural tumours
   5. Metastatic spinal disease

I.   Miscellaneous conditions

muscular condition, the quest has been for some neuromuscular difference between right and left sides. This work has encompassed electroencephalography, equilibrial function, and electromyography at one end of the spectrum to the structure and ultrastructure of the paraspinal muscles and the spinal cord at the other [7]. These investigations have shown that some evidence of abnormality can be demonstrated in some patients with idiopathic scoliosis, generally those with bigger curves, but not all patients, and indeed in many controls with straight backs. Thus these changes cannot be considered aetiological because if they were to be so then all patients with idiopathic scoliosis should have evidence of the abnormality. The correct inference from these studies is that such changes as have been demonstrated might be considered factors favouring progression of an established idiopathic deformity. Indeed it would be quite reasonable to imagine that if there was some subtle alteration in a spinal balance mechanism then the spine would be less able to resist buckling deformation.

Many studies, such as those concerned with electromyography or the structure of the paraspinal muscles, have demonstrated that whatever changes have been shown are secondary to the presence of the curve. This again is not surprising in the presence of a significant deformity of the axial skeleton. Moreover, none of these workers has produced any evidence of how a structural spinal deformity can be caused by, for example, a bit of equilibrial dysfunction.

Proponents of neuromuscular factors in the aetiology of idiopathic scoliosis have conveniently ignored the extensive literature on this subject dating from the beginning of the nineteenth century. The classic work of Adams in 1865 [6], and indeed other workers before him, indicated that the primary lesion of idiopathic scoliosis was a lordosis at the curve apex. Adams stated that 'lordosis plus rotation equals lateral flexion'. This statement was the result of his clinical observations as well as his dissections of individuals with idiopathic scoliosis. It was abundantly clear to him that once a lordosis developed in the thoracic spine, which should normally be kyphotic, then with both growth and forward flexion it would readily buckle round to the side to produce the appearances of a lateral curvature of the spine.

This lordosis theory can be readily confirmed by two simple observations. First, the PA radiograph of any patient with any form of structural scoliosis shows a lateral curvature of the spine with rotation such that the posterior elements lie in the curve concavity while the anterior vertebral bodies twist into the curve convexity (Fig. 7.2). As Roaf later pointed out, a line conjoining the tips of the spinous processes will thus pursue a shorter distance through the curve than a line conjoining the middle of the anterior bodies. The back of the spine is therefore shorter than the front and this elementary geometrical point confirms that every structural scoliosis, including the idiopathic variety, is lordotic. Second, it is a standard clinical observation since the time of Adams that the rotational deformity is much less obvious in the erect position than leaning forward. This is why the forward bending position is used in scoliosis clinics as well as in the field for epidemiological purposes. On forward flexion the over long front of the spine is forced to buckle to the side in order to be accommodated. The deformity of kypho-scoliosis does not therefore exist [5] and, as Steindler later pointed out [8], 'kyphosis is a condition which counteracts and not facilitates the presence of a lateral spinal curvature.'

If, however, the coronal and sagittal planes of the patient, and not the rotated deformity, are selected for X-ray purposes then both the PA and lateral views will therefore be oblique views of the apical region (the obliquity being dependent upon the degree of apical rotation). Stagnara demonstrated that by turning the patient or X-ray beam according to the amount of apical rotation a true PA view of the apex could be obtained and in this line of projection the deformity was maximal [9]. He referred to this as the 'plan d'election'. More importantly, if a true lateral view of the curve apex is obtained (90° to the plan d'election) then every structural scoliosis can be demonstrated to be lordotic over the apical three or four vertebral bodies (Fig. 7.3a). In Leeds we have now taken true planar views of more than 300 patients with idiopathic thoracic scoliosis and have also studied sagittal profile in the areas above and below the curve apex. The apical three or four vertebrae are always lordotic and this lordosis is at bone level, the disc height not contributing to spinal shape.

The appearances on the true lateral view are

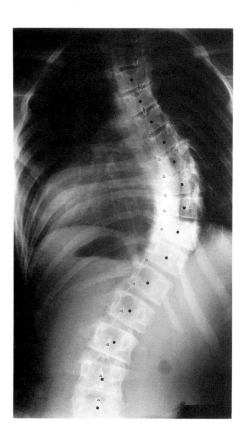

Fig. 7.2 PA radiograph of an idiopathic thoracic scoliosis. The tips of the spinous processes have been marked with hollow triangles and the centre of the anterior bodies with black dots. Therefore a line drawn through the curve along the posterior elements can be seen to be shorter than a line drawn down the vertebral bodies. The back of the spine is shorter than the front in every structural scoliosis and these deformities are therefore lordotic.

exactly the opposite of the other idiopathic deformity of childhood, Scheuermann's kyphosis (Fig. 7.3b). In the former the vertebral bodies are wedged, with anterior height being greater than posterior and any Schmorl node formation and end-plate irregularity being sited posteriorly. In Scheuermann's kyphosis, however, the bodies are wedged kyphotically with anterior height being reduced in comparison to posterior and any Schmorl's nodes or end-plate irregularity more anteriorly. Thus both idiopathic thoracic scoliosis and Scheuermann's kyphosis are principally concerned with shape in the sagittal plane over the three or four apical vertebrae. All that matters now is the position of this apical region in relationship to the axis of spinal column rotation, which normally passes anterior to the thoracic kyphosis and posterior to the cervical and lumbar lordoses. As the thoracic spine is normally kyphotic and lies behind this axis then it is under tension and will not therefore buckle to the side under the influence of either growth or forward flexion. Any excessive degree of thoracic kyphosis, as in Scheuermann's disease, puts the

thoracic kyphosis even further behind this axis while any degree of flattening of the thoracic spine brings the vertebral bodies closer to the buckling point. In the presence of a frank lordosis, as occurs in idiopathic scoliosis, then the front of the thoracic bodies at the curve apex lies anterior to the axis of spinal column rotation and on growth and forward flexion must mechanically buckle to the side to be accommodated.

These changes in the sagittal plane are not as gross as might be considered. The normal thoracic kyphosis extends from D3 to D10 (the upper and lower most thoracic vertebrae belonging to the cervical and lumbar lordoses, respectively). If we say that the degree of normal thoracic kyphosis from D3 to D 10 is of the order of 24° (this figure being selected for arithmetic ease principally) then the eight thoracic vertebrae between D3 and D10 would normally be kyphotically wedged by some 3° or so. Scheuermann's disease is diagnosed radiographically by three consecutive thoracic vertebrae being wedged by 5° or more [10]. Thus normal sagittal spine shape only has to increase over three vertebrae by 2° to be

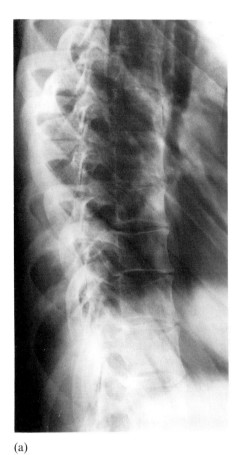

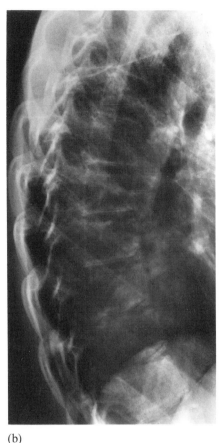

Fig. 7.3 (a) True lateral of the apex of an idiopathic thoracic curve showing lordotic vertebrae. (b) Lateral radiograph of the apex of idiopathic thoracic hyperkyphosis (Scheuermann's disease) which is the opposite deformity in the sagittal plane to idiopathic scoliosis.

(a)   (b)

diagnosed as Scheuermann's disease. Reciprocally, reduction of the normal thoracic kyphosis by just over 3° will produce an area of lordosis, the patient then developing idiopathic scoliosis.

Meanwhile children and adolescents are growing in three dimensions at the same time and it is an established fact that the normal thoracic kyphosis of late childhood flattens during early adolescence while again increasing just before maturity [11]. If the thoracic kyphosis flattens excessively during early adolescence and becomes frankly lordotic then the patient develops idiopathic scoliosis, a condition typically presenting in early adolescence [5]. On the other hand, if the patient's thoracic kyphosis becomes increased beyond the norm during later adolescence then the patient develops Scheuermann's disease, a condition characteristically appearing within 2 years of maturity. Both idiopathic scoliosis and Scheuermann's disease occur in otherwise entirely normal healthy children, occur at the same site with the D8–9 region being principally

affected, have a similar familial trend and community prevalence rate [10]. The familial trend has nothing whatever to do with a 'gene for idiopathic scoliosis or Scheuermann's disease' but reflects the familial trend in sagittal spine profile which has already been demonstrated in anthropometric studies. It is therefore quite unnecessary and indeed illogical to propose a primary neuromuscular cause.

However, should the neuromuscular balance mechanisms of the spine be in any way deficient then progression of this unstable deformity will be favoured. It is well known that in early onset idiopathic scoliosis the great majority of children have resolving curves. These children are characterized by being of normal birth weight, normotonic, and of normal neurological development scores. By contrast, the less common infantile malignant idiopathic progressive curve, while having exactly the same lordo-scoliotic deformity, is characteristically found in low birth weight, floppy, hypotonic babies with low neurological development scores [12]. In this situation progression of the deformity is strongly enhanced. Thus, as regards idiopathic deformities, they are divisible into two primordial types – lordosis (which buckles to the side to produce a secondary scoliotic deformity) and kyphosis (a deformity which is rotationally stable and stays in the sagittal plane). True sagittal plane views of the vertebrae above and below the apical region of an idiopathic scoliosis demonstrate that these vertebrae are truly kyphotic. Indeed this can be clearly seen on the PA radiograph of the patient (Fig. 7.2). Vertebral rotation, with the posterior elements being directed towards the curve concavity, persists into the upper and lower compensatory curves. If the scoliosis was of the typical right thoracic variety then above and below the apical region the compensatory curves are convex to the left, while the posterior elements are still rotated towards the left. This implies that

these areas of so-called 'compensatory scoliosis' are indeed asymmetric kyphoses restoring three dimensional spinal balance. In the infantile idiopathic malignant progressive curve the asymmetric kyphosis above the area of buckled lordosis can progress in its own right to produce a combination of deformities of angular kyphosis above and buckled lordosis below (Fig. 7.4).

Meanwhile in the patient with Scheuermann's kyphosis this area of deformity is balanced by lordoses above and below. The hyperlordosis below the apex of a Scheuermann's kyphosis may then buckle to the side to produce a secondary scoliotic deformity, as in idiopathic scoliosis. This accounts for why more than 60% of patients with Scheuermann's kyphosis have evidence of idiopathic scoliosis four or five segments below the apex of their kyphosis [13] (Fig. 7.5). It would be nonsensical to talk about two different pathological processes four or five vertebrae apart in an

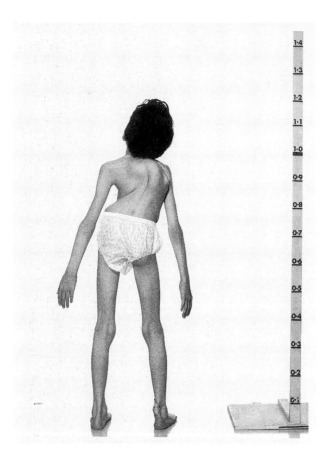

Fig. 7.4   The angular kyphosis above an area of lordo-scoliosis is typical of the child with infantile progressive scoliosis.

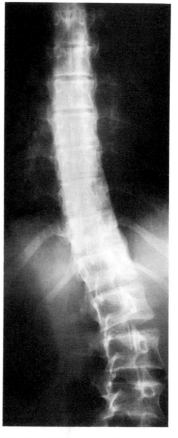

Fig. 7.5   PA spine radiograph in a case of Scheuermann's thoracic hyperkyphosis showing the associated lordo-scoliosis in the lumbar region.

otherwise normal, healthy adolescent [5]. The idiopathic scoliosis below the Scheuermann's kyphosis seldom, however, achieves clinical significance. This is because the deformity of Scheuermann's kyphosis does not develop until much closer to skeletal maturity and because the area of kyphosis, so close to the area of buckled lordosis, protects from significant rotation.

The above analysis of idiopathic spinal deformities would reduce the average engineer to a state of boredom. He would readily confirm that his beam, or more strictly speaking cantilever, can in fact only fail in one of two ways – simple angular collapse (kyphosis) or beam buckling (lordo-scoliosis) [14]. He would also say that not only the development but also the subsequent behaviour of these two primordial deformity types is governed by elementary mechanical principles. This is where the rest of the aetiological classification of spinal deformities comes in. As regards beam buckling, this is governed by Euler's law and of the various parameters incorporated in this law some are more obviously relevant to spinal deformities.

If there is intrinsic weakness of the cantilever or, in this case spinal column, then beam buckling is facilitated. At bone level this weakness occurs in Von Recklinghausen's disease with its typical dystrophic vertebral form, osteogenesis imperfecta, the mucopolysaccharidoses, and skeletal dysplasias. Although the structural scoliosis in Von Recklinghausen's disease is of the same lordo-scoliotic type as seen in the idiopathic patient, the usually sharp, angular, dystrophic vertebral shape in association with an earlier onset deformity and more progressive one testifies to nothing more than the principles of Euler's law. Similarly in brittle bone disease, the worse the degree of the underlying condition, the more prevalent and progressive the spinal deformity associated with it. At soft tissue level, intrinsic spinal load is increased by soft tissue weakness of the cantilever or spinal column. Thus in Marfan's syndrome, homocystinuria, and Ehlers–Danlos syndrome, buckled lordo-scolioses are both more prevalent and progressive than in the idiopathic patient. At neuromuscular level, again Euler's law has to be obeyed. Patients with cerebral palsy, poliomyelitis, and the true neuromuscular conditions of childhood (e.g. the peripheral neuropathies, Friedreich's ataxia, and the muscular dystrophies) all have a higher prevalence

rate and progression potential of buckled lordo-scolioses; the more severe the neuromuscular failure the more prevalent and progressive the spinal deformity. These neuromuscular deformities are generally long C-shaped collapsing deformities extending through the thoraco-lumbar region down to an oblique pelvis. Here the lumbar lordosis is often exaggerated as a part of the primary condition and once asymmetric paraspinal muscle action is applied then the deformity readily buckles (Fig. 7.6).

Simple angular collapse implies true material failure, either of the anterior column under compression, as in trauma, tumours, or infection, or the posterior elements under tension, as in flexion injuries of the spine, or post-laminectomy. As with the idiopathic counterpart, these deformities are behind the axis of spinal column rotation and do not rotate. In the trauma patient with para-

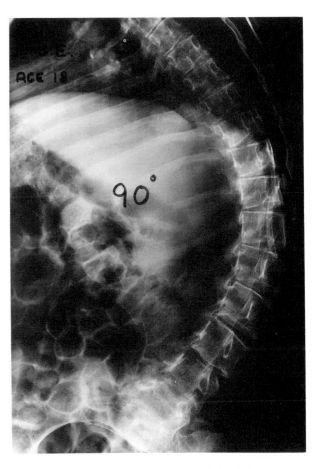

Fig. 7.6 The long c-shaped lordo-scoliosis with associated pelvic obliquity typical of the neuromuscular deformity.

lysis there is often an area of angular kyphosis where the bony injury occurred and below this an area of collapsing paralytic lordo-scoliosis secondary to neuromuscular failure in the region of a primary lordosis. If, however, paralysis is superimposed on an area of the spine which is primarily kyphotic, such as occurs with the congenital kyphosis of myelomeningocele, then the thoraco-lumbar spine is protected from buckling because the spine is behind the axis of spinal column rotation. Thus in the spina bifida kyphosis patient the spine remains in the sagittal plane (Fig, 7.7).

It can therefore be seen from the pathogenesis of idiopathic and other types of spinal deformity that these deformities can, and indeed must, be explicable on the basis of simple mechanical principles. Superimposed upon this is the biology of the situation and the more severe the underlying condition, the more its effect will be on increasing the intrinsic load to the spine. Meanwhile the idiopathic deformity, whose prevalence rate and progression potential is least obvious, must still obey Euler's law. The longer the cantilever or spinal column the more the centre of it will buckle, and it is interesting to note that patients with idiopathic scoliosis are marginally but significantly taller than their straight-backed counterparts [15]. Whether this merely implies a period of accelerated growth, the spine is still obeying Euler's law. Another important factor in this law is that the bigger the deformity the more likely it will be to progress. Thus a deformity of 40° is more progressive than a deformity of 20° on purely mechanical terms.

There are therefore two primordial types of spinal deformity – lordosis and kyphosis. The former can buckle to the side to produce the appearances of a structural scoliosis, while the latter remains in the sagittal plane. These two principal deformity types are seen throughout the classification of spinal deformities where the local biological situation dictates the severity of the mechanical response.

Management strategy

It is important to have an overall management strategy to which only detail needs to be added for the particular case or condition. There are four principal factors in this strategy – curve size, progression potential, the presence of paralysis, and the underlying condition.

Curve size

For centuries it has been recognized that the bigger the curve the more likely is the risk of subsequent cardiopulmonary dysfunction. Studies of untreated scoliosis patients have shown two to three times higher mortality and morbidity rates, as well as significant social and psychological impairment, with curves at the more severe end of the spectrum [16]. A figure of 60° has been bandied about as a threshold for thoracic curves at or above which it has been deemed necessary to prescribe surgical treatment in order to mitigate the future pulmonary consequences. This strategy, based upon curve size alone, is totally incorrect. The patients who form the basis of these long term studies were a hotchpotch of diagnoses, although usually idiopathic,

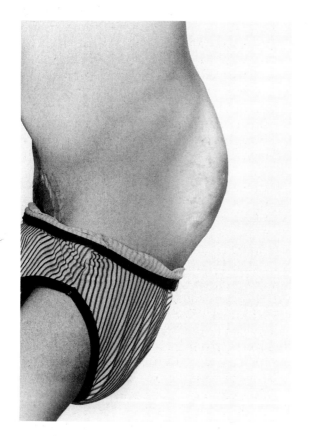

Fig. 7.7   The congenital lumbar kyphosis of myelomeningocele.

and had a very wide range of curve sizes. What was ignored in these studies was the age of onset of the curve. Clearly, all other things being equal, a curve of 130° must have started earlier than a curve of say 65°. The correct inference from these studies is that it is age of onset that matters rather than the actual curve size. Indeed in Nachemson's study he was able to identify a group of patients whose curves definitely started early in adolescence and these patients showed no differences whatever as regards organic ill health from control date [16].

More importantly Reid, the principal pathologist at the Brompton Hospital in London, had already performed autopsy studies on children with scoliosis who had died from other reasons and found that provided the curve was not considerable, not more than 60°, during the phase in which the pulmonary alveoli are developing, up to the age of 5, then there was no risk of severe pulmonary dysfunction no matter what size the curve ultimately achieved [17]. This largely ignored work has been recently confirmed by Branthwaite who surveyed all of Zorab's cases in the Brompton Hospital. She clearly demonstrated that late onset thoracic scoliosis, beyond the age of 5 years, was not associated with any risk of cardiopulmonary dysfunction in the future, while the much less common early onset progressive case, with an appreciable curve size during the phase of pulmonary alveolar development, was accountable for all the mortality and morbidity in thoracic scoliosis. It is therefore only necessary to consider two types of scoliosis – early onset and late onset. The former is a matter of great concern to organic ill health, while the latter is solely a question of deformity. Of course, the bigger the deformity, the more unfair life is to patients, with lower marriage rates, higher divorce rates, lower numbers of children per marriage, higher psychiatric consultation rates, and higher suicide rates, but this must be clearly demarcated from true organic ill health.

The majority of patients coming to surgical treatment are of the late onset variety and thus what matters is the deformity and what the patient and family's assessment of it is. If the deformity is deemed acceptable by the patient and family, and not by the surgeon whose opinion of somebody else's deformity is quite irrelevant, then preservation of acceptability is the aim. If, on the other hand, the deformity is

deemed unacceptable then treatment should be directed towards making it acceptable again. The management strategy for late onset scoliosis, as regards curve size, is therefore straightforward. If the deformity is acceptable then this would be the place for conservative treatment so that the deformity would never become unacceptable during growth. Thus far, bracing has been the mainstay of conservative treatment, although the French have used serial casts as an alternative and there has been some dabbling with electro-spinal stimulation. The first popular brace was the Milwaukee brace [18] developed, not for the idiopathic patient, but for the poliomyelitis patient whose spine required support postoperatively. With the end of the great poliomyelitis epidemics the Milwaukee brace was soon used for idiopathic curves as a conservative measure. Although it enjoyed popularity for more than 2 decades, proponents never challenged its efficacy against untreated controls. There was therefore no scientific evidence that it either corrected the deformity or prevented its progression. A recent trial, albeit of a small number of patients, showed that there was no significant difference in the progression rates whether the brace was worn or not [19], while a recent study from Oxford showed that, even in the most apparently compliant patients, the brace was only worn for less than 20% of the time that it should have been. Meanwhile natural history studies have demonstrated that many fewer curves than formerly thought actually progress. For 30° curves in early adolescence one-third progress, one-third stay the same, and one-third actually improve somewhat. Against these natural history figures there is no evidence that either Milwaukee (or Boston) bracing is effective. Similarly, electro-spinal stimulation is ineffective and that has also been demonstrated by a controlled study [20].

It is not difficult to appreciate why the deformity of lordo-scoliosis cannot be treated nonoperatively [21]. The opposite deformity of kyphosis, being a uniplanar deformity in the sagittal plane, requires extension and a patient with Scheuermann's disease can rapidly reduce their kyphosis wearing an extension brace or cast. This is because the deformity is rotationally stable. If, therefore, kyphosis requires extension then the opposite deformity of lordosis requires flexion and that is when it is rotationally unstable, buckling out to the side to enhance the rib

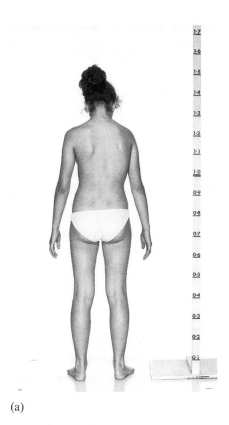

(a)

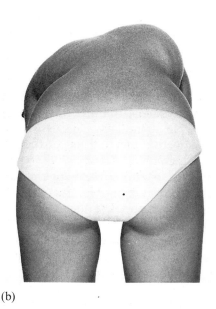

(b)

Fig. 7.8   (a, b) Erect and forward bending views of a girl with idiopathic thoracic scoliosis showing that the rotational prominence is enhanced on forward bending.

hump (Fig.7.8). It might, however, be conceived that imprisoning a patient in some form of erect orthosis or cast would at least minimize the number of flexion cycles during the day and thus attenuate progression but there is no evidence that this is so. If the curve is going to get worse then it will do so whether it is surrounded by a brace or not.

Another common misunderstanding is the duration of spinal growth. It has been assumed that the spine stops growing at the same time as the extremities and pelvis [22]. This would be at about 15 years in girls and between 16 and 17 years in boys. As a result, inspection of the status of ossification of the vertebral ring apophyses or the iliac crest apophysis is used as an assessment of adolescent growth and fusion is believed to imply the attainment of spinal maturity. Anatomists in previous centuries, have however clearly shown that the vertebral end-plate epiphyses, not the ring apophyses which have nothing whatever to do with spinal growth, do not fuse on average until the 25th year [23]. This does not mean that the spine grows inches between 15 and 25 but that change of shape is still possible until these end-plate epiphyses fuse. While this may not have very much import to the straight spine, it may be crucial for the deformed spine whose buckling tendency will continue to be accommodated until the middle of the third decade. It is not therefore surprising to find evidence that curves continue to deteriorate until the mid-20s although suppositions concerning the effect of pregnancy have been shown to be erroneous. Thus, even if a conservative treatment measure could be devised which prevented progression, it would have to be prescribed for a time period not commensurate with patient compliance. No 10-year-old girl would be prepared to wear a contraption 23 hours a day for 15 years.

If the deformity is acceptable at presentation then the patient should be observed at intervals during the phase of spinal growth in order to determine what the future has in store. The majority will stay the same or regress and thus no treatment will ever be required. The minority will progress, but only some of them will progress sufficiently to achieve unacceptability. These require surgical treatment.

For those that present with an unacceptable deformity then correction is inherent in the management strategy. This is the place of operative treatment. The earliest corrections were obtained pre-operatively using a localizer or turn-buckle cast but in the 1950s Harrington instrumentation was developed [24]. This system of distraction on the concave side combined with compression on the convex side was introduced for the poliomyelitis patient without fusion, but the metalwork rapidly failed without biological support. It was soon used for the idiopathic patient and although considerable spinal stability was achieved, such that the previously high pseudarthrosis rate was considerably reduced, the degree of correction was no better than that achieved by former casting methods. This is because the method of correction is by distraction at the top and bottom of the curve and cannot be expected to have any influence over the rotational disposition of the curve apex (Fig. 7.9). The rib hump therefore remained essentially unchanged.

The addition of wires attached to the posterior elements of the spine and tightened round the longitudinal metalwork enabled the apical region to be influenced, but the direction of pull was necessarily sideways [25]. Although the Cobb angle over the apical region was seen to be improved, there was no alteration of the rotational prominence because the metalwork was pulling behind the axis of spinal column rotation. Indeed in some cases rotation was made worse, while in others some cosmetic improvement occurred as a result of the rib hump being pulled more closely towards the midline. Like Harrington instrumentation, this technique of sublaminar wiring was developed for the poliomyelitis spine but soon found its greatest usage in the idiopathic case. In February 1982 in Leeds, following several years of clinical, mechanical, radiological, and animal experimentation [5], a technique was developed whereby the rib hump could be appreciably reduced by derotation. A longitudinal Harrington distraction rod was bent into 20° of kyphosis and segmental wires under the concave laminae were then tightened. The direction of the pull of these wires was thus more backwards than sideways so that the concave side was elevated and the convex side reciprocally depressed with a reduction in the rotational prominence (Fig. 7.10). As a result, there was not only an enhanced correction in the coronal plane but an average 50% correction of the rotational disposition of the apical vertebra [26]. Then, 1 year later, Cotrel

and Dubousset developed a similar system of derotation and thoracic kyphosis restoration by bending a longitudinal rod favouring the lateral curvature and then rotating it round 90° into the sagittal plane with the spine attached to it (Fig, 7.11). The addition of a convex rod, slightly less bent, applied downward pressure on the convex side. For mild, flexible curves only a 40% derotation was achieved [27]. None the less, it is the rotational prominence with which the majority of patients present and which in turn these patients wish corrected and these are the only two methods which will do so.

Then in the 1960s Dwyer, in Australia, developed his system of anterior spinal instrumentation, this time for the idiopathic thoracolumbar or lumbar curve [28]. Screws are passed transversely through the vertebral bodies from convex to concave sides and then a braided metal cable is passed through holes in the screw heads. Using a special cable tightener, followed by crimping the screw heads over the cable, the convex side was shortened and correction facilitated by excision of the intervertebral discs in the curve. Good corrections were observed in the coronal plane but the complication rate was high. More recently this instrumentation has been upgraded by Zielke and the German instrument school [29]. The metalwork is superior but the technique and results similar. Although popularized for the idiopathic case these instrumentation systems are more often used for paralytic thoraco-lumbar and lumbar curves with pelvic obliquity, as a preliminary first stage (Fig. 7.12).

The method by which all of these instrumentation techniques achieve a correction is by taking up the natural flexibility of the curve. If a curve measures say 60° standing and 30° on side bending or under maximum traction then the instrumentation will correct the curve down to 30° but seldom any further. The bigger a curve gets the more rigid it becomes and flexibility correspondingly reduces. Thus for the more severe and less flexible curve little is achieved by instrumentation alone. In order to enter this rigid phase spinal traction was devised so that before the instrumentation stage as much pre-operative correction as possible was obtained. Unfortunately there is no evidence that any form of traction enters this rigid phase, and one study comparing Cotrel dynamic traction versus localizer casting versus halo-pelvic traction showed

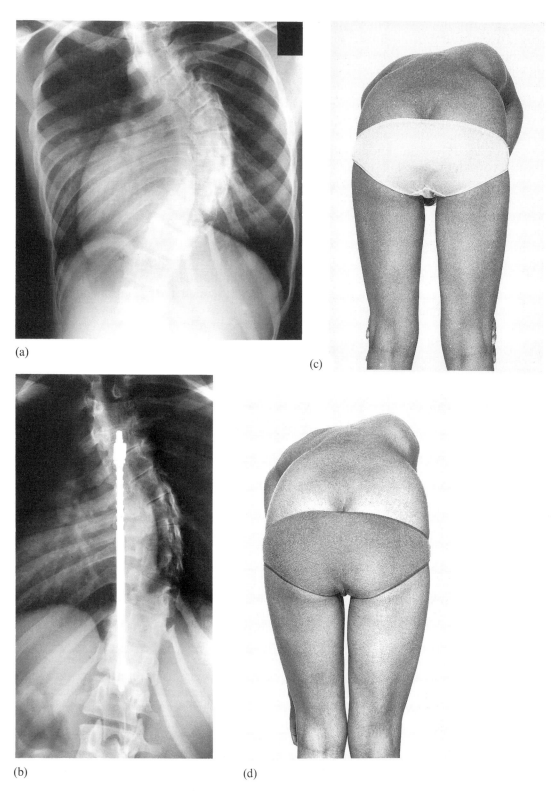

(a)

(b)

(c)

(d)

Fig. 7.9 (a) PA radiograph of an idiopathic thoracic scoliosis before surgery. (b) PA radiograph after Harrington distraction instrumentation and fusion showing a seemingly good correction. (c) Forward bending view of this girl before surgery. (d) Forward bending view 2 years after surgery showing no change whatever in the rotational prominence with which she presented.

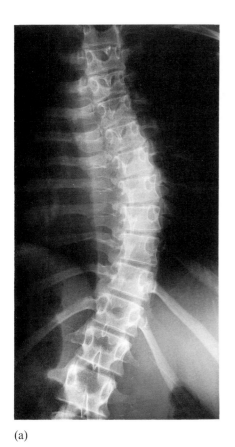

(a)

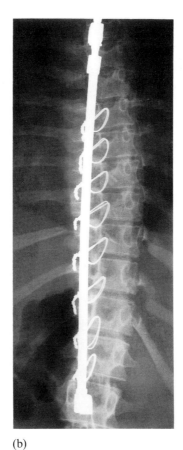

(b)

Fig. 7.10   The Leeds procedure – segmental derotation combined with thoracic kyphosis recreation. (a) PA radiograph of an idiopathic thoracic curve before surgery. (b) PA radiograph after the Leeds procedure. (c) Forward bending view showing the obvious rib hump before surgery. (d) Forward bending view 2 years after surgery showing an almost complete correction of the rotational element of the deformity.

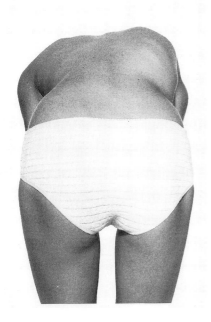

(c)

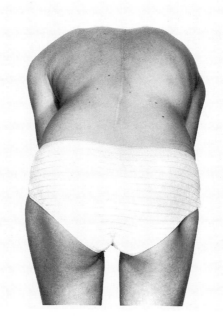

(d)

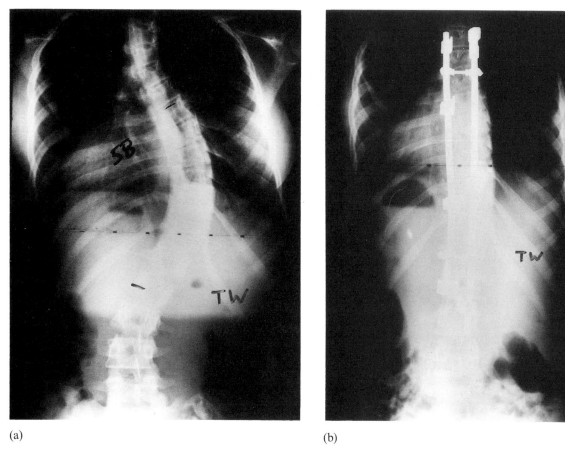

(a)   (b)

Fig. 7.11   Cotrel–Dubousset (CD) instrumentation. (a) PA radiograph of a thoracic idiopathic curve before surgery. (b) PA radiograph after surgery. The improved rib symmetry indicates appreciable derotation.

no significant differences with none of the treatment modalities able to enter the rigid phase [30].

The only effective way to enter this phase is by surgical intervention [26]. For curves that are not excessive, but are beyond a one posterior instrumentation stage, flexibility can be achieved by way of a preliminary soft tissue release. As the back of the spine is shorter than the front and is therefore the compression side, it would appear logical to release the relatively tighter posterior soft tissue structures, but this would lead to unacceptable lengthening of the curve with an increased risk of tension paralysis. The soft tissue release should therefore be performed anteriorly by way of multiple discectomies of the apical region. Then in the second posterior instrumentation stage, the same instrumentation procedure as is performed for the more mild and flexible curve, there is room for the over long front of the spine to be pulled through without causing undue

lengthening (Fig. 7.13). Moreover, and very importantly, along with the discs are removed the vertebral growing end-plates so that the front of the spine will not overgrow in the future.

For the most severe and rigid curves, of whatever aetiology, even anterior discectomy is insufficient. The only satisfactory solution to this problem of straightening a rigid, bent pipe which contains the vital spinal cord is to shorten the apex of the pipe itself. This is achieved by way of two stage wedge resection, a technique devised and popularized by Leatherman [31]. When rigid congenital curves were first dealt with it was by way of either one stage hemivertebrectomy or by opening wedge osteotomy. The complication rate, and in particular the paralysis rate, was unacceptably high because too much surgery was done at one sitting, shortening was not a feature of the procedure, and there was little stability available as Harrington instrumentation had not

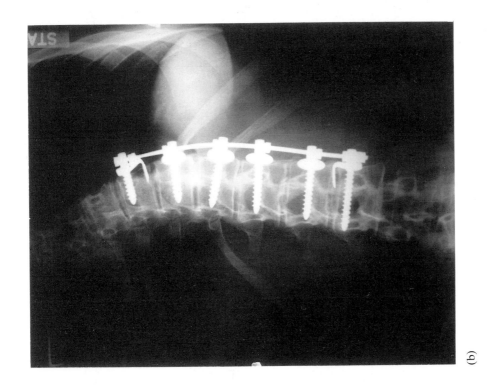

(b)

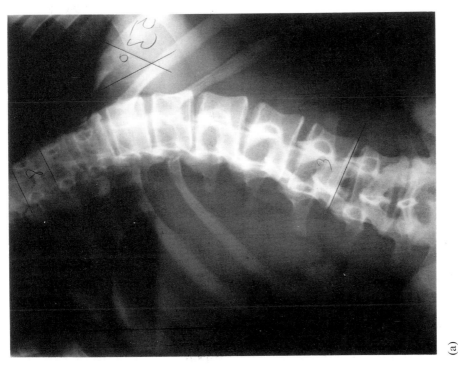

(a)

Fig. 7.12 The Zielke procedure. (a) PA radiograph of a thoraco-lumbar idiopathic curve before surgery. (b) PA radiograph after anterior segmental Zielke instrumentation showing a good correction.

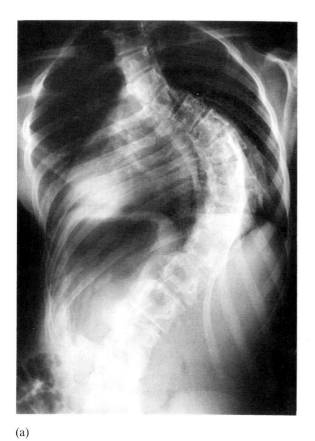

(a)

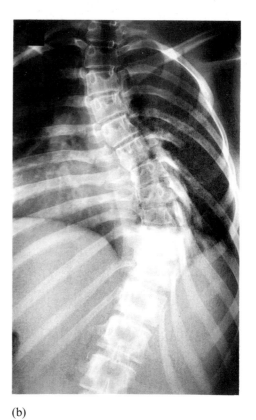

(b)

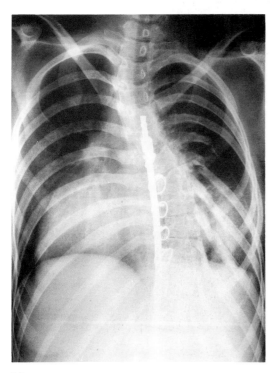

(c)

Fig. 7.13 Two stage anterior and posterior Leeds procedure. (a) PA radiograph of a severe thoracic idiopathic scoliosis before surgery. (b) PA radiograph a few days after anterior multiple discectomy. The deformity has collapsed into itself spontaneously without instrumental correction. (c) PA radiograph just after second stage posterior Leeds instrumentation showing further improvement but the great majority of the correction has occurred between stages spontaneously.

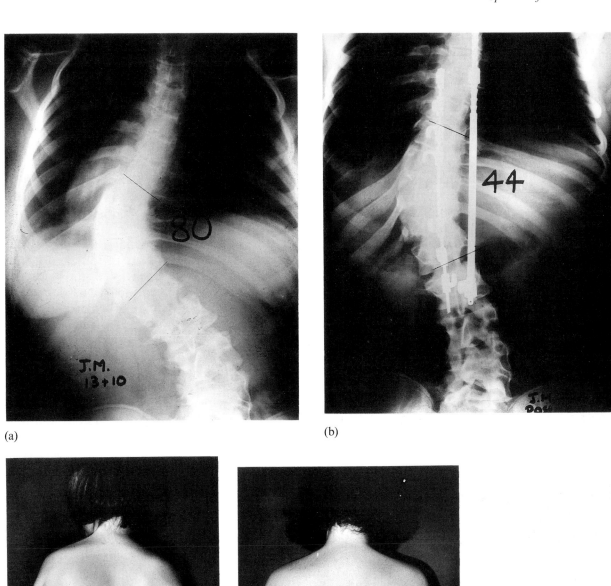

(a)

(b)

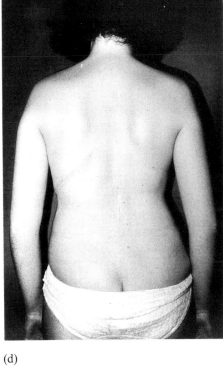

(c)

(d)

Fig. 7.14 Leatherman's two stage closing wedge osteotomy and fusion for severe rigid curves. (a) PA radiograph of a severe lower thoracic curve before surgery. (b) PA radiograph postoperatively. (c) Back view of this girl before surgery showing a severe deformity. (d) Back view 2 years after surgery showing no appreciable torso asymmetry. Radiographs say little about surface shape.

yet been devised. Two stage wedge resection fulfils these criteria and in the first stage the anterior vertebral body, which is always wedge shaped in three dimensions, is resected. In the second stage the posterior elements are resected to complete the wedge excision. Then a Harrington compression system is applied to the convex side and tightened so that the wedge is closed. Only then is a distraction rod inserted on the concave side to aid stability and to gain some correction in the upper and lower compensatory curves (Fig. 7.14). This procedure has stood the test of time and is the safest way of dealing with a severe rigid curve. It is always far better to plan two stages, although this means more surgery for the patient, than to take on too big and rigid curves by means of one instrumentation stage only.

The early onset curve is undoubtedly the most difficult to treat. Fortunately more than 90% of early onset idiopathic curves resolve spontaneously, but those that do not are as progressive as their congenital and Von Recklinghausen's counterparts. If the rib vertebra angle difference is in excess of 20° or rises on sequential measurements, particularly in the low birth weight hypotonic baby, then action must be taken immediately. Serial EDF casting has been shown to convert curves with all the hallmarks of progression into resolving or static ones [12]. This is infinitely preferable to having to tackle these curves surgically at such an early age. Unfortunately many do not present until curve size is excessive, and so of course is rigidity, in which case a preliminary anterior stage is very often necessary.

Progression potential

During the phase of spinal growth, i.e. the first 25 years of life, spinal deformities have progression potential. Thus for curves which have been seen to progress during the phase of observation, or those which have been corrected surgically, it is necessary to prevent subsequent progression with growth. This is the place for spinal fusion operations. At the beginning of this century when spinal fusion was first carried out it was performed posteriorly principally for the convenience of the surgeon. It was not, however, clear at that time that the essential lesion of structural scoliosis is an apical lordosis [5] and thus posterior fusion would not appear to be the most logical solution to progression potential. It is rather akin to performing a postero-medial fusion for talipes equinovarus instead of the postero-medial release which is obviously to be preferred. None the less, the great majority of patients being treated were adolescents with idiopathic curves whose growth velocity was waning and for whom posterior fusion did appear to stop or minimize progression subsequently. With the development of Harrington instrumentation it became standard practice to correct the curve with the instrumentation and at the same sitting perform a posterior spinal fusion in order to prevent progression. Long term studies of this procedure have demonstrated that, despite an initial correction due to the instrumentation, the fusion of the over short back of the spine does lead in most cases to subsequent further buckling so that 2 or 3 years from surgery the deformity is very much the same as that pre-operatively.

The younger the child in whom posterior fusion is performed the greater is the risk of tethering the back of the spine in bone and thus allowing the anterior bodies, which are already overgrowing, to buckle round to the side (Fig. 7.15). Thus purely posterior fusion for young patients is positively harmful [32] and for early onset curves the spine must be fused front and back in order to both attenuate spinal growth locally and stabilize the deformity from progression. The opinion is still widely held that as soon as an early onset curve has demonstrated progression it should be forthwith dealt with by posterior fusion, but long term studies of this approach testify to its harmful effect. The strategy as regards progression potential is therefore simple. If the curve is late onset it can be held by a posterior fusion, but only reliably so if the thoracic kyphosis is recreated during the instrumentation procedure so that the spine is now put in its right position in relationship to the axis of spinal column rotation [26]. For young patients with progressive curves the spine must be fused front and back. Furthermore, for curves of greater progression potential than idiopathic ones, e.g. those in Von Recklinghausen's disease or the heritable disorders of connective tissue, posterior fusion is never sufficient to mitigate progression and an anterior fusion should always be performed.

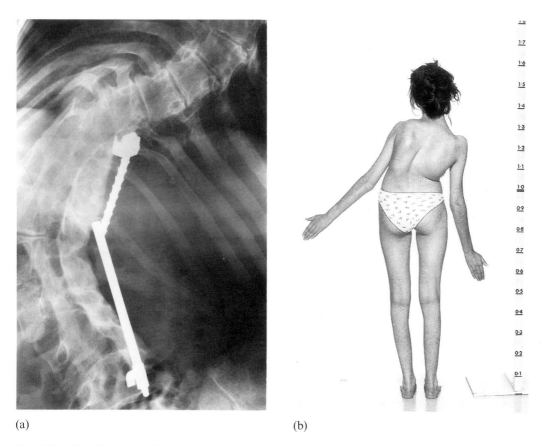

(a)   (b)

Fig. 7.15 The disastrous effects of posterior tethering fusion on the young spine. (a) & (b) PA radiograph and appearance in the erect position showing an idiopathic lumbar scoliosis with a tethered posterior fusion, a broken rod, and almost 90° of apical rotation.

The presence of paralysis

There are two important factors here – the presence of a neuromuscular condition, or the presence of a structure which may itself induce paralysis. For the typical paralytic lordo-scoliosis with pelvic obliquity it has become quite clear that the spine cannot be reliably propped up by posterior instrumentation and fusion alone. Anterior instrumentation and fusion should always be insisted upon as a preliminary first stage. Moreover, the indications for operating on the paralytic spine have also become quite clear. It was generally accepted that if either walking potential or sitting stability were being jeopardized by the presence of the scoliosis then surgery was indicated. However, Lonstein, when he looked at the results of surgery in more than 100 cases of cerebral palsy scoliosis, showed the futility and harm of operating on the walking patient [33]. The great majority of these patients do require a mobile lumbar hyper-lordosis in order to walk at all to counter gluteal muscle weakness. If the lumbar spine is then flattened and made rigid as a result of surgery, many of these patients, who still had walking potential were rendered wheelchair bound. Therefore the only indication for operating on the paralytic spine with pelvic obliquity is loss of sitting stability. If the patient is unable to sit in a wheelchair without the use of their arms for support then the spine should be stabilized surgically which will liberate the hands for prehensile function.

It is important to be aware of conditions associated with a high risk of paralysis by way of natural history or treatment. There is a high incidence of spinal dysraphism in patients with

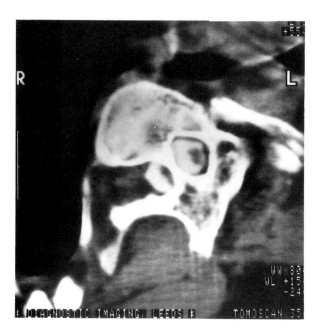

Fig. 7.16 CT myelogram showing a diastematomyelia, a bony spur splitting the cord.

congenital spine deformities and thus all patients should be assessed pre-operatively by way of spinal cord imaging (Fig. 7.16). Should the cord be cleaved by a diastematomyelia, or compressed locally by an intradural lipoma, or be associated with a tethered filum terminale then surgical treatment is extremely dangerous without the offending structure being removed by way of a preliminary laminectomy. In any event the spinal deformity must always be shortened during straightening in these rigid deformities [31].

If the patient with the seemingly typical idiopathic deformity is troubled by spinal pain, particularly at night, then this should raise suspicion of spinal tumour. Some will be found on technetium bone scanning to have an osteoid osteoma/osteoblastoma, but others will be shown by spinal cord imaging to be associated with an intradural neoplasm or syrinx. This latter group are particularly important. Spinal cord tissue is already embarrassed by the space occupying lesion and if this is not recognized and the spine is corrected by way of distraction instrumentation the paralysis rate is in excess of 50%. Such spines should therefore be dealt with neurosurgically and then stabilized by spinal fusion but no attempt at correction of the deformity should be made.

The underlying condition

Under no circumstances should the spinal deformity be divorced from the underlying condition. In patients with Duchenne dystrophy, homocystinuria, Ehlers–Danlos syndrome, and many other conditions associated with a spinal deformity there are matters of much greater import to the patient than the spinal deformity. Although most patients with Duchenne dystrophy develop a significant paralytic scoliosis while sitting in their wheelchair, death is inevitable from an underlying cardiomyopathic or pulmonary event by the end of their teens. While it may seem beneficial for these patients to have a stable spine during their terminal years the mortality rate of 10% from simple posterior spinal instrumentation and fusion is unacceptable.

Patients who demonstrate generalized ligament laxity and have features of the Marfan's syndrome should be very carefully assessed by clinical experts in this field. If the patient has true Marfan's syndrome, or a forme fruste thereof, then surgery is not contraindicated. If, however,

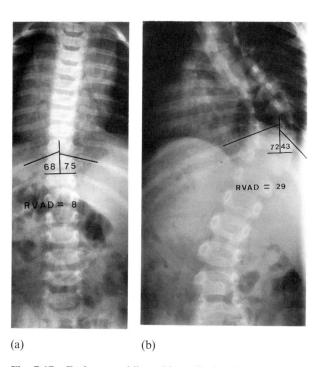

(a)   (b)

Fig. 7.17 Early onset idiopathic scoliosis. (a) PA radiograph of a resolving curve with a small Cobb angle and small/rib vertebra angle difference (RVAD). (b) PA radiograph of a progressive infantile curve with a large Cobb angle and RVAD.

the patient has homocystinuria then intravascular coagulation is very prevalent following surgical intervention such that the mortality is unacceptable high. Similarly if the patient has the type of Ehlers–Danlos syndrome which is associated with blood vessel fragility then excessive haemorrhage during surgical intervention is the rule rather than the exception. Again the mortality rate is too high to contemplate surgical intervention here.

Although these conditions are nowhere near as common as idiopathic scoliosis, knowledge of the important aspects of the underlying condition is crucial to the appreciation of when and when not to operate. With so many powerful weapons in our surgical armamentarium the most important decision a surgeon can reach is when not to operate.

Types of spinal deformity

Idiopathic deformities

Idiopathic scoliosis

Early onset idiopathic scoliosis

The much more common resolving form is differentiated from the progressive form by clinical and radiographic examination (Fig. 7.17). The resolving variety is found in normal birth weight healthy looking babies whose deformities are completely correctible during side bending over the examiner's knee. Curve size is modest and the rib-vertebra angle difference (RVAD) less than 20°. The progressive variety occurs in low birth weight floppy babies with rigid deformities which show no correction on side-bending. Curve size is greater and the RVAD is in excess of 20°. Both types share the same body moulding features of plagiocephaly, plagiopelvy, bat ear, and sometimes a torticollis [12]. This is attributable to lateral decubitus cot positioning, whereas prone cot positioning seems to prevent such moulding. The moulding features are more obvious in the progressive case.

Resolving scoliosis merely requires serial observation to ensure regression although the rotational prominence is often the last clinical feature to disappear, sometimes taking as long as 10 years. Progressive curves require immediate treatment by way of serial EDF casting and this can be performed under very light general anaesthesia [12]. The cast is changed every 3 or 4 months according to the growth of the child. By this means some are converted to 'resolvers', but some remain static and may form the template for subsequent progression during adolescence. Although it is traditional to apply a spinal brace after, say, 2 years of casting there is no evidence that this alters the natural history of the condition. Clearly, the static curves may require surgical treatment for progression during adolescence. For those who present too late for effective cast treatment, or for those who fail to respond to cast treatment, surgical intervention is necessary. If the deformity is acceptable then anterior and posterior spinal fusion should be performed. If the deformity is unacceptable then correction is necessary. Moderate curves with some flexibility respond well to multiple anterior discectomy followed by posterior spinal fusion with Harrington instrumentation, trying as far as possible to create some degree of thoracic kyphosis [26]. For those with the most rigid curves there is no substitute for two stage wedge resection [31].

Late onset idiopathic scoliosis

If the deformity is acceptable then preservation of acceptability is the aim. Unfortunately no non-operative method alters the natural course of this form of scoliosis and thus a period of observation is necessary [21]. Should the deformity be unacceptable, or achieve unacceptability during observation, then surgical correction is necessary. It should be emphasized that unacceptability is a matter for the patient and family and not for the orthopaedic surgeon. Obviously if the patient is young with the curve progressing during observation then the surgeon can advise the parents that the deformity may finish up two or three times as bad as it is at present and this may influence in favour of early surgical intervention. However, if the patient is beyond skeletal maturity, or indeed in their early twenties, then progression potential is generally insignificant. Surgical intervention, therefore, is a matter solely for the patient and family to decide upon.

Thoracic curves should be dealt with by recreation of the thoracic kyphosis and in Leeds we favour a kyphotic distraction rod using sublaminar wires on the concave side to derotate [26] (Figs 7.10 and 7.13). If the convex rib prominence appears obvious following instrumentation then further correction of the rib hump can be achieved by dividing the apical ribs just beyond the transverse processes and tucking the lateral end under the medial. This is a minor procedure and is performed subperiosteally and extrapleurally. It adds little to the operative time and postoperative discomfort is minimized by infiltrating bupivacaine into, or cryoprobing, the local intercostal nerves. Posterior spinal fusion out to the tips of the transverse processes is then performed and homograft cancellous bank bone laid into the bed. It is quite unnecessary to remove bone from the patient's pelvis which adds to the scarring, operative time, blood loss, and postoperative discomfort.

It is preferable to perform this, and all other types of, instrumentation under continuous spinal cord monitoring and a 50% change in amplitude or latency demands an immediate 'wake-up' test to ensure that the spinal cord is not jeopardized by tension. The use of a combination of Harrington distraction instrumentation with sublaminar wiring is associated with a higher neurological complication rate but this is not due to the sublaminar position of the wires but rather what is done with them. If the Harrington rod is first maximally distracted before the wires are tightened then the spinal deformity is made rigid under tension. The wires will then almost certainly not be able to bring the spine in contact with the rod but more important the bony spine will be further lengthened, thus incurring the risk of paralysis. The correct method of performing this procedure is therefore to distract the rod sufficiently to engage the hooks only. Then the sublaminar wires are tightened. Further distraction is then only permissible when all the wires are tight and the spine is in contact with the rod throughout [26]. It is usually found that the rod will not distract any further after the wires have been tightened. It is therefore attention to operative detail in relationship to an understanding of the three dimensional nature of the deformity of structural scoliosis which minimizes neurological complication rather than having to rely on spinal cord monitoring or the 'wake-up' test.

It is probably unnecessary to support the spine postoperatively when there is a combination of rods and sublaminar wires, but in Leeds we prefer to apply a lightweight zippable polyurethane (Neofract) support for the first 6 months. For those who have undergone convex rib division we apply a Cotrel EDF cast with a pull strap over the rib prominence for the first 6 weeks until these iatrogenic rib fractures unite. This allows the rib hump to be favourably influenced until rib union.

Thoraco-lumbar and lumbar idiopathic curves require much thought before surgical intervention. Long term studies of these lower curves when dealt with by posterior spinal instrumentation and fusion have demonstrated a high incidence of the ugly flat back deformity with spinal pain, presumably from overloading the lower lumbar discs. This is in many situations a worse deformity than the patient had preoperatively. In Leeds we would endorse Nachemson's view that lumbar curves should not be operated upon and that a mobile lumbar spine, albeit deformed, is better than a straighter, flatter, rigid one [34]. Thoraco-lumbar curves can be managed by anterior Dwyer or Zielke instrumentation because it is not necessary to incorporate so many vertebrae in the fusion. None the less, some degree of flattening of the upper lumbar spine will occur. For double structural curves with a thoracic and thoraco-lumbar/lumbar component the same strictures apply. The lower curve should not be operated upon but, as is often the case, it is the thoracic component with its rib hump that is the more significant. This should be dealt with as for a single thoracic curve leaving a mobile, albeit somewhat deformed, lower spine. For a thoracic double structural curve, with two apices, one at D3 and one at D8/9, it is important that the rod crosses the spine to be inserted on the upper concave side of the upper curve. In this situation it is advisable not to use sublaminar wires but to perform convex rib division of the lower curve.

It is therefore thoracic curves with their associated rib hump which are most suitable for surgery. One stage posterior instrumentation and fusion is satisfactory for curves that are relatively mild and flexible but bigger curves, i.e. those with a Cobb angle between 65° and 90° do require anterior multiple discectomy in order to allow some flexibility and shortening [14,26]. For curves in excess of 90° or those which have undergone a previous fusion, there is no substitute for the safety and correctibility of two stage wedge resection [31] (Fig. 7.14).

Idiopathic kyphosis

This is the opposite deformity to idiopathic scoliosis and there are two types. Type I occurs in the thoracic region at the T8–9 level during late adolescence and is much the more common. Type II (apprentice's spine) occurs in the thoracolumbar or upper lumbar regions and is thought to be an epiphyseal response to strenuous activity.

Type II presents as a result of lumbar spine pain and the deformity is never considerable. By contrast, Type I presents with an increased thoracic kyphosis and local discomfort. On physical examination the deformity is rigid and this differentiates it from postural round back deformity. Radiographs demonstrate the opposite lesion to idiopathic scoliosis with an increased kyphotic wedging over the apical three vertebrae. There is often a mild idiopathic scoliosis four or five segments below the apex of the kyphosis and this is due to the compensatory lordosis buckling to the side [13]. Treatment is nearly always conservative and any form of extension orthosis or cast leads to a rapid correction of this rotationally stable deformity (Fig. 7.18). Because spinal maturity does not occur until the middle of the third decade, conservative treatment should always be prescribed up to this age. Only if the deformity is excessive in the older individual should surgery be considered. Anterior multiple discectomy with interbody and strut grafting followed by a second stage posterior instrumentation using rectangular segmental instrumentation is required to correct and stabilise

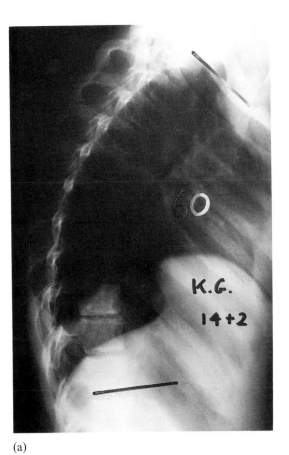
(a)

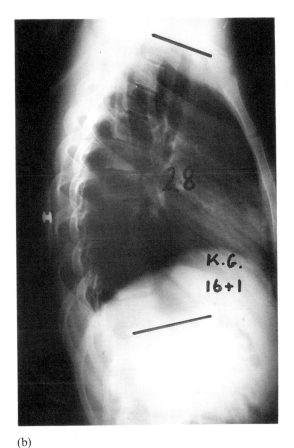
(b)

Fig. 7.18   Extension brace treatment for thoracic Scheuermann's disease. (a) Before treatment showing 60° of kyphosis. (b) After a year's extension bracing showing a more than 50% correction.

these deformities and this is not inconsiderable surgery while achieving a less than 50% correction of the degree of kyphosis. The real indication for surgery is the rare case with such a severe degree of kyphosis as to be jeopardizing neurological function in which case anterior dural decompression is additionally required in the first stage.

Congenital deformities

Congenital bony deformities

The offending congenital anomaly is either a failure of formation (hemivertebra) or a failure or segmentation (bar). There are two principal deformity types according to direction – scoliosis or kyphosis. If the hemivertebra or bar is on one side of the spine (unilateral) then a scoliosis develops, whereas if the growth discrepancy occurs

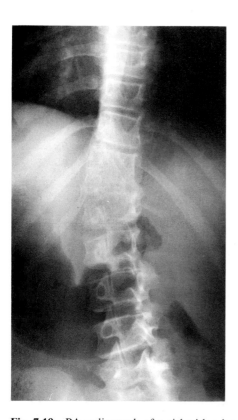

Fig. 7.19   PA radiograph of a girl with a lumbo-sacral hemivertebra on the right tilting the lumbar spine to the left. A T11–12 hemivertebra on the left helps to restore balance.

in the sagittal plane an angular kyphosis develops. The progression potential is worst when there is a bar on one side and a hemivertebra on the other, there being no growth plates on one side of the spine and too many on the other. Thus prognosis can be estimated according to the nature of the underlying anomaly [35]. Solitary hemivertebrae do not give rise to a significant progressive deformity and occurs solely in the coronal plane (the only true progressive scoliosis). If the hemivertebra occur in the lower lumbar region in the presence of a sacral tilt towards the side of the hemivertebra (a bad lumbo-sacral offshoot) then a progressive list can develop which can produce an ugly deformity (Fig. 7.19). By contrast, unilateral bars affect the back of the spine as well and thus the typical structural lordo-scoliosis is produced which progresses both by way of growth asymmetry and mechanical buckling. A rotational prominence is thus generated [14] (Fig. 7.20).

In the sagittal plane kyphoses usually occur at the thoraco-lumbar region. Anterior bars seldom produce a kyphosis of significance but the dorsal hemivertebra (anterior failure of formation) is notorious in producing an angular progressive kyphosis with neurological signs.

The intradural anomalies of spinal dysraphism are common in association with a congenital spine deformity and should be excluded by myelography, CT, or both. In addition, there is also a high prevalence rate of urinary anomalies and these should be assessed routinely by intravenous urography.

Treatment is a question of either progression potential or the presence of neurological signs. A thoracic or thoraco-lumbar hemivertebra requires observation only and the less segmented the hemivertebra the less is the progression potential and therefore the likelihood of the need for treatment [35]. Failures of segmentation are dangerous in terms of progression potential and while they should also be observed with the passage of time surgical intervention is frequently required. If the deformity is acceptable then preservation of acceptability is the aim and for this anterior and posterior fusion is required. If the deformity is unacceptable then the only safe solution to this problem is by way of two stage wedge resection of the curve apex [31]. For the lower lumbar/lumbo-sacral hemivertebra no action is required if the sacrum is horizontal. In the pres-

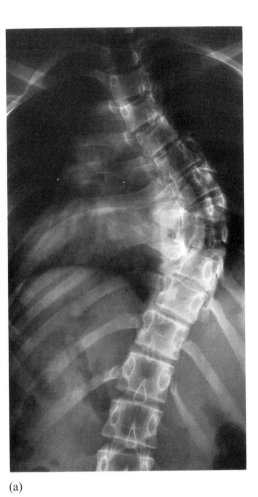

(a)

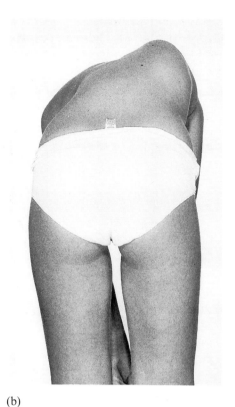

(b)

Fig. 7.20 (a) PA radiograph of a girl with a congenital thoracic scoliosis due to a unilateral unsegmented bar. (b) Forward bending view of this girl showing the significant rotational prominence associated with this lordo-scoliosis.

ence of an offshoot progression is inevitable and an early fusion does protect against progression. Because of the difficulties of anterior fusion in the lumbo-sacral region a posterior fusion suffices. For those presenting with an unacceptable deformity two stage hemivertebra resection is required [31]. In the second stage the lumbar lordosis must be maintained by contoured posterior metalwork and the entire structural curve should be fused. There is a considerable danger of L5 nerve root damage during hemivertebra removal and thus prophylactic fusion while the deformity is still acceptable is to be preferred.

Kyphoses should not be treated for cosmetic reasons only. The dorsal hemivertebra with the sinister neurological effects must be watched carefully (Fig. 7.21). There is a definite place for prophylactic anterior and posterior fusion for the progressive case. If neurological signs are already present (leg weakness, hyperreflexia, and clonus) then the spinal canal must be decompressed

anteriorly by removal of the offending hemivertebra followed by anterior strut grafting 31]. The problem is pressure from the front and thus laminectomy is not only futile but positively harmful by way of removing the integrity of the posterior column.

If an intradural tethering structure is present then there is usually cutaneous evidence (tuft of hair, naevus, dimple, or sinus) and the patient may have already presented with either incomplete control of micturition or an attenuated lower limb, often with an associated club foot deformity. Opinion varies concerning the need for treatment but a consensus opinion would be to remove the offending structure by way of laminectomy to deter neurological deterioration in the future. If corrective surgery is contemplated on a congenital spinal deformity in the presence of an intradural tethering lesion, then the tether should be removed by a preliminary laminectomy [31].

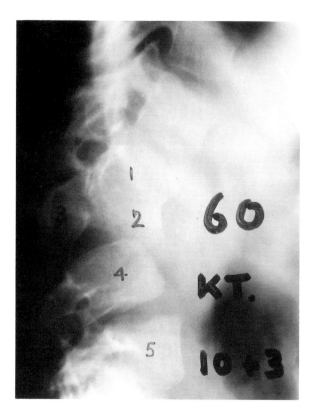

Fig. 7.21   Lateral radiograph showing a congenital dorsal hemivertebra. Cord compression commonly ensues.

Congenital cord deformities

These represent the spina bifida syndrome where there is evidence of myelodysplasia and neurological dysfunction. The more severe the neurological dysfunction the more the likelihood of a significant collapsing lordo-scoliosis with pelvic obliquity. This is difficult surgery with potentially serious complications (pseudarthrosis and sepsis being the most relevant). The walkers should not be treated lest a rigid and flat lumbar spine militates against ambulation. It is the wheelchair sitter who is losing sitting stability that merits surgical intervention and this must be in the nature of both anterior and posterior instrumentation and fusion [14] (Fig. 7.22).

Forty percent of progressive scolioses in the spina bifida syndrome are due to congenital bony anomalies in the thoraco-lumbar region with a relatively straight lumbar spine below. These should be dealt with by two stage wedge resection of the curve apex, again for sitting stability reasons [14].

Ten percent of deformities in association with myelodysplasia are lumbar kyphoses (the congenital lumbar kyphosis of myelomeningocele). The problem here is of kyphotic vertebral wedging at the curve apex, present since birth, associated with anterior soft tissue contracture (annulae fibrosi), anterior longitudinal ligament, diaphragmatic crura, iliac psoas, and even the anterior abdominal wall. Again treatment is for sitting stability that is being lost. Two-stage surgery is again required and in the first stage a thorough anterior division of all tight structures is required, followed by second stage posterior instrumentation and fusion [36] (Fig. 7.23).

Neuromuscular deformities

Cerebral palsy, poliomyelitis, and the true neuromuscular disorders of childhood (spinal muscular atrophy; the peripheral neuropathies, Friedreich's ataxia, and arthrogryposis; the muscular dystrophies) are all associated with a tendency towards a paralytic thoraco-lumbar collapsing scoliosis with pelvic obliquity. The prevalence rate and progression potential of these deformities correlates well with the degree of neuromuscular deficiency. Thus a scoliosis of significance occurs in 75% of patients with Friedreich's ataxia but only 10% of patients with the peripheral neuropathies. Similarly, the early onset (Werdnig–Hoffman) spinal muscular atrophy is notorious in comparison with the later onset (Kugelberg–Welander) variety. The underlying condition is also important. The more severe the neurological dysfunction in the cerebral palsy patient, the greater the degree of mental impairment, such that these children are often not able to capitalize on treatment programmes. The more severe the condition (e.g. Werdnig–Hoffman spinal muscular atrophy or Duchenne dystrophy) the shorter the life expectancy and while surgery may be clearly indicated for spinal reasons this must be balanced against the future for the child. By contrast, the congenital myopathy varieties of muscular dystrophy are stable and non-progressive conditions but surgery is often poorly tolerated because of cardiac and pulmonary dysfunction. All these matters must be taken into consideration before a decision is reached in favour of surgical intervention [14].

As for other paralytic spinal deformities it is

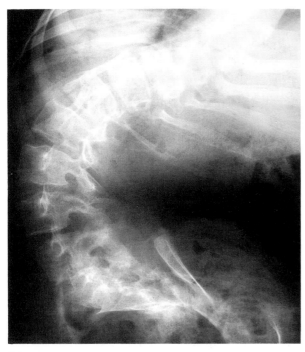

(a)

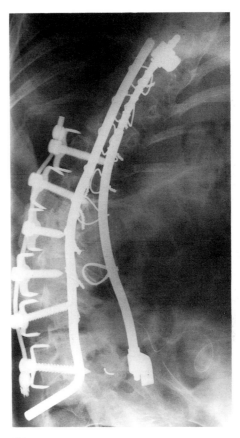

Fig. 7.22 (a) PA radiograph of a boy with a severe collapsing lordo-scoliosis in association with spina bifida. (b) After anterior segmental Dwyer instrumentation and posterior Harrington and Luque instrumentation and fusion. Segmental posterior wires can only be attached where there is a sufficiency of bone stock.

(b)

injudicious to contemplate surgery on the walker. A feature of the progressive types of neuromuscular condition is increasing gluteal muscle weakness with the development of a compensatory functional lumbar hyperlordosis above. If this is flattened or made rigid the patient is promptly converted from being a walker to a wheelchair patient [33]. Thus, again, surgery is principally indicated for the wheelchair patient who is losing sitting stability. Both anterior and posterior instrumentation and fusion is wherever possible to be preferred, but in conditions associated with cardiac and pulmonary dysfunction anterior surgery is usually contraindicated. Segmental spinal instrumentation combined with fusion may be strong enough to support the less severe and more flexible deformity, but these have not yet manifested themselves by way of loss of sitting stability. This surgery must therefore be regarded as prophylactic rather than immediately therapeutic and has to be balanced by a high

mortality rate combined with high morbidity rate involving preoperative tracheostomy in many severe cases [14].

Deformities associated with neurofibromatosis

Von Recklinghausen's disease is an autosomal dominant condition but at least 50% of cases are spontaneous mutations. The diagnosis is made by the presence of any two of the following clinical features – a positive family history, a positive nodule biopsy, six café au lait spots, and multiple nodules. The condition affects all components of the musculoskeletal system but the spine is most commonly involved, in more than 50% of cases. There is, however, a spectrum of spinal involvement which mirrors the degree of severity of the condition. At one end of the spectrum the spine appears clinically and radiographically normal while at the other there is evidence of severe dystrophic change with attenu-

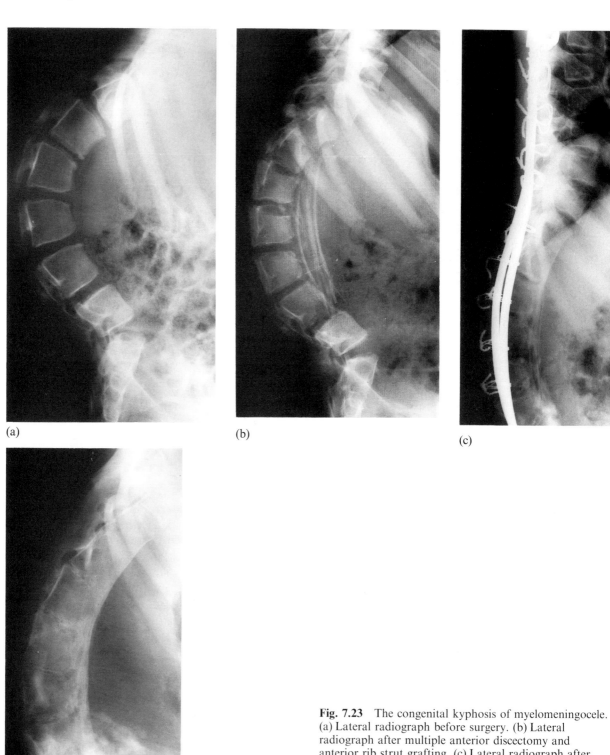

(a)

(b)

(c)

(d)

Fig. 7.23 The congenital kyphosis of myelomeningocele. (a) Lateral radiograph before surgery. (b) Lateral radiograph after multiple anterior discectomy and anterior rib strut grafting. (c) Lateral radiograph after second stage posterior Harrington–Luque instrumentation. (d) Lateral radiograph 5 years after surgery. The instrumentation was removed because of prominence under the skin. A solid spinal fusion has resulted except at the lumbo-sacral area where there is a hypertrophic non-union which was fortunately stable. The lumbo-sacral region is difficult to fuse in this condition.

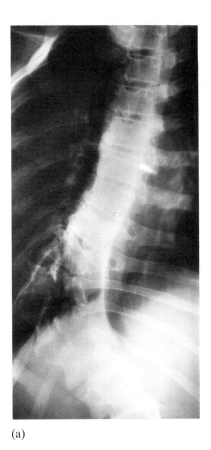

(a)

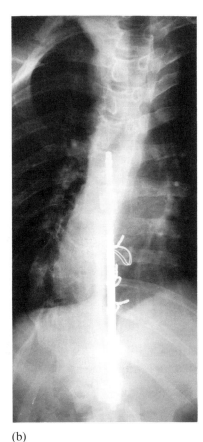

(b)

Fig. 7.24 (a) PA radiograph of a lower thoracic curve in association with Von Recklinghausen's disease. (b) After two stage anterior and posterior fusion showing a solid spine with some improvement. Even prevention of progression is an achievement in this unpredictable condition.

ated ribs, enlarged intervertebral foramina, and scalloped vertebrae. The prevalence rate and progression potential of spinal deformities reflect the degree of dystrophic change. At the mild end of the spectrum children have deformities indistinguishable from idiopathic ones and are treated accordingly. At the severe end of the spectrum, however, early onset, severely progressive, short angular curves are the rule rather than the exception. As in the idiopathic deformity, there are two types – buckling lordo-scolioses or kyphoses – and both may be present in the same spine, although several segments apart. The obviously dystrophic early onset curve will progress and if the deformity is still acceptable then anterior and posterior fusion should be prescribed to halt progression and thus to obviate the cardiopulmonary consequences of these progressive early onset curves. All too frequently patients do not present until the deformity is severe and again two stage surgery is necessary with preliminary anterior soft tissue release or apical

wedge resection according to the degree of severity [14] (Fig. 7.24).

Kyphoses are much less common than generally considered because of failure to appreciate that most deformities which appear kyphotic are in reality severely buckled lordo-scolioses. None the less, pure kyphoses do exist and in dystrophic spines have a severe progression potential with a strong likelihood of neurological dysfunction. Prophylactic anterior and posterior fusion should be prescribed for the early deformity but in the presence of neurological signs anterior decompression and strut grafting is essential [14]. The cervical spine is not uncommonly involved and deformities here should be promptly fused front and back lest neurological signs develop which are extremely hazardous if not impossible to treat satisfactorily. Occasionally neurological signs arise from intraspinal neurofibromata but are much less commonly encountered than generally considered. Laminectomy followed by tumour removal is the treatment of choice.

Mesenchymal deformities

Here there is a wide spectrum of underlying conditions including the heritable disorders of connective tissue, the mucopolysaccharidoses and the skeletal dysplasias.

The heritable disorders of connective tissue comprise osteogenesis imperfecta, Marfan's syndrome, homocystinuria, and the Ehlers–Danlos syndrome. Osteogenesis imperfecta is a group of disorders arising from inherited defects in collagen synthesis, with the common feature of bone fragility. Cases at the most severe end of the spectrum are not compatible with longevity and it is the milder forms which come to clinical attention as regards the spine, the changes in which are indistinguishable from those in juvenile osteoporosis with multiple compression fractures and biconcave vertebrae. Anterior chest wall deformities are also common. As in Von Recklinghausen's disease the prevalence rate and progression potential of spinal deformities correlates well with the severity of the underlying condition, and in those with the type I mild tarda form scoliosis is not common, whereas those with the type II severe congenita form invariably have a spinal deformity. Again these deformities are of two types – lordo-scolioses or kyphoses (Fig. 7.25) and the indications for surgical intervention are not easy to define [14]. Posterior instrumentation and fusion has an extremely bad record, with high pseudarthrosis and other complication rates. Sublaminar wires are tolerated poorly because of weak bone and Harrington hooks often have to be supported by methyl methacrylate cement. For a severe early onset life threatening case two stage wedge resection is probably the best treatment.

Marfan's syndrome with its arachnodactyly, dislocated lenses, aortic dilatation and skeletal problem is associated with a scoliosis in about 50% of cases. Attention must be paid to the very delicate heart and great vessel status, but experience shows that this has not been a problem in spinal surgery. Treatment of the spinal deformities in association with Marfan's syndrome is along the same lines as that recommended for idiopathic scoliosis at the same site.

Homocystinuria is similar to Marfan's syndrome but mental impairment is common in the majority. The danger to surgery here is vascular damage leading to thrombosis in both arterial

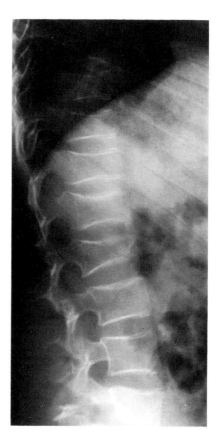

Fig. 7.25   Lateral radiograph showing a smooth kyphosis with platyspondyly typical of brittle bone disease.

and venous systems. The pattern of scoliosis is similar to that encountered in Marfan's syndrome but because of the thrombotic risk surgical treatment should be withheld. The Ehlers–Danlos syndrome of fragile, bruisable skin with loose-jointedness is also associated with the same type of spinal deformity. Biochemical advances have delineated several different types of this syndrome and it is essential to ensure that vessel friability is not a feature of the particular type of Ehlers–Danlos syndrome otherwise surgical treatment is most definitely contraindicated because of the haemorrhagic risk [14].

The mucopolysaccharidoses are skeletal disorders due to a failure of normal breakdown of complex carbohydrates which accumulate in tissue and appear in the urine. There is a range of severity with the Hurler syndrome, fatal before the age of 10 years, the milder Hunter syndrome with survival through to the second or third decades, the Morquio syndrome and the

Maroteaux–Lamy syndrome with moderate longevity. The Morquio syndrome is most commonly encountered and there are skeletal deformities in association with short-trunked dwarfism but intelligence is normal. Death occurs from cardiorespiratory dysfunction or spinal cord compression. It is the latter which is the real worry in patients with the Morquio syndrome and can occur from a progressive thoraco-lumbar kyphosis, or atlanto-axial instability as a result of a deficient odontoid (Fig. 7.26). The thoraco-lumbar kyphosis can respond to extension bracing and this should certainly be prescribed first. Should neurological signs develop then anterior resection of the bullet-shaped apical vertebra, followed by strut grafting, should be performed [14]. Because of the high incidence of neurological problems from atlanto-axial instability, many experienced surgeons recommend prophylactic fusion as soon as the patient is encountered.

The skeletal dysplasias represent a wide variety of conditions with disordered development and growth in some part of the skeleton. Some are common, but most are rare, and classification is generally by the skeletal site involved, e.g. epi-

physis, metaphysis, or spine [37]. The same two primordial types of spinal deformity can occur, i.e. lordo-scoliosis or kyphosis, but it is the latter which is the more common [14].

In multiple epiphyseal dysplasia, one of the more common types, in addition to hip, knee, and elbow epiphyseal dysplasia the spine is not severely involved, but most children have a thoracic kyphosis similar to Scheuermann's disease. The autosomal dominant achondroplasia has two important spinal features—spinal stenosis and a thoraco-lumbar kyphosis – both of which can give rise to neurological problems. A thoraco-lumbar kyphosis is the rule and develops early due to a thoraco-lumbar bullet shaped vertebra. More than 90% resolve spontaneously with growth and there is therefore no urgent therapeutic need. For the uncommon patient with a progressive kyphosis and neurological deterioration there is no substitute for anterior decompression and strut grafting. Although the entire spine is affected in achondroplasia the lumbar region most commonly produces symptoms and often requires decompressive laminectomy. Fortunately most patients have reached maturity by the time this posterior de-stabilizing procedure is required. In the adolescent, however, there is a real risk of producing a kyphosis by laminectomy such that prophylactic segmental rectangular support with fusion should be performed at the same time (Fig. 7.27).

The spondylo-epiphyseal dysplasias have both disordered epiphyseal growth and flattened vertebrae. The X-linked tarda variety is characterized by flat vertebrae which are humped posteriorly and this differentiates from multiple epiphyseal dysplasia and the Morquio syndrome. Kyphosis is common but scoliosis rare. Extension bracing can be effective but there is sometimes local instability at the site of the bullet-shaped vertebra in which case anterior strut grafting is required. The rare, but severe, congenita variety has irregular platyspondyly and a Scheuermann's-type kyphosis. Treatment is similar. In diastrophic dysplasia there are three spinal problems – odontoid hypoplasia, cervical kyphosis, and a structural scoliosis. Odontoid hypoplasia gives rise to atlanto-axial stability which frequently requires reduction, halo-cast stabilization and posterior fusion. Cervical kyphosis is more neurologically worrying and if progression is observed anterior and posterior

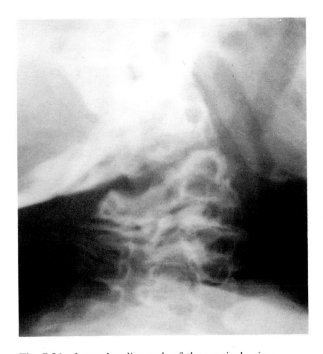

Fig. 7.26 Lateral radiograph of the cervical spine showing the typical odontoid aplasia of Morquio's syndrome.

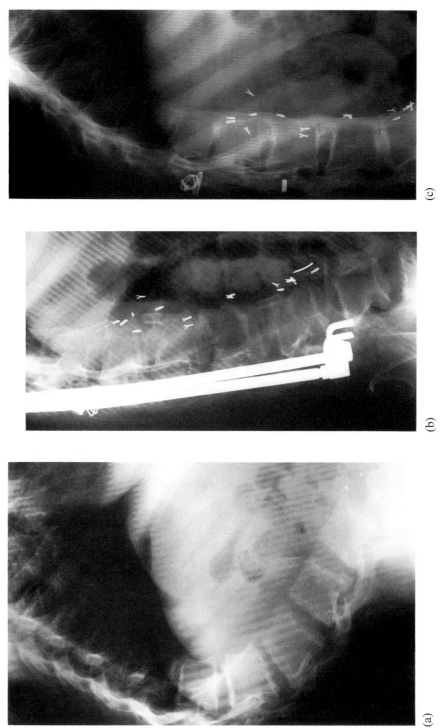

(c)

(b)

(a)

Fig. 7.27 The thoraco-lumbar kyphosis of achondroplasia compounded by posterior decompressive laminectomy. (a) Lateral radiograph showing a severe thoraco-lumbar kyphosis. (b) After two stage anterior and posterior fusion. (c) Three years after surgery showing a solid fusion with a gratifying correction.

fusion should be prescribed. A significant structural scoliosis is not a constant finding but is present in about 50% of cases. It is uncommon, however, for these scolioses to be severe. They should be dealt with as for any progressive scoliosis in association with a dystrophic bone situation – anterior and posterior fusion for milder curves, and two stage wedge resection for the more severe categories [14]. Spina bifida in the cervical or lumbar region, or both, is the rule in diastrophic dysplasia and if distraction instrumentation is contemplated CT myelography is essential to exclude spinal cord tether in these sites.

Included in the mesenchymal disorders are some metabolic conditions and it is probably true that rickets is the commonest cause of scoliosis worldwide. The deformity is indistinguishable from idiopathic scoliosis but the more severe the rachitic problem the earlier the onset and the more progressive the curve. Treatment is similar to the idiopathic counterpart.

Deformities due to trauma

These can be either spinal or extraspinal, with the former being much more common. Most spinal injuries are of the vertical loading with flexion variety, so typically characterized by Holdsworth. The anterior column fails under compression, while the posterior column fails under tension, and the axis of the injury is somewhere in between. The more anterior the axis, the more the spinal cord will be behind it and therefore vulnerable to tension insult. There are two principal spinal deformities resulting from spinal injuries of this nature – a kyphosis at the level of the bony injury and a lordo-scoliosis below in those who suffer a neurological insult [14] (Fig. 7.28). The progressive kyphosis is probably underestimated in its prevalence and generally results from inadequate initial management of the bony injury. It is debatable, however, whether this forms an indication for initial surgical stabilization as experienced spinal injuries centres show that the great majority of the acute kyphoses can be reduced and stabilized by hyperextension conservative treatment. The same can be said for injuries which are deemed radiographically 'unstable'. The only absolute indications for the fixation of a spinal fracture initially are three [38]

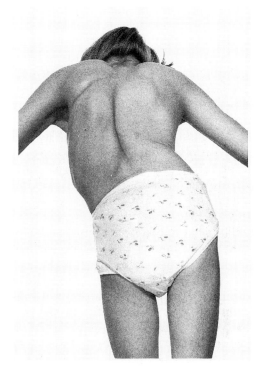

Fig. 7.28 Back view of a young girl with a progressive lordo-scoliosis secondary to a spinal cord tumour with radiotherapy.

– when there is total loss of spinal continuity at the level of injury (i.e. total dislocation), in the presence of multiple injuries, and in the presence of a significant head injury. In the former situation no conservative measure can reliably realign the spine. For the patient with multiple injuries the spine should be stabilized surgically lest treatment of other injuries and the nursing thereof impairs spinal stability. The patient with a severe head injury often goes through a phase of considerable cerebral irritability and an unstable spinal injury will not tolerate such vigorous body movements. None the less, there is an epidemic of early fixation of spinal fractures for which there is no clinical or scientific justification. Certainly there is no evidence whatever that the neurological situation is improved by any form of surgical intervention.

There is, however, perhaps due to orthopaedic surgeons not learning the lessons from spinal injuries centres, a rising prevalence rate of progressive and often painful local kyphosis. This can be most distressing to the patient and spinal stabilization should be performed. As in all kyphoses, the spine must be stabilized anteriorly using a strong cortico-cancellous strut graft.

Despite the fact that the great majority of spinal injuries are in effect acute kyphoses, laminectomy is still far too commonly performed. This destabilizes the spine by removing the integrity of the posterior column while doing nothing for the spinal cord pressure which, of course, is at the front. What is the inevitable result is progressive kyphosis often with its own neurological trouble in the future. Again anterior strut grafting is the treatment of choice with anterior dural decompression for the patient whose neurological signs are deteriorating.

In the child, what may appear simply to be an acute flexion spinal injury, without any neurological signs, frequently represents a Salter–Harris type V growth plate injury. Progressive kyphosis during growth is therefore not uncommon and must be watched for in the immature [14]. Any tendency towards progression should be countered by an anterior and posterior spinal fusion. If there has been lateral end-plate pressure then a true scoliosis can occur, but this is uncommon.

The higher the level of the spinal cord lesion following trauma the greater the potential for deformity as well as widespread spasticity. In children, the younger the child the more the tendency toward a progressive deformity. If the spinal cord damage is at the level of T12 or below there is no spinal deformity, but if the neurological lesion is at T10 or above then a progressive collapsing lordo-scoliosis is the rule. If this is impinging upon sitting stability then it should be dealt with by anterior and posterior spinal instrumentation and fusion as for any paralytic spine deformity.

Extraspinal causes of deformities due to trauma are much less common. Decades ago empyemas following pneumonia before the antibiotic era often gave rise to long, but relatively mild, spinal curvatures due to fibrotic pleural thickening, while thoracoplasty in relation to pulmonary tuberculosis also produced a relatively mild deformity. There does, however, appear to be an increasing prevalence rate of idiopathic-type scoliosis in association with thoracotomy, either for a cardiac problem or for a tracheo-oesophageal fistula. The deformities should be dealt with as for their idiopathic counterpart.

Rarely, retroperitoneal fibrosis, either idiopathic or as a result of trauma, or following the insertion of the old fashioned theco-peritoneal shunt for hydrocephalus, can give rise to a progressive and rigid lumbar hyperlordosis by way of soft tissue tether.

Deformities due to infection

Two-thirds of spinal infections are pyogenic and one-third tuberculous, and in both types there is potential for progressive deformity. Infection commences in the vascular end-plates which, untreated, show evidence of destruction along with the intervening disc. The majority of pyogenic infections are due to the *Staphylococcus aureus* and respond to anti-staphylococcal antibiotic therapy along with symptomatic treatment. Only in the florid case with abscess formation or neurological impairment is surgical treatment indicated and this is in the form of anterior decompression and strut grafting. Even untreated, pyogenic infections seldom produce a significant kyphosis.

Tuberculous spinal disease is, however, more insidious and produces a more significant local deformity with the gibbus being diagnostic. Treatment is contentious. The Medical Research Council, as a result of their controlled trials and other studies over the past 2 decades, preach that any degree of severity of tuberculous spinal disease can be managed by anti-tuberculous chemotherapy alone and they recognize no role for surgical intervention. This conservative approach also encompasses total tuberculous paralysis. Against this view is that of Hodgson [39] and other anterior spinal surgical experts. If there is abscess formation or neurological impairment then anterior surgical decompression and excision of all diseased tissue followed by strut grafting is not only therapeutic but curative (Fig. 7.29). Such treatment is only applicable where such anterior surgical expertise is available. None the less, as a result of anterior surgical intervention, the sinister progressive kyphosis is obviated. Once established and progressive it is very difficult to treat satisfactorily. Anterior decompression is only indicated for the subsequent development of neurological impairment but the anterior decompression is difficult to perform and is very dangerous, with many of these

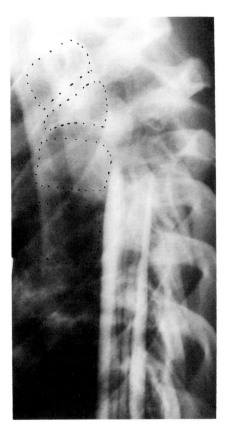

Fig. 7.29 Lateral myelogram of the upper thoracic spine showing an angular kyphosis with a block to the passage of dye in tuberculous spinal disease.

patients having a rigid chest and little pulmonary reserve. Accordingly, treatment should be reserved for the patient with frank neurological deterioration. This is more commonly encountered in children where even anterior surgical decompression and strut grafting cannot be expected to completely prevent progression of the kyphosis as the end-plates are involved in the fusion process.

Deformities due to tumours

As with infections, it is the anterior column which fails under compression with extradural tumours. However intradural tumours, and syringomyelia, as well as the paravertebral tumours of childhood, can produce spinal deformities. Any patient presenting with a seemingly idiopathic deformity but accompanied by pain, particularly at night, should be considered as having an intradural tumour or syringomyelia until proven otherwise (Fig. 7.30). The diagnosis is clinched by spinal cord imaging. While meningiomas and neurofibromas are the commonest intradural tumours in adults, it is malignant astrocytomas and neuroblastomas which are prevalent in children. Many of the latter present very late and are considered as having other conditions such as poliomyelitis, muscular dystrophy, or postural torticollis before the diagnosis is eventually made. Surprisingly, the prognosis is not bad and with surgical removal, even though it is often incomplete, followed by radiotherapy and chemotherapy the survival rate is in excess of 50%.

The problem for spinal stability is as the result of either the laminectomy approach for these lesions or the subsequent radiotherapy. The radiation changes to the vertebrae are usually minimal, although some degree of platyspondyly and a thoraco-lumbar kyphosis are not uncommon. If more than 5000 rad have been administered there is a rising prevalence rate of radiation myelopathy which can itself produce a paralytic curve due to spinal cord embarrassment. It is, however, the necessary laminectomy, which may have to be widespread, as an approach to the extirpation of these intradural tumours, which can produce in the immature a very progressive kyphosis. If the facet joints have not been sacrificed then a long rounded kyphosis, similar to Scheuermann's disease, develops and this may respond to extension brace treatment. With removal of the facet joints an angular kyphosis develops and this may produce its own neurological signs in the future. Should this occur, then anterior decompression and strut grafting must be performed.

The paravertebral tumours, Wilms' tumour and neuroblastoma, produce their deformities by way of local irradiation and these are seldom considerable.

Extradural tumours inevitably produce a local kyphosis, even in the lumbar region, as the line of the centre of gravity of the body passes anterior to the body of L4. Although these can occur in childhood, with Ewing's sarcoma, the malignant lymphomas, aneurysmal bone cyst, and eosinophilic granuloma, the majority are metastatic problems in the adult. The importance of these kyphoses is two fold – local pain and the poten-

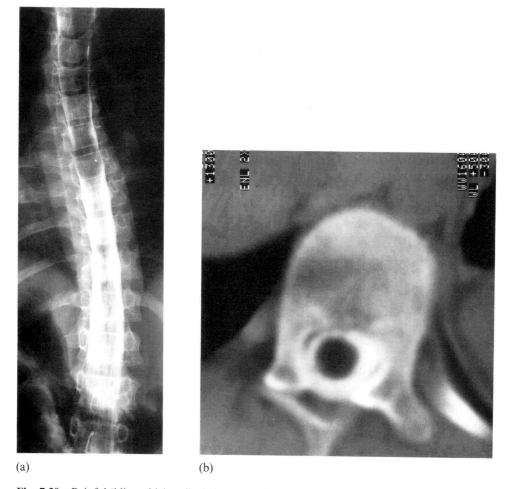

(a)   (b)

Fig. 7.30   Painful 'idiopathic' scoliosis in association with syringomyelia. (a) PA myelogram showing the deformity and the widened canal. (b) CT myelogram showing the typical appearance of a syrinx.

tial for neurological impairment. Both can be extremely distressing to the patient with metastatic disease. The great majority will, however, succumb within a matter of months, but those with breast or prostatic lesions can have some longevity. It is these patients to whom therapy should be particularly addressed. If the metastasis is solitary and painful or the source of a neurological insult, then anterior vertebral body excision followed by strut grafting is indicated. In these patients it is advisable to add posterior stabilization and fusion using rectangular segmental wiring. Although the prognosis is clearly limited it is most undignified and distressing for the patient to perish in a prolonged paraplegic state and thus surgery should always be prescribed where indicated [14] (Fig. 7.31).

Other spinal deformities

Some spinal deformities do not belong to any of the above categories and these can be encountered in both children and adults. In children idiopathic-type deformities are more prevalent with congenital heart disease, ocular and visual problems (blind children, ophthalmoplegia, and congenital strabismus) and in association with congenital anomalies of the upper extremity. These should be treated as for their idiopathic counterpart. A mild spinal deformity is also prevalent in juvenile chronic arthritis but these are nearly always non-structural, and thus non-progressive.

In the adult spinal deformities occur as a result of Paget's disease, ankylosing spondylitis, and

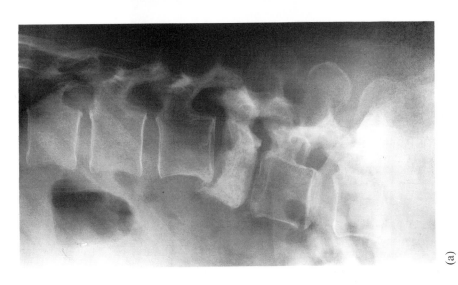

(a)

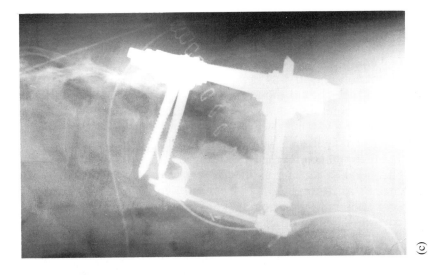

(b)

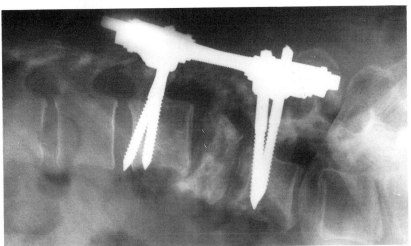

(c)

Fig. 7.31 Metastatic spinal disease with intractable pain and progressive paraparesis. (a) Lateral radiograph of a woman with breast cancer with a metastatic deposit in L3. (b) Lateral radiograph after first stage posterior transpedicular fixation using the AO fixateur interne. (c) Lateral radiograph after second stage anterior dural decompression, the resultant gap being replaced with methyl methacrylate cement and a Harrington compression system operating in distraction mode.

osteoporosis or osteomalacia. In Paget's disease the vertebrae and pelvis are the commonest sites of skeletal involvement. Multiple vertebral involvement can cause a kyphotic deformity with pain and even neurological compression. Neurological embarrassment generally occurs as a result of vertebral collapse, which should therefore be dealt with by anterior decompression and strut grafting. However, there is a vascular steal syndrome whereby a vertebra magna can take blood preferentially so that the spinal cord vascularity is jeopardized. This steal syndrome can respond to diphosphonates or calcitonin.

Patients with ankylosing spondylitis, particularly of the more aggressive variety, can develop a progressive spinal kyphosis. This is most common in the thoraco-lumbar region, but also can occur in the cervico-thoracic area and it is most important to differentiate the true site of the deformity. If the kyphosis has progressed to the extent where the patient cannot see forward then osteotomy is indicated. If the area of kyphosis is thoraco-lumbar then the site of osteotomy is at the L2–3 level, just below the conus where the spinal canal is capacious. If however the area of maximum kyphosis is in the cervico-thoracic region then osteotomy at the C7–T1 level is necessary lest the spine be unbalanced. Many patients have concomitant hip disease and much of their kyphosis can be apparent due to a flexion contracture of the hip joints. In this situation total hip replacement should be prescribed before any considerations of spinal osteomy.

Spinal osteotomy is dangerous in the an-

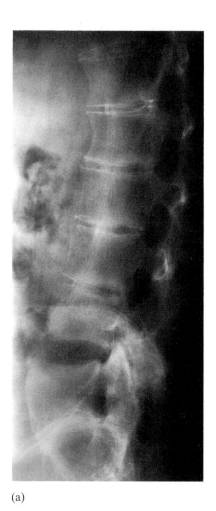
(a)

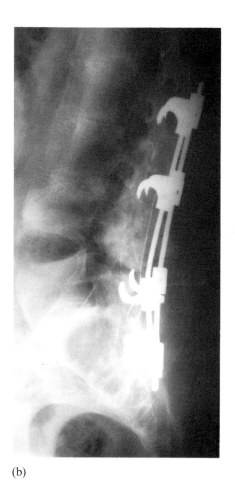
(b)

Fig. 7.32   (a) Lateral radiograph of the lumbar spine in a man with ankylosing spondylitis with a spontaneous pseudarthrosis at the L4/5 level. (b) Lateral radiograph after extension osteotomy at the site of the pseudarthrosis.

kylosing spondylitis patient and every series of any size reports anaesthetic problems, vascular problems from stretching or tearing of the aorta or its branches, and neurological impairment. Certainly anaesthesia is hazardous and often requires a preliminary tracheostomy. Patients should not be placed prone for surgery as this markedly hinders any form of access to the airway in case of emergency. For the patient with a cervico-thoracic kyphosis osteotomy is performed in the sitting position, under local anaesthesia, by the method of Simmons. For a thoraco-lumbar kyphosis the patient should be treated in the lateral decubitus position. Both techniques employ removal of a wedge of bone based posteriorly and apical at intervertebral foraminal level. In the thoraco-lumbar region the technique of McMaster is recommended whereby the posterior wedge is closed by double Harrington compression systems [40] (Fig. 7.32). This obviates the sudden correction achieved by a sudden manual pressure.

There are two other areas of spinal interest in the ankylosing spondylitis patient – spontaneous pseudarthroses and traumatic fractures. It is not uncommon in the spine which appears to be fused from top to bottom to have an area of instability due to a spontaneous pseudarthrosis (an area of the spine which has not completely ossified). These are potentially dangerous and represent a point of maximum mobility during spinal stress. Patients often present as a result of local pain or even neurological deterioration and spinal fixation and fusion is urgently required. Similarly, patients with true traumatic fractures of their ankylosed spine have the same neurological vulnerability. Conservative treatment is not adequate, as these patients can sustain severe neurological or even complete damage by standard nursing care. Fixation is urgently required.

There is a vogue for applying instrumentation to any spine and the osteoporotic/osteomalacic spine is no exception. Segmental instrumentation is increasingly prescribed for the kyphosis, often painful, of these elderly female patients. Certainly this condition is difficult to treat and these generally lightweight ladies do not tolerate at all well an orthosis of the sufficiency required to either abolish their pain or prevent progression of their kyphotic deformity. None the less, the application of segmental instrumentation throughout the whole thoraco-lumbar spine must be viewed with considerable suspicion and this highlights, par excellence, the concept of knowing when and when not to operate.

References

1. Goldstein, L. A. and Waugh, T. R. (1973) Classification and terminology of scoliosis. *Clin. Orthop.*, **93**, 10–22

2. Cobb, J. R. (1948) Outline for the study of scoliosis. *American Academy of Orthopaedic Surgeons Instructional Course Lectures*, **5**, 261.

3. Perdriolle, R. (1979) *La scoliose – son etude tridimensionnelle.* Maloine, Paris.

4. Bunnell, W. P. (1984) An objective criterion for scoliosis screening. *J. Bone Joint Surg.*, **66A**, 1381–1387.

5. Dickson, R. A., Lawton, J. O., Archer, I. A. and Butt, W. P. (1984) The pathogenesis of idiopathic scoliosis. Biplanar spinal asymmetry. *J. Bone Joint Surg.*, **66B**, 8–15.

6. Adams, W. (1865) *Lectures on the Pathology and Treatment of Lateral and Other Forms of Curvature of the Spine.* J. Churchill & Sons, London.

7. Zorab, P. A. (ed.) (1974) *Scoliosis and Muscle.* William Heinemann Medical Books Ltd., London.

8. Steindler, A. (1929) *Diseases and Deformities of the Spine and Thorax.* C. V. Mosby, St Louis.

9. de Peloux, J., Fauchet, R., Faucon, B. and B. Stagnara, P. (1965) Le plan d'election pour l'examen radiologique des cypho-scolioses. *Rev. Chir. Orthop.*, **51**, 517–524.

10. Sorensen, K. H. (1964) *Scheuermann's Kyphosis. Clinical Appearances. Radiograph, Aetiology and Prognosis.* Munksgaard, Copenhagen.

11. Willner, S. and Johnsson, B. (1983) Thoracic kyphosis and lumbar lordosis during the growth period in boys and girls. *Acta Pediatr. Scand.*, **72**, 873–878.

12. Mehta, M. H. and Morel, G. (1979) The non-operative treatment of infantile idiopathic scoliosis. In *Scoliosis.* Proceedings of the Sixth Symposium (eds P. A. Zorab and O. Siegler). Academic Press, London, pp. 71–84.

13. Deacon, P., Berkin, C. R. and Dickson, R. A. (1985) Combined idiopathic kyphosis and scoliosis: an analysis of the lateral spine curvature associated with Scheuermann's disease. *J. Bone Joint Surg.*, **67B**, 189–192.

14. Leatherman, K. D. and Dickson, R. A. (1987) *Management of Spinal Deformities.* Wright, Bristol.

15. Archer, I. A. and Dickson, R. A. (1985) Stature

and idiopathic scoliosis. A prospective study. *J. Bone Joint Surg.*, **67B**, 185–188.

16. Nachemson, A. (1986) A long term follow up study of non-treated scoliosis. *Acta Orthop. Scand.*, **39**, 466–476.

17. Reid, L. (1971) Lung growth. In *Scoliosis and Growth* (ed. P. A. Zorab), Proceedings of a Third Symposium. Churchill Livingstone, Edinburgh.

18. Blount, W. P. and Moe, J. H. (1973) *The Milwaukee Brace*. Williams and Wilkins, Baltimore.

19. Miller, J. A., Nachemson, A. L. and Schultz, A. B. (1984) Effectiveness of braces in mild idiopathic scoliosis. *Spine*, **9**, 632–635.

20. Bradford, D. S., Tanguy, A. and Vanselow, J. (1983) Surface electrical stimulation in the treatment of idiopathic scoliosis: preliminary results in 30 patients. *Spine*, **8**, 757–764.

21. Dickson, R. A. (1985) Conservative treatment for idiopathic scoliosis. *J. Bone Joint Surg.*, **67B**, 176–181.

22. Risser, J. C. (1958) The iliac apophysis, an invaluable sign in the management of scoliosis. *Clin. Orthop.*, **11**, 111–119.

23. Deacon, P. and Dickson, R. A., Spinal growth. *J. Bone Joint Surg.* (in press).

24. Harrington, P. R. (1962) Treatment of scoliosis. Correction and internal fixation by spine instrumentation. *J. Bone Joint Surg.*, **44A**, 519–610.

25. Luque, E. R. (1982) The anatomic basis and development of segmental spinal instrumentation. *Spine*, **7**, 256–259.

26. Archer, I. A., Deacon, P. and Dickson, R. A. (1986) Idiopathic scoliosis in Leeds – a management philosophy. *J. Bone Joint Surg.*, **68B**, 670.

27. Dubousset, J., Graf, H., Miladi, L. and Cotrel, Y. (1986) Spinal and thoracic derotation with CD instrumentation. *Orthop. Trans.*, **10 (1)**, 36.

28. Dwyer, A. F., Newton, N. C. and Sherwood A. A. (1969) An anterior approach to scoliosis: a preliminary report. *Clin. Orthop.*, **62**, 192–202.

29. Griss, P., Harms, J. and Zielke, K. (1984) Ventral derotation spondylodesis (VDS). In *Management of Spinal Deformities* (eds R. A. Dickson and D. S. Bradford), Butterworths International Medical Reviews, London, pp. 193–236.

30. Edgar, M. A., Chapman, R. H. and Glasgow, M. M. S. (1982) Pre-operative correction in adolescent idiopathic scoliosis. *J. Bone Joint Surg.*, **64B**, 530–535.

31. Leatherman, K. D. and Dickson, R. A. (1979) Two-stage corrective surgery for congenital deformities of the spine. *J. Bone Joint Surg.*, **61B**, 324–328.

32. McMaster, M. J. and MacNicol, M. F. (1979) The management of progressive infantile idiopathic scoliosis. *J. Bone Joint Surg.*, **61B**, 36–42.

33. Lonstein, J. E. and Akbarnia, B. A. (1983) Operative treatment of spinal deformities in patients with cerebral palsy or mental retardation. *J. Bone Joint Surg.*, **65A**, 43–55.

34. Nachemson, A. (1987) Personal communication.

35. McMaster, M. J. and Ohtsuka, K. (1982) The natural history of congenital scoliosis. A study of 251 patients. *J. Bone Joint Surg.*, **64A**, 1128–1147.

36. Leatherman, K. D. and Dickson, R. A. (1978) Congenital kyphosis in myelomeningocele. Vertebral body resection and posterior spine fusion. *Spine*, **3**, 222–226.

37. Fairbank, T. (1951) *An Atlas of General Affections of the Skeleton*. Williams and Wilkins, Baltimore.

38. Gaines, R. W. and Humphreys, W. G. (1984) A plea for judgement in management of thoracolumbar fractures and fracture-dislocations. *Clin. Orthop.*, **189**, 36–42.

39. Hodgson, A. R. and Stock, F. E. (1960) Anterior spine fusion for the treatment of tuberculosis of the spine. *J. Bone Joint Surg.*, **42A**, 295–310.

40. McMaster, M. J. (1985) A technique for lumbar spinal osteotomy in ankylosing spondylitis. *J. Bone Joint Surg.*, **67B**, 204–210.

8

Lengthening of limbs by the Ilizarov method

R. Cruz-Conde Delgado and J. C. Marti Gonzalez

Ilizarov's external fixator was originally described in Kurgan, Siberia (USSR), in 1951 by Gavril Abramovich Ilizarov. The official title given by the Ministry of Health of the USSR was 'compression-distraction apparatus' [3,4], to encompass the idea of simultaneous or alternate distraction and compression which could be applied to a bone segment. The apparatus (Fig. 8.1) was developed at the Experimental and Clinical Institute of Scientific, Orthopaedic and Traumatic Studies (Kniiekot) in Kurgan, but introduced to the West in 1981 by ASAMI (the Italian Association for the study and application of the Ilizarov technique) [3,4].

It is basically a circular external fixator (Fig. 8.2) but also a complex system built with a limited number of parts yet able to provide a versatile construction capable of between 700 and 800 different combinations. As an external fixation device, it depends simply on the introduction of crossed Kirschner wires into the bone and fixed under tension to a ring, which in turn is secured to rods. A second ring is attached in a similar manner, thus allowing compression or distraction; additional forces of angulation or rotation can be applied by the use of multiple rings and crossed wires [3,4,15].

Osteogenesis

Ilizarov considered that his method not only allowed lengthening of a limb but induced new bone formation. Indeed, experimental evidence revealed that osteogenesis appeared to be stimulated by a combination of distracting forces on the periosteum and stability between the bone segments. Preservation of the blood supply is vital and is very dependent on the rate of length-

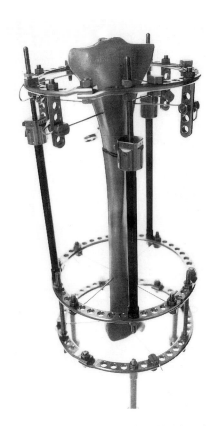

Fig. 8.1 Ilizarov's fixator for tibial lengthening with telescopic rods and corticotomy at the proximal end.

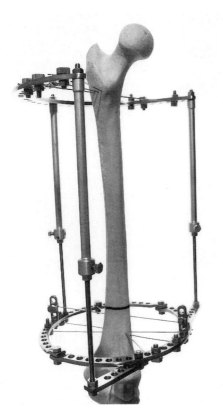

Fig. 8.2 Ilizarov's fixator for femoral lengthening with original set. (The site of corticotomy is marked with a black ring at the distal end.)

ening; and this also applies not only to the blood vessels but to all the surrounding connective tissue structures [15,16].

Stability

Perhaps the effect of weight bearing and exercise for the limb is another important factor in stimulating osteogenesis [3,4,15]; and the apparatus provides sufficient stability and strength to withstand full weight bearing. Initially the device was applied by inserting cross wires at either ends of the diaphysis but better stability is achieved by a four-level assembly; two in the proximal and two in the distal metaphysis.

Rate of lengthening

The studies carried out at the Kurgan Institute by Ilizarov were conducted in seven separate series

under varying conditions of stability, tension and rate of lengthening. They confirmed that the optimum rate of lengthening for osteogenesis was 1 mm per day, divided into 0.25 mm every 6 hours. These experiments, carried out on dogs, revealed that by increasing the rate to 1.5–2.0 mm per day caused thrombosis in the capillary vessels and subsequent necrosis in the regenerating bone; conversely, a slower rate of lengthening allowed early consolidation of new bone and prevented any distraction [4,16].

Preservation of blood supply to bone

The Ilizarov method tries to prevent any serious damage to the local blood vessels by (1) a delicate but accurate division of the cortical bone [3,4], (2) closed osteoclasis of the cancellous or medullary bone using minimal force and (3) minimal damage to the periosteum and surrounding tissues [2,3,4,10].

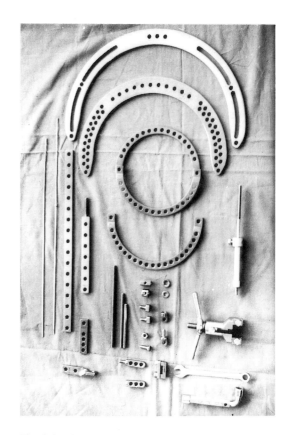

Fig. 8.3 Original set for Ilizarov's method.

Indications

Limb lengthening has been confined in the past to those limbs with acquired shortening due to trauma, poliomyelitis and infection causing arrest of growth. Recently there has been increasing interest in lengthening congenital short limbs due to achondroplasia, osteodystrophy, various forms of dwarfism, congenital shortening of the femur and agenesis of the long bones [2,6,7,8,9,17,21].

The apparatus

The component parts of the Ilizarov apparatus are illustrated (Fig. 8.3), and are translated from Russian with the help of the Italian (ASAMI) catalogue. There are two sets: (1) for bone anchorage and (2) for linkage [2,6,7,8,9,17,21].

Bone anchorage

(a) *Kirschner wires* in diameters of 1.5 and 1.8 mm with either three cutting edges for insertion into metaphysial bone or two cutting edges (bayonet) for penetration of the harder diaphysial cortex. This latter cutting edge is designed to reduce heat generated in their insertion into bone. They may support loads of up to 300 kg yet also provide some elasticity.
(b) *Tensor* is an essential component to be applied to the Kirschner wires so that they receive the correct tension. It is calibrated in kg [3,4].

Linkage

(a) Rings, half-rings and arches. They have many drill holes in various sites and angles to allow a wide choice of insertion of the Kirschner wires, and there are various sizes to accommodate the size of the limb.
(b) Bolts and clamps for securing the Kirschner wires to the rings and arches. They have drill holes and grooves to adapt to the position of the wires, rings and arches (Fig. 8.4) [3,4].

Rods

Threaded so that one complete turn equals 1 mm. There are various lengths from 60 to 200 mm.

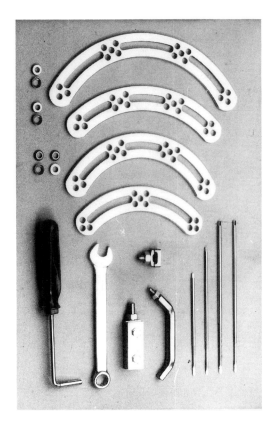

Fig. 8.4 Femoral set modified by Italian ASAMI.

Perforated for the Kirschner wires but only used for fractures.

Grooved for a more versatile fixation and again only used for fractures.

The Italian ASAMI has modified the original telescopic rods, as can be seen in Fig. 8.5, designed for monitoring the distraction as they are marked in millimetres and automatically lock at each quarter turn [3,4].

Preparation and maintenance

Before embarking on any application all the components must be checked. Sterilization can be carried out in a traditional autoclave; the use of gas (ethylene oxide) is preferred as it is less likely to affect the metal. Similarly, iodine and other corrosive materials should be avoided. It can be stored after cleaning with glycol [4].

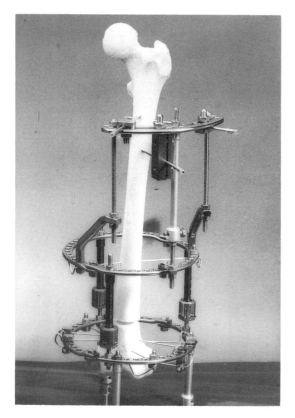

Fig. 8.5 Ilizarov's fixator modified by Italian ASAMI for femoral lengthening with telescopic rods and corticotomy at the distal end.

Application

The insertion of the wires and the construction of the external fixator may appear to be simple but unless the basic principles are carefully adopted complications may arise and ruin the result [4].

Insertion of the Kirschner wires

This requires a knowledge of the immediate important anatomical structures so that they can be avoided [24]. A low revolution drill is important in order to avoid any unnecessary burns to the skin and bone and the temperature can be reduced by frequent stops and irrigation with an antiseptic solution or saline. The wires should be inserted perpendicular to the long axis of the bone and the second wire should cross as near 90° as possible in order to achieve sound mechanical stability. Finally, the skin and soft tissues should

not be subjected to undue stress particularly near the joints because walking must be encouraged. The site of the wires in flexion and extension of the joints must not produce tension in these important soft tissues. When the wires are being inserted via the anterior aspect of the limb, the adjacent joint should be kept in flexion and vice versa [3,4].

Choice of rings

The size of the ring is determined by the maximum diameter of the limb but a clearance of at least 2.0 cm is necessary in order to avoid any pressure necrosis in the skin if there is any swelling of the limb during treatment [3,4,10].

Tension of the wires

This is a fundamental requirement so that the strength and elasticity of the apparatus is achieved. The optimum tension lies between 100 and 110 kg and should be tested at intervals. Excessive tension will reduce the elastic property of the steel and may result in a bad fixation [3,4].

Fixation of the rings

This is achieved by attaching three telescopic or threaded rods so that they lie in the long axis of the bone and form the pattern of an equilateral triangle. This is not always as easy as it sounds because different sized rings may have been used but a perpendicular system can be worked out by use of some of the accessory fixation components [3,4,10].

Technique

The first stage is the assembly of the apparatus and the pattern depends on the bone which has to be lengthened.

Fig. 8.6 (a–d) Bilateral tibial lengthening of 14 cm in an 11-year-old boy with achondroplasia (total period of treatment: 10 months). (a) Preoperative radiograph of lower limbs. (b) Immediate postoperative radiograph. (c) One and 3 months postoperative radiographs during lengthening. (d) Final result.

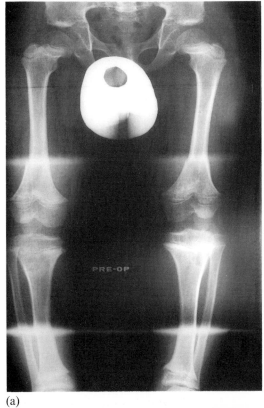

(a)

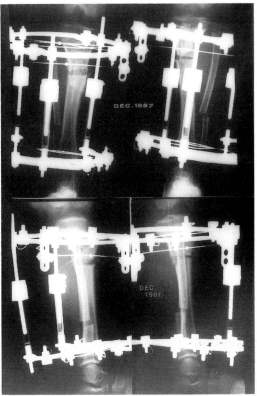

(b)

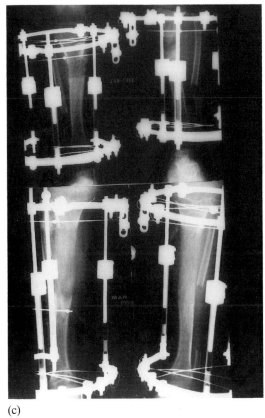

(c)

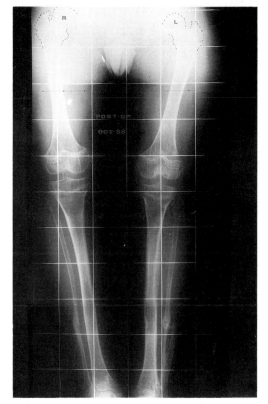

(d)

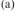

The *tibia* is the easiest of the bones to lengthen because it is not surrounded by bulky muscles and it is comparatively superficial [6,14,19]. A more ambitious programme of lengthening can be planned for the tibia compared with other long bones (Fig. 8.6a, b, c, d).

In the *proximal end* two rings are usually required, but one ring and a third or supplementary wire through the anterior cortex may be sufficient. This will tend to control the tendency of anterior bowing which may occur if it has been necessary to perform an anterior division of the cortex in the proximal metaphysis. One of the wires must pass through the head of the fibula in order to prevent dislocation of the superior tibiofibular joint during lengthening [14].

In the *distal end*, one ring should be at the level of the junction between the middle and distal thirds, and the second is usually a half-ring placed on the anterior surface to allow access to the Achilles tendon which may require lengthening. A tenotomy is usually performed by the authors when they consider it necessary but a prophylactic tenotomy is described. This half-ring is placed in the distal metaphysis and one wire should penetrate both the tibia and the fibula just above the syndesmosis which should prevent any proximal migration of the lateral malleolus and any subsequent valgus deformity of the ankle and foot [19].

An *osteotomy of the fibula* is carried out through a small incision in the distal third of the leg.

Corticotomy, or division of the cortex, is performed at the junction between the metaphysis and the diaphysis. If extensive lengthening is planned, for example in achondroplasia, a double corticotomy is performed in the proximal and distal halves of the bone [5,12,13,14,21,25].

The *femur* requires a different assembly because of the problems involved and dangers of introducing wires through the proximal thigh. The Italian (ASAMI) team have designed an anchorage system using threaded pins which are inserted in different planes and then joined to an arch at the level of the greater trochanter. This arch is joined to two distally placed rings by using angled rods, thus providing an uniform force surrounding the femur and soft tissues (Fig. 8.7a, b, c) [4].

Corticotomy is performed just below the lesser trochanter which is preferable to the distal but

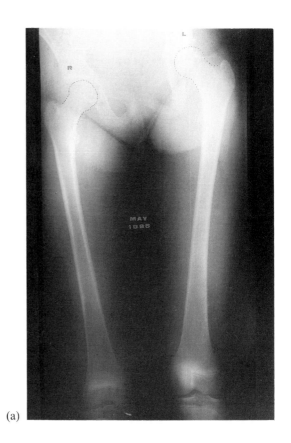

(a)

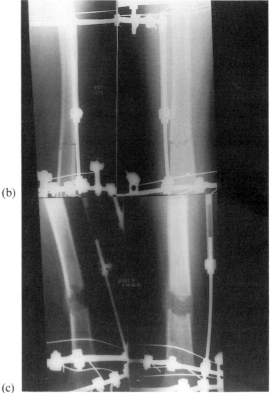

(b)

(c)

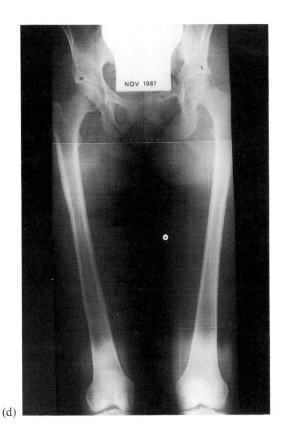

(d)

Fig. 8.7   (a–d) Femoral lengthening of 4 cm in a 14-year-old girl with idiopathic right femoral shortening (total period of treatment: 5 months). (a) Preoperative radiograph of lower limbs. (b) Corticotomy and (c) 2 months postoperative radiograph. (d) Two and a half years after lengthening (R) femur.

more accessible metaphysis where there is a danger of producing stiffness of the knee joint.

The *humerus* requires a two half-ring assembly; one in the proximal and the other in the distal third [9].

Corticotomy is performed in the proximal third.

Corticotomy

This technique is important and unique to the Ilizarov method and implies division of the cortical bone but with sparing of the cancellous or medullary bone and most of the surrounding periosteum [19]. The bone is finally broken by osteoclasis.

The tibia, for example, is approached by an incision 1.5 cm in length at the level of the proximal metaphysis and just below the tubercle. A very small and thin osteotome, 1.0 cm wide, is used to divide the periosteum which is carefully elevated on the antero-medial and lateral surfaces. The anterior crest of the tibia is cut to a depth of 5 mm using the small osteotome and mallet. The cortex on the antero-medial and lateral surfaces is also divided by lifting or depressing the handle of the osteotome, and this can all be performed through the 1.5 cm skin incision. The postero-medial cortex is divided in the same way. Finally, a force is applied to the bone by internally rotating the proximal and externally rotating the distal part until the bone breaks. The rotation is advised in this manner in order to prevent damage to the external popliteal nerve [23]. Radiographic control is made after the osteoclasis by using an image intensifier or conventional films in order to check the position of the divided bone. The lengthening rods are then applied. When a double level of lengthening is planned the central segment of bone has to be secured by an intermediate ring and wires in the bone.

Postoperative management

For 3 days the patient remains in bed with the limb elevated (the arm supported on pillows). Active exercises can be encouraged but are restricted by pain.

On the fourth day, walking and weight bearing is encouraged using crutches but preferably ordinary walking sticks.

On the fifth day, distraction starts at the rate of 0.25 mm every 6 hours.

On the eighth day, the patient may return home with instructions how to proceed with the distraction. Walking is to be encouraged.

On the tenth day, the patient is checked as an out-patient and radiographs are taken of the osteotomy site.

Physiotherapy may be required in order to encourage the patient to move the joints and to regain confidence in walking. If the femur has been lengthened it is unwise for the knee to be actively flexed more than 30° because further flexion may increase the tension on the ilio-tibial tract, which in turn may cause posterior subluxation of the knee.

Care of the wounds

The patient may have a shower every day and the entry and exit wounds of the wires need to be cleaned with soap and water. If any minor sepsis occurs it will usually clear up by applying an antiseptic solution; any obvious purulent discharge may require systemic antibiotic cover after taking a swab and culture assessment. If the local infection fails to clear up it may be necessary to replace the affected Kirschner wire in another site nearby.

Dismantling the apparatus

Osteogenesis and consolidation of the lengthened segment of bone will depend on the age of the patient and the distance that the bone has been lengthened. When the correct distance has been achieved and there is radiographic evidence of new bone filling the entire gap then the distraction nuts may be loosened. This will mean that the bone will be taking weight but not all the external stress. The apparatus can be removed when there is sound evidence of consolidated new bone (Fig. 8.8a, b) but activity will have to be restricted for at least 6 months.

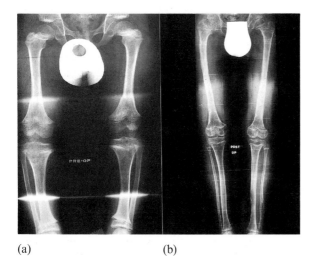

(a)   (b)

Fig. 8.8 The same patient as Fig. 8.6. (a) Preoperative radiograph of lower limbs. (b) At the end of treatment: both tibia and femur have been lengthened; total lengthening = 29 cm.

Complications

Generally there were few complications and they could be divided into three groups: (1) soft tissues, (2) bone and (3) apparatus [22].

Soft tissues

Skin may split occasionally when the lengthening exceeds 3.0 cm but it heals quickly without causing any problems. The main concern was pin-track infection which was fairly common, and minor infection occurred in 30% but cleared up after cleaning with an antiseptic solution. In 10% there was more persistent infection which responded to systemic antibiotic cover; two pins had to be repositioned. Slackening of tension in the pins was the main cause of skin irritation and local sepsis.

Pressure necrosis occurred on two occasions and in both the supporting rings were too small and failed to accommodate the swelling and increased circumference of the limb.

Nerve damage occurred twice. The external popliteal nerve was stretched, which caused paresis of the dorsi-flexors of the foot. It was perhaps due to over-ambitious lengthening of the tibia and fibula but both recovered within 9 months.

Arterial injuries did not occur in this series. Swelling of the limb was not uncommon and occurred in 70% of femoral and 30% of tibial lengthening which has to be borne in mind when planning the size of component. The swelling was not a permanent problem and tended to resolve either as a result of walking or after the apparatus had been removed at the conclusion of the lengthening procedure.

Contractures. An equinus contracture of the foot was not uncommon but most resolved as a result of physiotherapy and weight bearing during the lengthening phase. A persistent flexion contracture or worse, a posterior subluxation, at the knee can be a serious problem and should be avoided. It is caused by a combination of tight hamstring muscles, a tight ilio-tibial band, a persistent tendency to hold the knee flexed beyond 30° and the inherent tendency of the tibia to displace posteriorly when the joint is held in a flexed position. The authors have overcome this problem by insisting on a course of physiotherapy after the apparatus has been dismantled and by restricting the range of flexion to 30° during the lengthening phase. There were no permanent contractures of the joints in this series [22].

Bone

Infection occurred in one patient as a result of pin-track sepsis. The localized area of osteomyelitis resolved after the pin track had been changed and the affected area curretted.

Delayed bone production occurred in one patient who had trophic changes in the limb. This delayed consolidation of the lengthened segment and a cancellous bone graft was required, but eventually sound union was achieved.

Malalignment of the malleoli at the ankle will result if the distal end of the fibular diaphysis is not transfixed satisfactorily by the distal pin. Failure to secure the fibula will cause proximal migration of the lateral malleolus and this occurred in one patient. It was a difficult problem to overcome and it required a complicated osteotomy because the tibia had been lengthened by 14 cm.

Apparatus

Metal fatigue, fracture and loosening of nuts and bolts are all possibilities but unlikely if the apparatus has been constructed correctly. Loss of tension in the pins has been mentioned already and this has to be checked not only at the time of application but also at 3-weekly intervals during the lengthening phase.

The patients

A total of 121 bones were lengthened in this series from Asepeyo Hospital in Madrid (tibia, 74 cases and femur, 47 cases). Congenital abnormalities provided the largest source including idiopathic causes, achondroplasia, Turner's syndrome, congenital hypoplasia and fibular agenesis. Achondroplasia played a relatively large part in this group. The maximum increase in length of the tibia was 17.5 cm.

Acquired conditions were caused either by trauma or infection. Again the tibia was the most commonly lengthened bone.

The time required to obtain the desired increase in length did not vary between the categories, and it was calculated at the rate of 1.0 month per 1.0 cm for patients under 10 years old and 1.5 months per centimetre for those older than 10 years.

Most patients were standing on the third day and walking on the fifth day.

The average time in hospital was 7 days.

Discussion

The method of limb lengthening as described originally by Ilizarov has been tried in Asepeyo Hospital and this chapter has hopefully confirmed the success which was claimed by the original author. There is no doubt that once the components of the apparatus have been mastered and the rules of its application are followed the variety of conditions which can be treated are enormous. It is fairly obvious that the acquired problems are more amenable to lengthening than the congenital, where soft tissues have not the advantage of genetic programming for normal bone growth. Nevertheless, the method can be adapted to more or less any long bone and Ilizarov has applied it successfully to feet.

The advantage that this method has over previous methods must include (a) the minimal operative exposure, (b) the minute division of periosteum, (c) the delicate division of cortical bone and preservation of vital structures such as blood vessels. Finally, the experience of using this method has not caused any serious complications but it has achieved a fair measure of success with a minimal stay in hospital and generally a painless experience. The patients are able to walk on the fifth day and do not find it difficult to master the technique of lengthening their limb at home.

References and further reading

1. Badelou, O. (1988) La technique d'Ilizarov chez l'enfant avec un fixateur externe radio transparent. *Rev. Chir. Orthop.*, **T.74 Sup. II**, 237–240.
2. Beguiristain, J. L., Oniaifo, A. and Cañadell, J. (1979) Consideraciones sobre nuestra experiencia en elongacion de femur y tibia, segun el metodo de Wagner. *Rev. Ortop y Traum.*, **23**, 227–230.

3. Bianchi-Maiocchi, A., Benedetti, G. B., Catagui, M., Cattaneo, R., Tentoni, L. and Villa, A. (1983) *Introduzione Alla Conoscenza Delle Metodiche d'Ilizarov in Ortopedia e Traumatologia.* Medi Surgical Video, Milano.

4. Bianchi-Maiocchi, A., Catagui, M., Cattaneo, R., Tentoni, L. and Villa, A. (1985) *L'Osteosintesi Transossea Secondo G. A. Ilizarov.* Medi Surgical Video, Milano.

5. Cañadell, J. and De Pablos, J. (1985) Breaking Bony Bridges by Physeal Distraction: A New Therapeutic Approach. *Int. Orthop. S.I.C.O.T.*, **9**, 223–229.

6. Catagni, M. A. and Villa, A. (1988) *Allungamento di Gamba Secondo la Metodica di G. A. Ilizarov.* Medi Surgical Video, Milano.

7. Cattaneo, R. (1985) Traitement des pseudo-arthroses diaphysaires – septiques ou non septiques selon la methode d'Ilizarov en compression monofocale. *Rev. Chir. Orthop.*, **T-71**, 223–229.

8. Cattaneo, R. (1986) Traitement des inegalites du femur par la methode d'Ilizarov. *Rev. Chir. Orthop.*, **T-72**, 203–209.

9. Cattaneo, R. (1986) Application de la methode d'Ilizarov dans l'allongement de l'humerus. *Rev. Chir. Ortop.*, **T-72**, 203–209.

10. Forum sur la Methode d'Ilizarov. *Rev. Chir. Orthop.*, **T-73, Sup. II**, 29–70.

11. Cattaneo, R. (1988) La methode d'Ilizarov dans le traitement des grandes déviations axiales des membres. *Rev. Chir. Orthop.*, **T-74, Sup. II**, 237–240.

12. De Bastiani, G. B., Aldegheri, R., Renzi-Brivio, L. and Trivela, G. (1986) Limb lengthening by distraction of the epiphyseal plate. *J. Bone Joint Surg.*, **68-B; 4**, 545–549.

13. De Bastiani, G. B., Aldegheri, R., Renzi-Brivio, L. and Trivela, G. (1986) Chondrodiastasis: controlled symmetrical distraction of the epiphyseal plate. *J. Bone Joint Surg.*, **68-B: 4**, 551–556.

14. De Pablos, J., Villas, C. and Cañadell, J. (1986) Bone lengthening by physeal distraction: an experimental study. *Int. Orthop.*, **10**, 163–170.

15. Ilizarov, G. A. (1981) Personal comunication. XII Italian A.O. Club Convention Bellagio, Italia.

16. Ilizarov, G. A. and Y Soybelman, L. M. (1969) Some clinical and experimental data on the bloodless lengthening of lower limbs. *Exp. Chir. Anest.*, **4**, 27–32.

17. Ilizarov, G. A. (1986) L'Osteossintesi Transossea Nelle Fractura e Pseuddartrosi Dell' Avambracio. Medi Surgical Video., Milano.

18. Lazo, J., Aguilar, F., Mozo, F., Gonzalez, R., Baquerizo, A. and Lazo, J. M. (1980) Biocompresion: un principio diferente en el tratamiento de fracturas. *Rev. Ortop. Traum.*, **24 1B**, 1–12.

19. Lee, D. Y., Choi, I. H., Chung, C. Y. *et al.* (1994) Experience with lengthening by the Ilizarov Technique. *Orthopaedics International*, **2(4)**, 349–359.

20. Mendoza, J. L. (1949) *Algunas Consideraciones y Experiencias Sobre Distraccion Osea. El Cálculo Matematico en la Reduccion de las Fracturas.* Comunicacion Primeras Jornadas Ortopedicas de la S.E.C.O.T. Julio, Bilbao.

21. Monticelli, G. and Spinelli, R. (1981) Limb lengthening by epiphyseal distraction. *Int. Orthop.* **5**, 85–90.

22. Paley, D. (1987) Hinges: theoretical aspects. *Abstracts from the International Conferences on the Ilizarov Techniques for Management of Difficult Skeletal Problems.* Hospital for Joint Diseases, New York, 1–3 Nov.

23. Paley, D. (1988) Current techniques of limb lengthening *J. Pediatr. Orthop.*, **8**, 73–92.

24. Pous J., Ruano, D. and Suso, S. (1988) *Atlas Anatomotopografico de las Extremidades y Fijacion Externa Anular* (ed. S. A. Jims), Barcelona.

25. Wagner, H. (1971) *Operative Beinverlangerung.* **42**, 260–266.

9

The multiply injured patient with musculoskeletal injuries

M. F. Swiontkowski

High velocity trauma is the number one cause of death in the 18 to 38-year age group worldwide. In the USA alone, loss of income due to death and disability resulting from high velocity trauma totals 75 billion dollars annually [1]. This is an economic loss of staggering proportions. The goal of all governmental agencies responsible for health care decisions must be to minimize mortality and maximize return to function in this large, productive segment of the population. In this light, difficult decisions must be made regarding funding of research into injury prevention and trauma management, and legislation must be passed which is designed to minimize road traffic accident morbidity and mortality. Within the health care system, much effort has recently been directed toward optimizing the care of the polytrauma victim to speed return of these individuals to productive life. These efforts must continue for the foreseeable future because of the enormous impact of this problem on the individual and society.

Philosophy

In the care of the multiply injured individual, the treatment of complex injuries in multiple organ systems demands a team approach. The team must be able to evaluate the patient swiftly, be willing to discuss the effect of the management of one problem on another and be able to arrive at decisions quickly in regard to performing life-saving procedures.

Every team must have a final decision-maker, the captain. In the case of the polytrauma patient, this should be the individual most experienced in performing procedures to maintain the airway, manage shock from multiple causes, manage emergent situations affecting cardiac output (i.e. cardiac tamponade or injury to the great vessels), diagnose and treat intrathoracic or intra-abdominal haemorrhage, and make appropriate decisions regarding the early management of central nervous system and extremity trauma. In most settings in the western world, this will be the general surgeon with an interest and background in the care of the multiply injured patient. This need not be the case, however, as a neurological, urological, or musculoskeletal trauma surgeon with the same qualifications may be the critical decision-making individual in some settings, especially in more rural areas. At a minimum, the definitive care setting must have adequate laboratory facilities to perform quick and accurate haematological and blood chemistry determinations, arterial blood gas analysis, and alcohol and drug screens, and to provide emergent blood product support services. The facility must have a radiological suite to provide high quality plain radiographs of the spine, abdomen, chest, pelvis, and extremities, as well as emergent angiography and computed tomography services. An operating room must be staffed and ready 24 hours a day to manage emergency chest, abdominal, head, pelvic, and extremity trauma. The hospital administration must be willing to support these services, expensive as they are, to deliver high quality care to the multiply injured patient. Equally important, the team captain must have the support of surgical specialists available to him or her at any hour. These individuals must be familiar with the problems unique to the multiply injured patient and be willing to work together to optimize the patient's recovery – that is, they must be 'team players'.

Transport

The multiply injured patient must reach the definitive care setting in a timely fashion. He or she must be appropriately cared for during extrication and transport to avoid a preventable death due to airway obstruction, and shock treatment should be initiated. The ambulance crews of the 1950s and 1960s who simply threw the individual into the back of the vehicle and drove to the nearest hospital have, for the most part, been replaced by skilled Emergency Medical Technicians (EMTs). The EMTs are generally affiliated with fire departments within the hospital and are dispatched by local emergency operators to reported accidents. The EMT is generally well trained in the initial management of the multiply injured patient, and arrives at the scene in a well-equipped vehicle which has the equipment needed for extrication, special support, airway management, vital sign monitoring, i.v. solutions administration, cardiac arrest management, and fracture splintage. Increasingly, the EMT may arrive in a similarly-equipped helicopter.

There exists a degree of controversy as to the function of the EMT in the United States today. On one side is the 'scoop and run' philosophy, which holds that EMTs should swiftly and safely extricate the patient with spinal precautions and place the victim on a backboard [2]. The airway should be cleared and if spontaneous respirations are occurring, the individual should be placed in the vehicle and transported to the definitive care unit designated by the dispatcher. En route, i.v. access should be obtained, vital signs checked, and fluid therapy initiated. In cases of absent spontaneous respirations, cardiopulmonary resuscitation should be initiated en route. With this theory, speed of transport is critical. Cowley reported a three-fold increase in mortality for every 30 minutes of elapsed time without care [3].

Table 9.1　Basic EMT skills

1. Perform technically sound CPR
2. Maintain an airway (endotracheal intubation?)
3. Obtain IV access and start Ringer lactate therapy
4. Reduction and splintage of fractures
5. Perform primary survey of patient and report findings to destination centre
6. Act in concert with MD in early treatment decisions (radio/telephone contact)

The second philosophy, held by Copass *et al.* [4], is that EMTs can be trained to do procedures which will begin the resuscitation efforts in the field. In cases where spontaneous respiration is absent or where there is profound hypovolaemic hypotension, EMTs can safely intubate the patient and start central lines. Flutter valve needles can be placed intrathoracically to temporarily manage tension pneumothoraces. These procedures are performed under MD supervision via radio contact. Copass' group has shown that significant improvements in morbidity and mortality rates can be expected with this system [4].

Regardless of the philosophy employed, all agree that EMTs should be able to perform certain basic tasks (Table 9.1). There must be frequent open-ended dialogue among the dispatchers, EMTs, and the director of the regional EMT program to improve skills of the EMTs and thus optimize the care of critically injured individuals.

Treatment plan

Wolff *et al.* [5] have identified five phases in the care of the multiply injured patient after arrival at the definitive care centre The five phases are:

1. Resuscitation.
2. Emergency procedures.
3. Stabilization.
4. Delayed operative procedures.
5. Rehabilitation.

Resuscitation

The goal of the resuscitation phase is to establish normal vital signs by dealing with all situations acutely affecting a clear airway, normal ventilatory response, normal blood pressure, pulse, and distal perfusion. In essence, this means establishing an airway by endotracheal intubation or tracheotomy, placing the patient on controlled ventilation, and treating shock. In most instances, this phase of treatment is initiated in the field by the EMTs and is continued upon arrival at the definitive care centre.

In the United States, regional trauma centres have been designed along strict lines. The criteria for a Class I Trauma Centre include thoroughly equipped operating rooms, in-house 24-hour-a-day trauma surgeon presence, surgical subspecialty consultation available within 15 minutes, and the presence of surgical housestaff. Class II criteria are the same, with the exception of the training requirement. In most trauma centres the resuscitation is carried out in the emergency department. These facilities, in general, are equipped for all emergent surgical procedures, standard radiographs, and the institution of ventilatory support. Blood bank support must be quickly accessible for the treatment of shock. The details of the management of shock are completely discussed in Chapter 10.

As long as adequate blood pressure can be maintained in combination with ventilatory support, diagnostic studies can be performed. In many instances, tube thoracostomy, placement of MAST trousers, and/or pericardiocentesis may be required to restore normal blood pressure. If normal blood pressure proves difficult to maintain with appropriate fluid management, abdominal peritoneal tap may be performed to rule out intra-abdominal haemorrhage. If the blood pressure is stable in a moderate range, abdominal CT scanning can be extremely helpful in establishing a diagnosis of a liver or splenic injury, ruptured viscus or renal injury. In the case of a head injury, midface injury, or cervical spine injury, CT scan of the head must be conducted during this phase as well, to rule out intracerebral haemorrhage. Plain radiographs of the entire spine should be obtained at this stage if indicated. These should supplement the initial lateral radiograph of the cervical spine (exposing down to C7), chest, and pelvis radiographs. If the patient's blood pressure is not maintained within a reasonable range at any point, there is no indication for further diagnostic studies and the patient must enter the second phase of treatment.

Immediate surgery

During this phase of treatment the patient is generally moved to the operating theatre. It is during this phase that all maximally invasive life-saving surgical procedures are performed. As noted above, an extremely unstable patient in whom an adequate systolic blood pressure (as indicated by capillary perfusion of the distal extremities and urinary output of 30 ml/h) has not been restored may have to be moved to the operating room before all diagnostic procedures have been performed. In rare circumstances, major surgical procedures may be instituted in the emergency room as typified by a thoracotomy for open cardiac massage. This manoeuvre, however, has generally only been successful for penetrating trauma, and its indications in blunt trauma are subject to debate.

Most patients are brought to the operating room having already been intubated and placed on a volume respirator, with two large bore i.v. access lines (volume replacement ongoing) and a urinary catheter in place. If there has been inadequate opportunity to obtain a clear lateral cervical spine radiograph all the way to C7, the patient must be assumed to have a cervical spine fracture, and a hard cervical collar should be in place. In most instances, trauma victims will have full stomachs and/or have ingested alcohol within 8 hours, and this must be taken into consideration for all victims who arrive in the operating theatre non-intubated. This complicates the situation, and techniques to apply cricothyroid pressure during intubation to minimize the risk of aspiration must be utilized. The trauma anaesthesiologist will generally choose shorter-acting intravenous and inhalation agents along with paralysing drugs for the multiply injured patient.

The majority of life-saving operations in this phase will be performed for ongoing haemorrhage (Table 9.2). This would include laparotomy for splenic, liver, or renal parenchymal injury or thoracotomy for injury to the aorta, vena cava, or pulmonary vessels. Penetrating trauma results in injuries to the same structures, but the types of lesion found will vary according to the type of projectile involved. Neurosurgical procedures for ongoing mass effect of depressed skull fractures or subdural haematoma are also indicated at this stage, and can be performed in

Table 9.2 Indications for immediate surgery

1. Haemorrhage secondary to:
   a. Liver, splenic, renal parenchymal injury – laparotomy
   b. Aortic, canal, or pulmonary vessel tears – thoracotomy
   c. Depressed skull fracture or acute subdural bleed – craniotomy
   d. Pelvic fracture – stabilization

2. Prevention of pulmonary failure:
   a. Femoral shaft fractures
   b. Pelvic fractures

Table 9.3 Evaluation of multiple trauma: patient injury severity score

AIS defined body areas
1. Soft tissue
2. Head and neck
3. Chest
4. Abdomen
5. Extremity and/or pelvis

Severity code
1. Minor
2. Moderate
3. Severe (non-life threatening)
4. Severe (life threatening)
5. Critical (survival uncertain)
6. Fatal (dead on arrival)

$ISS = A^2 + B^2 + C^2$ where A, B, C = individual regional injury severity code

concert with the abdominal or thoracic procedures. Rarely, ongoing haemorrhage due to extremity arterial trauma will require vascular repair in conjunction with stabilization of the fractures by the orthopaedist.

Recent data have indicated that stabilization of femoral and pelvic fractures prevent the pulmonary failure state in blunt trauma [6–8]. Therefore, after haemorrhage due to the above factors has been controlled, femoral shaft fractures and unstable pelvic injuries should be stabilized under the initial anaesthesia. Non-critical orthopaedic injuries to the tibia, foot and ankle, and upper extremities can await the next phase of treatment. If, however, the patient is haemodynamically stable, all open fractures and displaced fractures of the femoral or talar neck should be managed under the initial anaesthesia.

During this phase of treatment, the overall injury severity, age, premorbid nutritional status, and general medical condition of the patient must be taken into consideration. To this end, many systems of trauma scoring have been developed to aid in prognostic decisions in the multiply injured and to assist in research into the problem of polytrauma. These systems include the triage index (TI) [9], trauma score (TS) [10], abbreviated injury scale (AIS) [11], and the injury severity score (ISS) [11,12]. The last-mentioned grew out of the AIS and is the most widely used at this time. In this scale, a severity rating is applied to each injury within each organ system, and the results are squared and summed (Table 9.3). General condition and age cannot be taken into account in this system, but it has been demonstrated that the LD50 for the 15–44 age group is an ISS 40, for 45–64 it is 29, and for 65 and older it is 20. This information must be

considered during the phase of emergent surgery. As an example, a severe crush injury to a tibia associated with an ISS of 40 in a 19-year-old motorcyclist should be managed with debridement and application of an external fixator, while the same injury in a 70-year-old with an ISS of 40 should be managed with an immediate open below-the-knee amputation [13]. This illustrates the importance of communication on the part of the orthopaedist with the team captain general surgeon during this phase of treatment.

Stabilization

The goals for this phase of care of the multiply injured patient and the procedures subsequently performed depend to a large extent on the condition of the patient prior to entry into the phase of immediate surgery. If a stable blood pressure was maintained during the resuscitation and the majority of the major diagnostic work was completed, there will be far less diagnostic work to do during this phase than if the patient was rushed to the operating theatre. Claudi [14] has outlined the goals of this phase of treatment to include:

1. Restoration of stable haemodynamics.
2. Restoration of adequate oxygenation and organ perfusion.
3. Restoration of adequate kidney function.
4. Treatment of bleeding disorders.

This phase of treatment begins after the phase of immediate surgery and after the initial treatment of shock has proven effective. It may last hours to days. During this phase, all open wounds should be optimally managed and all fractures splinted in the position of function. In general, this phase of therapy is conducted in an intensive care unit under the continued direction of the trauma surgeon. In many settings, an intensive care specialist familiar with the evaluation and treatment of the polytrauma victim will take over the stabilization. The goal is to stabilize the patient rapidly to prevent parenchymal damage and to prepare as soon as possible for return to the operating room for other procedures.

In the restoration of stable haemodynamics, the usual monitoring tools are central lines or triple lumen catheters (for measuring pulmonary artery capillary wedge pressures and cardiac output), arterial lines (continuous measurement of arterial blood pressure and access for multiple arterial blood gas samples), and a urinary catheter. Appropriate crystalloid and colloid replacement therapy will be selected based on physiological parameters as well as on frequent packed red blood cell values, arterial blood gas levels, urinary output, cardiac output, wedge pressures, and arterial blood pressure.

For most trauma victims, volume-controlled mechanical ventilation will be selected for this phase. The early use of positive end expiratory pressure (PEEP) is extremely valuable in preventing pulmonary failure [15–17]. Frequent arterial blood gas analyses should direct changes in the mechanical ventilator and PEEP settings. Weaning from mechanical ventilation may be systematically conducted based on the patient's responses to intermittent assisted ventilation and trials of removal from ventilator support once the patient's blood pressure, oxygenation, and ventilation function have stabilized, and if, in the absence of facial or tracheal injury, extubation can safely be performed. Early stabilization of pelvic and femoral fractures to avoid traction is critical in this phase [8].

For the most part, adequate renal function can be maintained by appropriate management of shock. Maintaining adequate blood pressure and urinary output during the two preceding phases is nearly 100% effective in preventing renal failure. Diuretics should be used in a limited fashion in this phase only when sufficient volume has been documented by adequate cardiac output and pulmonary capillary wedge pressure (PCWP) and in general is only indicated in elderly patients. If hypovolaemic acute renal failure follows high output failure as documented by serum and urinary electrolytes, appropriate use of renal dialysis directed by a nephrologist during this phase is indicated.

Bleeding disorders in the multiply injured patient are nearly always due to haemodilution, i.e. inadequate transfusion of platelets and coagulation factors, and/or shock-related hepatic dysfunction, with the former being far more common. Occasionally, a transfusion reaction may be encountered when O negative or type-specific blood has been used during the resuscitation phase. Wherever possible, cross-matched blood should be used and 6 units of platelets should be given with every 8–10 units of blood transfused. Fresh frozen plasma should be used when prolonged PT and PTT times are evident in patients receiving massive transfusions. Disseminated intravascular coagulation (DIC) is best treated by prevention, as it is very difficult to reverse once the process begins. Adequate initial shock therapy is critical to avoiding these complications.

Delayed operative procedures

As the length of the preceding phase is highly variable, all open wounds must be optimally managed and all fractures splinted in the position of function. This is done in an attempt to minimize the complications of infection, and to offer the pain relief of fracture stability in order to decrease the use of narcotics, which act as CNS depressants as well as respiratory and gastrointestinal function depressants, and should be used as little as possible [13]. In most cases, however, the phase of stabilization is complete within 3–4 hours, and the patient can then be brought to the operating theatre for care of non-life-threatening problems.

As mentioned in the previous section, operative management of femoral fractures and pelvic fractures prevents the pulmonary failure state, and these fractures should be managed whenever possible under the initial anaesthesia. Several other musculoskeletal problems must be treated within the first 6–8 hours for avoidance of complications. Compartmental syndromes, most often associated with fractures of the tibia and forearm in the polytrauma setting, must be managed with fasciotomy early to prevent permanent muscle cell death and/or loss of nerve function. As noted previously, open fractures must also be managed with irrigation and debridement in this time frame to avoid higher rates of infection [18]. Similarly, fractures with associated vascular injury must be reconstructed within 6 hours to avoid loss of muscle and nerve function. When revascularization times are delayed beyond this range, compartmental syndromes distal to the lesion due to prolonged ischemia time must also be considered. There is some evidence to suggest that emergent capsulotomy, open reduction, and internal fixation with compression minimize the risk of late necrosis of the femoral head [19]. These fractures, along with displaced fractures of the talar neck, should be managed in this early acute phase to avoid the devastating complications of bone necrosis in these major weight-bearing joints.

Major fractures of the metaphyseal distal femur, proximal tibia, distal tibia, ankle and foot, and wrist and elbow should be considered in the next line of priority. Especially in the case of severe fractures around the elbow, ankle, and hindfoot, if management is not completed within 8–10 hours of injury, major swelling and fracture blisters ensue, making it wise to delay operative procedures to 8–12 days. Reduction in this time frame will be much more difficult, and therefore early intervention is recommended. Internal fixation of closed tibial fractures should be classed in the next, less-urgent group, especially when associated with an ipsilateral femoral fracture. Conservative treatment in this setting has been shown by Veith *et al.* to be associated with higher rates of nonunion and a greater loss of knee motion [20]. Operative fixation of upper extremity shaft fractures can be grouped here as well.

The management of unstable cervical and thoracolumbar spine fractures varies as to whether the patient is neurologically intact or not. Patients with complete loss of neurological function distal to the fracture who have return of cord level reflexes (i.e. bulbocavernosus reflex) are best managed with early stabilization to enhance the rehabilitation phase. Recumbent, conservative treatment is not indicated in this group. Operative stabilization, which for the most part will be posterior internal fixation and fusion, is best accomplished in the first 5–7 days in this phase to return the patient to the upright position and improve the ventilation–perfusion efficiency of the pulmonary circulation. These patients, because of their lack of motor function, are at risk for deep venous thrombosis and need to be mobilized early [21]. Patients with cervical, thoracic or lumbar spine fractures and no loss of neurological function should similarly be managed in the same time frame to allow early mobilization and to prevent the complications of prolonged recumbency. Patients with spine fractures and partial loss of neurological function represent a group of different considerations.

Careful attention must be paid to the nutritional status of the patient, as the multiply injured patient has extremely high caloric requirements at this juncture [22]. If the patient, due to head injury, loss of gut or maxillofacial injuries, is unable to take in 2000–3000 calories per day, parenteral nutrition must be initiated. This caloric intake may be accomplished by tube feedings whenever possible, but can be effectively delivered by the total parenteral nutrition (TPN) route. Nutritional consultation and a dietary plan based on calory counts, skin tests, and lymphocyte counts can be extremely useful where the proper nutritional course is in question. Of course, the patient can be weaned from enteral or TPN as head injuries, maxillofacial fractures, and general condition improves.

Recovery/rehabilitation

This is the phase during which musculoskeletal injuries play a critical role. The vast majority of permanent disability following multiple trauma is due to musculoskeletal or CNS trauma. These injuries must be optimally managed in the emergent and delayed operative procedures phases. Closed head injury and complete spinal cord injury are little affected by management, but major improvements can be made by optimum management of musculoskeletal injury. As indicated in prior sections, these injuries are best treated as soon as possible. Fracture reductions are much easier to perform if done before the healing process has begun. Intra-articular fractures are therefore best dealt with operatively in the first 24 hours after injury. Open fractures, fractures with vascular injury, femoral and talar neck fractures, femoral shaft fractures, unstable pelvic fractures and fractures of emergent nature are discussed in preceding sections.

The recovery/rehabilitation phase begins at the

conclusion of the operative phase. In cases of head injury, maxillofacial trauma, or genito-urinary injury, great care must be taken to assure optimal patient nutrition. Therefore, the input of the nutritionist becomes critical at this juncture. Similarly, because of post-trauma depression, the role of the consulting psychologist or psychiatrist becomes important. Physical and occupational therapists play a critical role in optimizing return of function.

In cases of severe multiple musculoskeletal injury, especially those which occur in conjunction with head injuries, transferring the patient to a rehabilitation centre is appropriate at this point. In this setting, a psychiatrist with specialized training in rehabilitation medicine serves as a critical team leader. This individual organizes the input of the rehabilitation nurse specialists, occupational and physical therapists, and the orthopaedists, urologists, and neurosurgeons. Those patients who do not require speech or occupational therapy, do not have a spinal cord injury, and do not have neurological injuries that would benefit from admission to a rehabilitation unit may be best treated at home. To obtain optimal functional results, the orthopaedist should supervise the physical therapists and visiting home nurses. Patients with severe musculo-skeletal injury must be seen by the treating surgeon fairly frequently in the first 6 weeks post-discharge, and at 3- to 4-week intervals thereafter until functional results have been maximized.

Critical musculoskeletal injuries

The patient is too sick!

This is the most common argument against aggressive early management of the multiply injured patient. Frequently, anaesthesiologists and surgeons unfamiliar with the care of this type of patient raise this objection when the ortho-paedist indicates his or her desire to, for example, place intramedullary nails in the femoral and tibial fracture, or to internally fix the intra-articular distal humerus fracture under the initial anaesthesia. Several authors have retrospectively reviewed the efficacy of aggressive early management in polytrauma, and have concluded that mortality and morbidity are significantly decreased by early operative intervention in the

management of long bone fractures [5,6,16]. Meek *et al.* reviewed a series of 71 patients with multiple long bone fractures who were assigned to one of two groups according to the treating physician who performed either rigid stabilization of long bone fractures within 24 hours or traction/cast treatment [23]. The cases were matched according to ISS scores. Of the 22 patients treated with early stabilization, one expired; and of the 49 treated in traction and casts, 14 expired, which represents a highly significant difference. Johnson and colleagues reviewed a series of 132 consecutive cases of patients with musculoskeletal injuries (minimum of two long bone fractures) and ISS scores greater than 18 [7]. They compared a group of patients in which all major fractures (long bones, pelvis, and spine) were stabilized in the first 24 hours ($N = 83$) to a group of patients who had their operative stabilization delayed ($N = 49$), basing their analysis of the effect of these treatment regimens on adult respiratory distress syndrome (ARDS). They concluded that there is a significant increase in the incidence of ARDS associated with a delay in operative stabilization of major fractures. This was most dramatic in the group with an ISS of greater than 40. Retrospective reviews addressing similar issues by Wolff *et al.* [5], Ruedi [24], Riska *et al.* [25], Goris *et al.* [16], Gustillo *et al.* [6] and others have confirmed the fact that early operative stabilization of major long bone and pelvic fractures decreases the pulmonary failure state, morbidity, and mortality.

Border's group in Buffalo, New York prospectively studied 56 patients with blunt multiple trauma (ISS 22–57) and evaluated the effect of three musculoskeletal injury management schemes on the pulmonary failure septic state [8]. One group had immediate internal fixation of long bone fractures and postoperative ventilatory support, a second group had 10 days of femur traction and postoperative ventilator support, and the third group was immediately extubated after surgery and had 30 days of femur traction. Ten days of femur traction doubled the duration of the pulmonary failure state, increased the number of positive blood cultures by a factor of ten, the use of injectable narcotics by a factor of two, and the number of fracture complications by 3.5. Thirty days of femur traction increased the duration of the pulmonary failure state by a factor of three to five (relative to group I), the number of positive blood cultures by a factor of 74, the use of narcotics by a factor of two, and the number of fracture complications by 17.

It is clear from this body of retrospective and prospective work that the concept of the patient being too sick for surgery is incorrect. The sicker the patient (in terms of ISS), the more he or she stands to benefit from immediate stabilization of long bone fractures and the sicker he or she will become if treated conservatively or with traction.

Long bone fracture management

The indications for fixation of long bone fractures are clear and the techniques for this type of management are worthy of discussion. For fractures of the femoral shaft, there is no doubt that closed intramedullary nailing is the procedure of choice. Winquist, in a series of 520 femoral shaft fractures, has demonstrated that the rate of infection is 0.9% and nonunion 0.9% – rates that have not been duplicated with any other method of treatment [26]. Previously, there was concern about increasing the risk of fat embolism in the multiply injured patient by reaming the femoral shaft fracture; however, there has not been any clinical increase in the incidence of ARDS following the nailing of femoral shaft fractures [26]. Bach *et al.* have shown that both in the laboratory and clinically (including 86 open fractures) the reaming of a fractured femur does not produce an increase in fat release [27].

Interlocking nailing has extended the use of the closed nailing technique to include very proximal and distal fractures, as well as highly comminuted fractures. In the vast majority of multiply injured patients, the side-lying position for intramedullary nailing of the femur can be used. After the surgical management of intrathoracic or intra-abdominal haemorrhage, the patient is generally stable once lost blood has been replaced. If the patient's blood pressure has been difficult to maintain, the supine position can be used. The affected limb must be adducted past the midline to allow ease of exposure of the greater trochanter in order to develop the starting point for the intramedullary nail. Another indication for the supine position in nailing the femoral shaft fracture is an associated pelvic

fracture. Placing the patient in the side-lying position places stress across the posterior elements of the pelvis and can restart bleeding from fracture surfaces or minor sacral venous plexuses. Many authors prefer the supine position for the nailing of comminuted fractures utilizing interlocking nails, as they feel that the techniques for inserting the distal locking screws are much easier to employ with the patient in this position. In either position, the C-arm must be utilized throughout the procedure for the closed intramedullary nailing technique. Another advantage of the supine nailing position is that surgical conditions of the abdomen, chest, and head can be more easily treated simultaneously by surgical teams working together to expedite the management of the patient.

The closed intramedullary nailing technique has been safely extended to grade I and grade II [26] open fractures in the multiply injured patient with no significant increase in the rate of chronic bone infection. For grade III fractures, however, this technique should generally not be used. To avoid the need for traction following debridement of the wound, external fixation should be employed to allow mobilization of the patient's chest. The fixation should be applied with the patient in the supine position, utilizing the C-arm for pin placement after a thorough debridement of the wound. In general, lateral pin placement is preferred to avoid scarring within the quadriceps muscle mass and subsequent loss of knee motion.

Of all fractures of the long bones, the femur fracture is the most critical. Conservative care of femoral shaft fractures requires the use of traction with the concomitant problems of poor chest position, difficulty with moving the patient for subsequent studies, and the inability to get the patient out of bed. The femoral shaft fracture must receive the orthopaedist's highest priority in the multiply injured and should be stabilized with an intramedullary nail whenever possible.

Occasionally, when a humeral shaft fracture is present, intramedullary nailing is indicated to allow axial weight bearing with crutches early on. This is generally done in the secondary phase of procedures but may be indicated when the patient is stable and tolerating the initial operative session well. Closed tibial fractures may be managed with closed intramedullary or interlocking nailing in the multiply injured patient. Closed fractures can be splinted to partially immobilize the fracture fragments so that stabilization procedures can be delayed to the second visit to the operating room. Reamed or unreamed tibial nailing may be used in this setting. For open fractures, external fixation is currently the procedure of choice. This must be done after the initial debridement during the first anaesthesia to allow for adequate wound care without compromising fracture stability. Half-pin fixation frames have proven to be far superior to the old through-pin Hoffman type of frames. This is because the pins do not impale the muscle–tendon units and allow early motion of the adjacent joints. The half-pin constructs have also proven to have superior biomechanical characteristics. In general, reamed intramedullary nailing has no place in open fractures because of the increased risk of chronic bone infection. Unreamed Enders or Lottes nail fixation may be advantageous, as they allow good care of the soft tissues without the disadvantages of the external fixator. These procedures carry an acceptable risk of chronic infection.

In general, once the femoral shaft fracture has been stabilized and the open long bone fractures debrided and stabilized, the decision to proceed with further intramedullary stabilization of other long bone fractures can be made. The factors to be considered must include expertise of the surgical and nursing staff, availability of implants, condition of the patient, and level of fatigue of the surgical and nursing staff. In most trauma centres, a second surgical or nursing team can be brought in if it is in the patient's best interest to stabilize all the long bone fractures in the first surgical sitting.

Pelvic fracture management

Pelvic fractures are frequently life threatening. Several reported series note mortality rates of 5–20% [28–31]. In reviewing these series, it becomes evident that there is an important difference between simple and complex fractures in terms of morbidity, mortality, and treatment techniques. Simple fractures include simple avulsion fractures of the anterior superior (or inferior) iliac spines, iliac ring fractures and minimally displaced pubic or ischial rami fractures. These are generally low velocity fractures and rarely occur in association with polytrauma.

It is important to classify the complex fractures, as this yields important information with respect to associated injuries, risk of bleeding and mortality.

Classification

Pennal *et al.* [28] have classified pelvic fractures according to the direction of the applied force. Antero-posterior compression fractures, lateral compression fractures, and vertical shear fractures are thereby defined. The anterior half of the pelvis (Table 9.4) includes the pubic and ischial rami, while the posterior portion includes the ilia, the sacroiliac joint, the sacrum and the strong posterior sacroiliac ligaments. In general, injury to the anterior structures is associated with bladder rupture and urethral tears, while injury to the posterior structures is associated with a higher incidence of severe haemorrhage, as well

Table 9.4 Abbreviated injury scale for injuries to the extremity and/or pelvis

Code	Injury
1. Minor	Minor sprains and fractures
	Dislocation of digits
2. Moderate	Compound fracture and digits
	Undisplaced long bone or pelvic fracture
	Major sprains of major joints
3. Serious, non-life-threatening	Displaced simple long bone fracture and/or multiple hand and foot fractures
	Single open long bone fracture
	Pelvic fracture with displacement
	Dislocation of major joints
	Multiple amputation of digits
	Laceration of major nerve or vessels of extremities
4. Severe, life-threatening survival probable	Multiple closed bone fractures
	Amputation of limbs
5. Critical, survival uncertain	Multiple open limb fractures
6. Fatal	Dead on arrival

as injury to the sacral nerve roots. A-P compression fractures include the so-called 'open book' fracture – the widened symphysis pubis, as well as the 'straddle fracture' – displaced fractures of all four anterior rami. A-P compression fractures are generally associated with a higher incidence of bladder and urethral injuries. The lateral compression group of fractures generally consists of an impacted sacral fracture or a fracture through the posterior ilium associated with an ipsilateral or contralateral pubic and ischial rami fracture. These fractures may be associated with injuries to the sacral nerve roots, as well as, less commonly, bladder or urethral injury. Because the critical posterior sacroiliac ligament complex is generally not violated, severe haemorrhage (more than four to six units) is generally not a problem. The vertical shear fracture includes a disruption through the sacroiliac joint, posterior ilium or sacrum associated with a disruption of the symphysis or an ipsilateral fracture of the ischial and pubic rami. The hemipelvis will frequently migrate superiorly and the posterior sacroiliac ligament complex is disrupted. These are the fractures most often associated with major haemorrhage as well as disruption of the sacral plexus.

Based on the initial radiographs, the orthopaedist can focus attention on the associated injuries. With the A-P compression injury, a more careful search for urethral disruption should be conducted if there is blood at the meatus (in the male) or gross blood in the urine. With vertical shear injuries, attention must be given to blood replacement early on [31].

Criteria for emergent fracture care

Patients with severe pelvic fractures may frequently be transported in MAST trousers on backboards. These trousers must be removed after the patient's blood pressure has been stabilized to allow for examination of the pelvis and limbs and for operative procedures to be performed. The use of MAST trousers is not a definitive treatment for pelvic fractures, and the trousers should not be left on the patient indefinitely. Open pelvic fractures carry a 50% mortality rate, as they are frequently the most high energy type of fracture, with the most displacement and

a high risk of deep infection [30]. Generally, the ischial rami produce the open wounds in the perineum. In the female, the pubic rami can produce an open wound into the vagina and a digital pelvic examination is therefore mandatory. In open fractures, a diverting colostomy is indicated, and if the anterior rami fractures are amenable to simple internal fixation with plates and screws and the surgeon has the skills to do so, this should be performed as stability of the fracture fragments will decrease the risk of infection. If the injury is not amenable to this type of management and instability is detectable on examination, an anterior external fixator should be applied.

In the case of continuing haemorrhage, aggressive management of the pelvic fracture is mandatory. If other sources of blood loss have been dealt with and the patient has lost more than four to six units of blood, stabilization of the pelvic fracture is indicated. The simplest way to accomplish this is by applying a bilateral long-leg spica cast with distal femoral pins [13]. This prevents motion of the pelvis when the patient is transported and turned in bed. A large abdominal hole must be cut out for continued observation of the abdomen. The critical point of this treatment is that the legs are stabilized and cannot put loads across the fracture surfaces.

The next simplest way to treat pelvic instability at the first operation is to apply an anterior external fixator. These frames do not offer tremendous support to the posterior disruptions in the case of the vertical shear fractures and cannot hold posterior reductions. They are useful, however, for stabilizing fracture surfaces to markedly decrease their motion and thereby aid in promoting clotting. Ultimately, displaced posterior disruptions should be reduced and internally fixed. The fixation may be accomplished with lag screws across the ilium and into the sacrum placed posteriorly or with small plates placed in screws across the fracture or sacroiliac joint from the anterior side. Although several groups are investigating the role of emergent internal fixation [32], these reconstructions should generally be done as delayed operative procedures, as they often will decompress tamponaded bleeding surfaces and promote further bleeding. As is the case with femoral shaft fractures, traction should play no role in the acute management of pelvic fractures because of the enforced recumbency of the patient and inadequate stabilization of the fracture [8].

Once the pelvis has been adequately stabilized by spica cast, external fixator, or, rarely, internal fixation, haemorrhage will usually cease. For the rare patient who experiences continuing blood loss, pelvic arteriography is indicated. Because only 10–15% of the sources of blood loss are minor arterial in nature, this technique is not indicated as a first-line management of haemorrhage secondary to a pelvic fracture [31]. Eighty-five percent of the sources of bleeding are fracture surfaces or minor pelvic or sacral veins, and the technique cannot address these. After stabilization of the pelvis has been performed, if blood loss continues with loss of six to eight more units over the next 12–24 hours and does not appear to be slowing, the patient should be returned to the radiology suite. Arteriography and embolization with gelfoam or coils can be very effective in experienced hands in controlling blood loss from gluteal or pudendal arteries. Throughout the early course of resuscitation and management, attention must be paid to appropriate replacement of platelets and clotting factors.

Spine fractures

Multiply injured patients with head injuries should be assumed to have a spine fracture until it can be proven otherwise. They should be transported with hard cervical collars and on backboards. The initial screening examination of every multiply injured patient must include a lateral cervical spine film down to C7–T1. In the case of a head injury, during the stabilization phase, complete thoracic and lumbar films must be obtained. Only when the spine films have been cleared should the cervical collar be removed and the patient taken from the backboard.

Patients with spinal cord injuries will have special requirements in regard to fluid replacement during resuscitation. This is due to autonomic dysreflexia and loss of vacular tone. Fluid requirements due to vasodilatation can be massive.

The initial survey in patients with spinal cord injury must include examination for the bulbocavernosus reflex. In the patient with quadriparesis or hemiparesis, the absence of this reflex indicates the presence of spinal shock. The final neurological status of the patient with complete paraplegia or quadriplegia cannot be determined until these cord level reflexes return. Individuals with paraparesis or quadriparesis must be carefully examined for any sign of residual motor or sensory sparing, as this function indicates a partial cord injury and has important prognostic and treatment significance.

Cervical spine fractures

The initial treatment of cervical spine fractures is similar with respect to presence or absence of cord injury. Patients with C1 or C2 fractures are generally neurologically intact on presentation. They should be left in a hard cervical collar until more definitive immobilization can be performed. In general, this means application of a Halo and placement in temporary traction or attachment to a vest or cast. For lower cervical fractures, the patient should remain in a hard cervical collar until a definitive diagnosis of the fracture can be made. Frequently, this will include a CT scan to determine the status of the neural canal. For most lower cervical fractures or single or bilateral dislocated facets, the patient should be placed immediately into a Halo or Gardner–Wells tongs as soon as it has been determined that the patient's other injuries do not require immediate operation.

The three column theory of Denis has been helpful in distinguishing stable from unstable fractures [33]. With an anterior body fracture (the anterior column) with disruption of the posterior wall of the vertebral body (the middle column) and the interspinous ligaments (the posterior column), the fracture is unstable. Disruption of two of the three columns at any single level also indicates instability. Instability implies the potential for further neurological injury. In the face of complete quadriparesis, stabilization of the spine with fusion to the intact levels above and below (generally posterior) is indicated to allow early rehabilitation. In this way, the recumbent position with the concomitant risk of pulmonary problems is avoided. With posterior wiring techniques to supplement bone graft arthrodesis, little more than a cervical collar is necessary for postoperative immobilization. In the instance of partial quadriparesis with distal sparing of function, the general course is a posterior cervical fusion followed by an anterior decompression of the canal (removal of bone fragments). This has been accompanied by an improvement of distal function in many cases.

Thoracolumbar fractures

Once these fractures are properly diagnosed with plain radiographs and CT scans, the patient must be log-rolled, maintaining spinal alignment until the fracture can be definitively treated. Stryker frames or Roto-kinetic beds can be helpful adjuncts, especially when there are associated injuries.

The general principles of treatment for cervical spine fractures apply for fractures of the thoracolumbar spine. If the patient has a complete paraplegia, posterior fusion with rod placement should be carried out to allow mobilization of the patient and a timely rehabilitation. The spine fusion is protected with a plastic thoracic orthosis until the fusion is solid. In the case of a partial injury, a two-staged procedure is preferred, with initial posterior rodding and fusion, followed by an anterior decompression shortly thereafter. Most authors believe that early fusion (within the first 48 hours) is appropriate for patients with partial paraplegia. The indication for an emergent stabilization and decompression is neurological deterioration.

References

1. Baker, S. P. (1987) Injuries: the neglected epidemic: Stone Lecture, 1985 American Trauma Society Meeting. *J. Trauma*, **27**, 343–348.
2. Smith, J. D., Bodai, B. I., Hill, A. S. and Frey, C. F. (1985) Prehospital stabilization of critically injured patients: a failed concept. *J. Trauma*, **25**, 65–70.
3. Cowley, R. A., Hudson, F., Scanlan, E. *et al.* (1973) An economical and proved helicopter program. *J. Trauma*, **13**, 1029–1038.
4. Fortner, G. S., Oreskovich, M. R., Copass, M. K. and Carrico, C. J. (1983) The effects of prehospital trauma care on survival from a 50-meter fall. *J. Trauma*, **23**, 976–981.
5. Wolff, G., Dittman, M., Ruedi, T. *et al.* (1978) Koordination von chirurgie und intensivmedizin zur vermeidung der posttraumatischen respiratorischen insuffizienz. *Unfallheilkunde*, **81**, 425–442.
6. Gustillo, R. B., Corpuz, V. and Sherman, R. E. (1985) Epidemiology, mortality, and morbidity in multiple trauma patients. *Orthopedics*, **8**, 1523–1528.
7. Johnson, K. D., Cadambi, A. and Seibert, G. B. (1985) Incidence of adult respiratory distress syndrome in patients with multiple musculoskeletal injuries: effect of early operative stabilization of fractures. *J. Trauma*, **25**, 375–384.
8. Seibel, R., La Duca, J., Hassett, J. M. *et al.* (1985) Blunt multiple trauma (ISS 36), femur traction, and the pulmonary failure-septic state. *Ann. Surg.*, **202**, 283–295.
9. Champion, H. R., Sacco, W. J., Hannan, D. S. *et al.* (1980) Assessment of injury severity: the triage index. *Crit. Care Med.*, **8**, 201–208.
10. Morris, J. A., Auerbach, P. S., Marshall, G. A. *et al.* (1986) The trauma score as a triage tool in the prehospital setting. *JAMA*, **256**, 1319–1325.
11. Baker, S., O'Neill, B. and Haddlon, W. (1974) The injury severity score: a method for describing patients with multiple injuries and evaluating emergency care. *J. Trauma*, **14**, 187–196.
12. Baker, S. P. and O'Neill, B. (1976) The injury severity score: an update. *J. Trauma*, **16**, 882–885.
13. Hansen, S. (1984) Concomitant fractures in long bones. In *The Multiply Injured Patient with Complex Fractures* (ed. M. Meyers), Lea and Febiger, Philadelphia, pp. 401–411.
14. Claudi, B. F. and Meyers, M. H. (1984) Priority in the treatment of the multiply injured patient with musculoskeletal injuries. In *The Multiply Injured Patient with Complex Fractures* (ed. M. H. Meyers), Lea and Febiger, Philadelphia, pp. 3–8.
15. Blaisdell, F. W. and Lewis, F. R. Jr (1977) Respiratory distress syndrome of shock and trauma. In *Post-Traumatic Failure* (eds F. W. Blaisdell and F. R. Lewis Jr), W. B. Saunders, Philadelphia.
16. Goris, R., Draaisma, J., Van Neikerk, J. *et al.* (1982) Early osteosynthesis and prophylactic mechanical ventilation in the multitrauma patient. *J. Trauma*, **22**, 895–903.
17. Schmidt, G., O'Neill, W., Kotb, K. *et al.* (1976) Continuous positive airway pressure in the prophylaxis of the adult respiratory distress syndrome. *Surg. Gynecol. Obstet.*, **143**, 613–618.
18. Gustillo, R. B. and Anderson, J. T. (1976) Prevention of infection in the treatment of one thousand and twenty-five open fractures of long bones. *J. Bone Joint Surg.*, **58A**, 453–458.
19. Swiontkowski, M. F., Winquist, R. A. and Hansen, S. T. (1984) Fractures of the femoral

neck in patients between the ages of twelve and forty-nine years. *J. Bone Joint Surg.*, **66A**, 837–846.

20. Veith, R. G., Winquist, R. A. and Hansen, S. T. (1984) Ipsilateral fractures of the femur and tibia: a report of fifty-seven consecutive cases. *J. Bone Joint Surg.*, **66A**, 991–1002.

21. Myllynen, P., Kammonen, M., Rokkanen, P. *et al.* (1985) Deep venous thrombosis and pulmonary embolism in patients with acute spinal cord injury: a comparison with nonparalyzed patients immobilized due to spinal fractures. *J. Trauma*, **25**, 541–543.

22. Jensen, J. E., Jensen, T. G., Smith, T. K. *et al.* (1982) Nutrition in orthopaedic surgery. *J. Bone Joint Surg.*, **64A**, 1263–1272.

23. Meek, R., Vivoda, E. and Crichton, A. (1981) A comparison of mortality in patients with multiple injuries according to the method of fracture treatment. *J. Bone Joint Surg.*, **63B**, 456.

24. Ruedi, T. (1985) Priorities in the management of multiple trauma. *Helv. Chir. Acta*, **52**, 331–335.

25. Riska, E., Von Bonsdorff, H. and Hakkinen, S. (1977) Primary operative fixation of long bone fractures in patients with multiple injuries. *J. Trauma*, **17**, 111–121.

26. Winquist, R. A., Hansen, S. T. and Clawson, D. K. (1984) Closed intramedullary nailing of femoral fractures: a report of five hundred and twenty cases. *J. Bone Joint Surg.*, **66A**, 529–539.

27. Manning, J. B., Bach, A. W., Herman, C. M. and Carrico, C. J. (1983) Fat release after femur nailing in the dog. *J. Trauma*, **23**, 322–326.

28. Pennal, G. F., Tile, M., Waddell, J. P. and Garside, H. (1980) Pelvic disruption: assessment and classification. *Clin. Orthop.*, **151**, 12–21.

29. Rothenberger, D. A., Fisher, R. P., Strate, R. and Perry, J. F. Jr (1978) The mortality associated with pelvic fractures. *Surgery*, **84**, 356–361.

30. Rothenberger, D., Velasco, R., Strate, R. *et al.* (1978) Open pelvic fracture: a lethal injury. *J. Trauma*, **18**, 184–187.

31. Slatis, P. and Huittinen, V. M. (1972) Double vertical fractures of the pelvis. *Acta Chir. Scand.*, **138**, 799–807.

32. Goldstein, A., Phillips, T., Sclafani, S. J. *et al.* (1986) Early open reduction and internal fixation of the disrupted pelvic ring. *J. Trauma*, **26**, 325–333.

33. Denis, F. (1983) The three column spine and its significance in the classification of acute thoracolumbar spinal injuries. *Spine*, **8(8)**, 817–831.

33. Weigelt, J. Mitchell, R. and Snyder, W. (1979) Early positive end-expiratory pressure in the adult respiratory distress syndrome. *Arch. Surg.*, **114**, 497–501.

10

Traumatic shock and the metabolic responses to injury

R. A. Little and M. Irving

Calls continue for the word 'shock' to be abandoned because it lacks clinical and scientific precision. However, we do not know of any other word which so well conveys the urgency of the clinical problem in the patient suffering from the multifactorial organ/system failure commonly called 'shock' and once graphically defined as a 'momentary pause in the act of dying'. We would, however, agree that the word shock, whilst undoubtedly confirming the seriousness of the clinical problem and indicating the need for urgent treatment, obviously fails to give a scientific dimension or indicate a cause for the problem.

The fundamental defect common to shock of all varieties and aetiologies is a failure of tissue perfusion and oxygen delivery commensurate with the body's needs. This failure of perfusion affects all the body's tissues and organs to a varying degree. The defect has many causes but three broad categories stand out, namely hypovolaemia, pump failure and stagnation. In surgical practice, the most important cause of shock is fluid loss supplemented by nociceptive stimuli from the traumatized tissue. In the case of the traumatized patient or those undergoing surgical operation the lost fluid is usually whole blood. Equally shock may result from loss of serum in the burned patient, water and electrolytes in obstruction of the gastrointestinal tract and third space losses into the retroperitoneum in acute pancreatitis. However, surgical patients are not immune from other causes of shock such as sepsis, myocardial failure, pulmonary embolism, anaphylaxis and neurogenic shock all of which may occur alone or in combination.

In the traumatized patient shock rapidly may supervene if the normal homoeostatic mechanisms that immediately follow injury are overwhelmed. These mechanisms are the starting process of a series of events which lead to restoration of physiological and metabolic normality and the repair of damaged tissues. The interrelationship of these events was described by Cuthbertson in terms of 'ebb and flow' [1]. He divided the responses into an early transient 'ebb' phase, characterized by a reduction in metabolic rate (or oxygen consumption, $\dot{V}o_2$) which was followed, in those going on to recover, by the 'flow' phase with an increase in metabolic rate (Fig. 10.1).

The 'ebb' phase is seen most clearly in experimental animals at ambient temperatures below the thermoneutral zone where it can be attributed to a central impairment of thermoregulation [2]. There is no unequivocal evidence that there is a reduction in metabolic rate shortly after injury in man other than when the injury is so severe that tissue oxygen delivery is compromised. However, there is evidence that both behavioural and autonomic thermoregulation are impaired in man at this time. On the other hand the increase in metabolic rate of the 'flow' phase is best seen in man. It is not a feature of most experimental studies which are of short duration [3,4].

The 'ebb' phase is not to be equated with shock

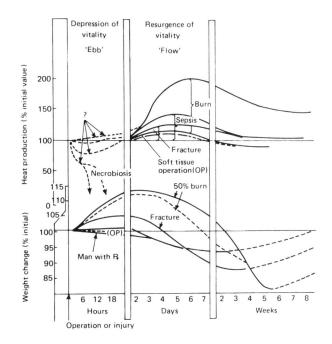

Fig. 10.1 The 'Ebb and Flow' response to injury.

for in this phase oxygen transport to the tissues is often adequate. Shock follows the ebb phase in those who are not resuscitated or who are so seriously traumatized that they will inevitably die. Such a downhill course has been designated necrobiosis (Fig. 10.1) and is characterized by a progressive failure of oxygen transport. In this chapter we will use the ebb and flow concept as a guide to the time course of the responses to injury.

Immediate response to injury

The immediate responses to injury mounted by the body are multifactorial but the most obvious of the responses are those due to activation of the neuro-endocrine system [5]. The principal stimuli of the neuro-endocrine responses are appreciation of danger, fluid loss and afferent nociceptive impulses resulting in, for example, severity related rises in adrenaline and noradrenaline. The former comes from the adrenal medulla and the latter from the sympathetic nerve endings. These hormones cause an im-

mediate response in the cardiovascular system with a tachycardia and a redistribution of the circulating blood volume from non-essential regions such as the skin to essential areas such as the heart, lungs and brain.

The combination of peripheral vasoconstriction and the translocation of interstitial fluid into the intravascular compartment means that arterial blood pressure may remain at near normal levels despite considerable fluid loss. However, when loss from the intravascular compartment exceeds 30% of the normal volume then hypotension supervenes.

Biochemical changes accompany the physiological and are also designed to meet the changed metabolic demands that follow injury. Prominent amongst the changes are measures to mobilize the body's energy stores of glycogen and fat, with the catecholamines, especially adrenaline, again having a major role. There is an injury severity related rise in plasma glucose concentration which is largely the result of a breakdown of liver glycogen and an increase in hepatic gluconeogenesis. This is fuelled by lactate release by skeletal muscle glycogenolysis and by glycerol arising from lipolysis of adipose tissue. Plasma glucose concentration continues to rise over the whole range of injury severity. On the other hand, although there is an increase in plasma nonesterified fatty acid concentrations after minor and moderately severe injuries there is no further rise with increases in severity, a finding which may be related to an increasing impairment of adipose tissue perfusion [6].

Vasopressin is released from the posterior lobe of the pituitary with the result that there is an increase in free water reabsorption from the distal tubules of the kidney. Aldosterone release ensures the retention of sodium and water and the production of ACTH by the anterior lobe of the pituitary leads to release of cortisol from the adrenal cortex. Initially the amount of cortisol in the circulation reflects the severity of the injury suffered by the patient but with increasing severity of injury (injury severity score > 12) the rise flattens off and indeed in the severest injuries the levels tend to fall. As ACTH levels continue to rise with increasing severity of injury it is possible that this failure of the cortisol response is due to a reduction in perfusion of the adrenal cortex.

The purpose of these changes from the teleological point of view is defensive, but when protracted, for example by prolonged inadequate treatment, there is a possibility that aspects of the responses may be harmful.

Clinical picture of shock

The clinical picture of shock is one of a low flow state characterized by skin pallor, sweating, mental confusion, oliguria, tachypnoea and usually, but not always, hypotension and tachycardia. In the early phases of hypovolaemic shock the arterial blood pressure may be raised due to an overvigorous response of the resistance side of the circulation to the evoked sympathetic nervous responses. Although the immediate response to hypovolaemia is a tachycardia this can be followed, as the magnitude of fluid loss increases, by a vagally mediated bradycardia elicited by stimulation of cardiac distortion receptors [7].

Although there may be minor variations in the clinical picture depending upon the cause of the shock state, the basic picture is essentially the same irrespective of the cause. A patient with septic shock may be pyrexial and initially have a warm periphery whilst a patient with cardiogenic shock may have irregularities in the heart rhythm and a raised central venous pressure.

In all types of shock the key to a successful outcome is early reversal of the physiological and biochemical changes by vigorous and adequate treatment.

Pathophysiology of the low flow state

If the changes that occur following injury are not reversed rapidly and thoroughly by treatment then the body enters the downward path to necrobiosis and the patient suffers increased tissue damage.

The deleterious changes possibly have a common pathway through the cardiovascular system. Early in the course of shock changes occur in the characteristics of the blood. Platelets and leucocytes are released into the bloodstream and red cells form rouleaux and begin to sludge. The intrinsic and extrinsic clotting mechanisms and complement are activated with consequent changes in the coagulation/fibrinolytic mechanisms. If normal flow characteristics are not re-

stored by repletion of the fluid volume the changes progress further. There is increased viscosity of the blood and thromboplastins are released from damaged cells and hypoxic endothelium. Thrombin is formed with consequent aggregation of platelets leading to intravascular fibrin deposition. The scene is set for the development of disseminated intravascular coagulation with all the consequences of impaired tissue perfusion.

Although the acute fall in peripheral perfusion triggers many of the changes characteristic of shock, it is important to realize that these are not necessarily reversed by restoration of tissue blood flow. There is increasing recognition that the reflow state is itself associated with adverse changes such as the generation of oxygen free radicals which can exacerbate tissue damage.

One of the principal organs to manifest the changes in tissue perfusion is the lung and indeed in the injured, postoperative or septic patient pulmonary failure is often the cause of death. Innumerable terms have been advanced to describe this heterogenous problem but none is more adequate than the presently accepted ARDS – adult respiratory distress syndrome [8].

Pulmonary responses to injury and shock can be seen immediately after the event. The pulmonary contusion resulting from the direct damage, lung collapse due to air or fluid in the pleural cavity and pulmonary oedema following head injury can all cause respiratory insufficiency.

With the passage of time from the moment of the accident, especially if shock persists or infection supervenes, the full clinical picture of ARDS can arise. The actual pathogenesis of this condition is unclear but the result is an increased vascular permeability in the lung with the accumulation of protein rich fluid in the interstices of the lung which then spills over into the alveoli.

Other organs are similarly affected by the shock state and the effects of DIC and other perfusional changes may be witnessed in the heart, liver, kidneys and brain. Sustained falls in perfusion pressure whilst capable of being tolerated for short intervals will, if sustained, cause permanent cellular damage.

Renal insufficiency in the early stages of shock is a homoeostatic mechanism but if the low flow state is sustained proximal and distal tubular necrosis occurs. In patients with crush injuries myoglobin casts may be present within the tubules. In sustained severe low flow states intestinal mucosal necrosis may be a problem, particularly in the colon. Lesions are also seen in the small intestine; these are thought to be due to hypoxia which can occur, perhaps surprisingly, without a reduction in total blood flow. The hypoxia is a result of the vascular anatomy of the mucosal villi which encourages the exchange of oxygen between the ascending and descending limbs of the mucosal countercurrent exchanger, making the villi very susceptible to a reduction in blood flow velocity [9] A loss of mucosal integrity has been associated with increased translocation of microorganisms and endotoxin into the vascular and lymphatic drainage from the gut, thereby initiating a systemic inflammatory response. Other splanchnic organs can also be adversely affected by hypovolaemia. The pancreas may be especially sensitive releasing, for example, cardiotoxic factors and proteolytic enzymes. The liver can also suffer, despite receiving an increase in the proportion of cardiac output after injury, with an impairment of reticulo-endothelial activity, and whole body energy substrate and metabolite homoeostasis.

The interest in myocardial depressant factors might suggest that the heart is the most susceptible organ in traumatic shock. However, there is little evidence that cardiac performance is impaired in such cases unless there has been direct myocardial injury, although this may not be so in sepsis. Indeed the early response to trauma is often associated with an increase in cardiac contractility. The most important determinants of cardiac function at this time are ventricular preload (end diastolic volume) and afterload (vascular resistance to ejection).

Cerebral blood flow is normally well protected by efficient autoregulatory mechanisms but these too may be impaired by injury. For example, the responsiveness of the cerebral vasculature to carbon dioxide is often lost after head injuries. The impairment of autoregulation may not be limited to direct head injuries. There is experimental evidence that the pattern of change in regional cerebral blood flow produced by haemorrhage can be affected by afferent nociceptive stimuli mimicking injury to peripheral tissues [10]. However, the major threat to cerebral blood flow is a rise in intracranial pressure due to an increase in intracranial mass.

Diagnosis and management of shock

Hypovolaemic shock

Of all the causes of shock, that of most concern to the surgeon is hypovolaemic shock resulting singly or in combination from loss of whole blood, plasma, or water and electrolytes.

The diagnosis of hypovolaemic shock is often, but not always straightforward. The previously mentioned clinical picture is usually apparent and the cause obvious. However, it has to be recognized that the extent of concealed fluid loss can be much more extensive than is clinically appreciated. Thus in traumatized patients a litre of blood can easily surround a fracture of the femur with little obvious swelling and 2 litres of blood can surround a fractured pelvis. Similarly in cases of acute traumatic pancreatitis following blunt abdominal injury large quantities of fluid can be sequestered in the retroperitoneal space – so called third space losses – without any palpable abnormality being apparent.

Today it is almost inevitable that the shocked patient will be subject to intensive clinical monitoring from the moment he presents. However, in most cases of straightforward hypovolaemic shock such measures are unnecessary and all that is usually required is measurement of the pulse rate and arterial blood pressure (perhaps combined to give the Shock Index) together with observation of the state of the superficial veins, skin colour and urine output. However, there is no doubt that in complicated patients, i.e. those with multiple injuries involving the trunk, those with cardiac disease and pulmonary disorders and those who develop complications additional monitoring is required. This will include direct measurement of the arterial blood pressure, right atrial and wedge pressures and estimation of cardiac output. The recording of cardiac output (and hence of oxygen delivery) is important to ensure that $\dot{V}o_2$ is not limited by an inadequate oxygen delivery (Do_2); indeed, improved outcome has been associated with increases in $\dot{V}o_2$ and Do_2 to supra-normal levels.

The interpretation of changes in pulse rate must take into account the biphasic nature of the pulse rate response to haemorrhage (*vide supra*). Also, it should be borne in mind that the persistence of a tachycardia after fluid resuscitation might be due to the inhibition of cardiac vagal activity by trauma and the defence reaction (preparation for fight or flight) rather than to persisting hypovolaemia. A danger here, especially in the elderly, is that attempts to 'titrate' the patient back to a normal pulse rate can lead to fluid overload with all its attendant problems.

Management of hypovolaemic shock

It should not be necessary to emphasize that the priority in hypovolaemic shock is to stop the source of fluid loss. In the case of external bleeding this can be accompanied by pressure and ligation. Bleeding around fracture sites can be lessened by immobilization of the bones. The use of MAST trousers, although superficially logical, has now been shown not to confer any benefit and is not recommended. Internal bleeding usually requires operative intervention but fluid loss from the obstructed gastrointestinal tract may be slowed down by aspiration of the stomach.

Replacement of the lost fluid should proceed at the same time as the loss is being stopped. Fluid should be infused through large cannulae at a rate necessary to reverse the hypovolaemia. Suitable fluids for this are:

1. electrolyte solution – crystalloids;
2. plasma substitutes;
3. blood.

The choice of fluid varies with national opinion. Crystalloids tend to be the preferred choice in the United States whilst colloids are used more frequently in the United Kingdom and Europe [11].

In patients in whom there is continuing loss of blood whole blood should be infused, but the administration of erythrocytes is, perhaps, less important than the maintenance of volume.

Septic shock is treated along similar principles, although in such patients it is necessary to evacuate any abscesses which may be the source of infection and to administer antibiotics. It is now generally accepted that steroids do not have a place in the management of the patient with septic shock or after trauma [12,13] although they may have a role in the acute management of spinal injuries.

Nutritional support for the injured patient

It has long been recognized that following even moderately severe injury patients lose weight, mainly as a result of reduction in the muscle bulk. The loss of weight occurs even in the presence of an apparently normal intake of food. The problem is compounded if, for any reason, the patient cannot eat, for example if he or she is being mechanically ventilated or if the gastrointestinal tract has been injured and requires resting. Yet it is the experience of clinicians dealing with the injured patient that the majority of patients do not require any special nutritional support to recover from their injuries and that the lost weight is soon regained following resumption of normal activity. However, some patients continue to lose weight and progress poorly and in such cases nutritional support has to be considered.

At the present time there is little evidence on which to decide the place of enteral or parenteral nutritional support in the injured patient [14, 15]. However a recent meta-analysis suggests that early enteral feeding reduces postoperative septic complications, when compared with parenteral feeding, in high-risk surgical patients: an effect which was most marked for those patients with trauma [16]. Unlike in general surgery, where there has been considerable interest in the indications for, and value of, nutritional support accidental injury remains a relatively unexplored area despite one or two good publications on the subject (e.g. [15]). On the other hand, enteral nutritional support using defined formula diets is now technically feasible and is administered more readily, especially in the elderly injured patient.

Metabolic consequences of injury

In the early phase of the response to injury there is a mobilization of energy substrates as already described. At this time fat is the main fuel for oxidation and most glucose oxidation can be accounted for by the brain. This preferential oxidation of fat is also seen in other 'stress' states such as sepsis. The early pattern of response is followed by the flow phase characterized by an increase in oxygen consumption which is fuelled by increases in the oxidation of both fat and carbohydrate with only a small contribution from protein [17]. Although glucose is being oxidized in the flow phase there are marked changes in the control of its metabolism, plasma insulin concentrations being much higher than expected from the prevailing glucose levels. The high insulin levels occur at the time of maximum nitrogen excretion. The excreted nitrogen is derived from the breakdown of tissue at the site of injury as well as the generalized wasting of skeletal muscle. Additionally, injury and sepsis appear to be associated with a reduction in protein anabolism.

The hormonal basis of the flow phase and more particularly of insulin resistance is unclear. Attempts at understanding the mechanisms involve using 'triple hormone' infusion of cortisol, adrenaline and glucagon which mimics many of the features of the flow phase [18]. However, the hormone concentrations used in such studies more closely resemble those found in the ebb phase than in the flow phase where the levels of such hormones have almost returned to normal. The monokines interleukin-1 and tumour necrosis factor (cachectin) released from phagocytes may also be involved in the flow phase, although there is no firm evidence for this.

Consequences of malnutrition

It is reasonable to question whether the state resembling malnutrition which follows severe injuries confers any serious disadvantage on the patient. However, there is little doubt that the morbidity and mortality in malnourished patients undergoing major surgery are higher than expected [19]. Malnutrition of moderately severe degree affects virtually every major system in the body [14]. The diminution of muscle bulk, which is due not only to muscle breakdown but also to lack of synthesis, has an adverse effect on respiratory function. Both the vital capacity and the resting minute ventilation are decreased resulting in a greater susceptibility to respiratory infection. Cardiac muscle is also affected, with a reduction in cardiac contractility and therefore reduced arterial pressures. In chronic malnutrition, renal function may also deteriorate as a result of a fall in glomerular filtration rate. The effective surface area of the gastrointestinal tract is decreased and the intestinal transit time increases, resulting in bacterial overgrowth. The

effect of both changes is to reduce absorption of nutrients. Malnutrition results in a greater risk of developing infection. Cell-mediated immunity is affected, with a reduction in the numbers of the T cells. Humoral immunity is also affected despite the fact that the B-cell levels are not significantly reduced.

In summary, prolonged malnutrition slows healing and increases morbidity, particularly from infection. Even if the patient should escape these problems, convalescence is likely to be prolonged.

Who needs nutritional support?

Before a decision is made to institute nutritional support, the patient must be resuscitated. The restoration of circulating blood volume to normal is of paramount importance in maintaining perfusion of both the vital organs and the fat depots since free fatty acids released by lipolysis are used as substrates for energy production. The stress caused by pain and fever must if possible be reduced because it results in impairment of mobilization of substrates. In particular, every effort should be made to decrease the size of the injury by, for example, an early decision to amputate a badly damaged limb. Sepsis must be vigorously sought and aggressively treated, for no amount of nutritional support will redress the negative nitrogen balance if infection is allowed to continue unchecked [20].

There are two broad indications for the use of nutritional support in injured patients. First, are those patients in whom malnutrition can be anticipated from the nature and/or the severity of the injury. Second, are patients developing serious complications after initially straightforward injuries. In general terms, the more severe the injury, the more likely will be the need for nutritional support. An objective measurement of the severity can be made using the injury severity score (ISS) [21]. It is recommended that unless the nature of the injury dictates otherwise, nutritional support is likely to be required in patients with an ISS of greater than 14 and is mandatory for those with scores exceeding 20 [22]. Injury of the gastrointestinal tract, and particularly injuries of the pancreas and extensive intestinal injuries, may lead to a prolonged ileus with a diminished appetite and diminished absorption.

The need for mechanical ventilation for any length of time also constitutes an indication for active nutritional support though mechanical ventilation may be beneficial in reducing the patient's energy requirements by taking over the work of breathing.

The patient who develops serious sepsis after an injury, which on its own was not such as to merit nutritional support, must none the less be considered for feeding. The reason for this is that sepsis will lead to further loss of nitrogen with a loss of muscle bulk and a fall in the serum albumin levels.

Indications for parenteral nutrition

It makes sound sense to feed enterally if at all possible. Parenteral feeding is expensive and potentially hazardous, and should be reserved for certain categories of patients. An absolute indication for its use is major gastrointestinal injury from which return of function may be slow. Some patients do not tolerate enteral nutrition despite gradual building up to full-strength solutions and they may have to receive parenteral nutrition. Because of the risk of aspiration, a patient whose level of consciousness is depressed should not be fed enterally unless there is a cuffed endotracheal tube in place.

The advantage of parenteral nutrition over enteral feeding is that it need not be discontinued for surgical procedures or investigations – a distinct benefit for the patient with multiple injuries whose feeding would otherwise be discontinuous because of the many journeys to the operating room for changes or dressings and plasters and other procedures.

It has been shown that the mortality of head injury is reduced by early institution of parenteral nutrition [23]. Rapp and colleagues also showed that parenterally fed patients had a better nitrogen balance and higher albumin levels that enterally fed patients. Considering that the volume of tissue damaged in even a serious head injury is small, such patients have surprisingly high resting metabolic rates. One explanation for this is the spasticity which accompanies serious head injury and another is an increase in metabolism by the central nervous system which, even under normal circumstances, makes up 20% of the total resting metabolic expenditure. Evidence for this comes from Dempsey and associates [24], who showed a considerable reduction in the resting metabolic expenditure by the administration of barbiturates to patients with severe head injury. The case for nutritional support in head injury is further strengthened by the observation that a considerable proportion of such patients ultimately die from infection [25], which, as has been discussed earlier, may be a consequence of malnutrition. Finally, an occasional patient will have such high energy requirements that it is impossible to meet these with conventional enteral feeding formulae.

Which nutrients and how much?

It is possible for a patient to maintain some oral intake, in which case he or she may be able to meet the requirements for electrolytes, otherwise they must be supplied parenterally. The amounts required are calculated from knowledge of normal daily requirements and losses in the urine and any other body fluids. As the patient moves from a catabolic to an anabolic phase, the requirements for potassium, magnesium and phosphorus rise.

Energy requirements are based on resting energy expenditure, which in turn depends on age, sex, size and severity and nature of injury. There are a number of reliable formulae by which the calorie requirements of injured patients can be calculated [26], although it is better, where possible, to measure an individual's energy expenditure by calorimetry. In this way, not only can the optimal level of calories be supplied, but also the form in which they should be taken can be determined. The respiratory quotient will indicate whether fat or carbohydrate is being oxidized [27]. In the past the energy needs of injured patients have been grossly overestimated. In fact, few patients need more than 2000 kcal/day [28]. Even in patients with multiple organ failure the resting energy expenditure rarely exceeds 2500 kcal/day. Only seriously burned patients require more [29]. To give more calories than the patient needs is not only wasteful but may be harmful. Additionally, glucose which is surplus to needs is converted into fat with the generation of 'excess' carbon dioxide, which has to be excreted by the lungs and this requires extra respiratory effort. In a patient with compromised respiratory function this may be enough to precipitate respiratory failure [30].

Calories must be supplied as a mixture of fat and glucose, with about one-third as fat. However, should the patient be septic or have a respiratory disorder, the ratio can, with benefit, be reversed.

Protein requirements are not difficult to assess if facilities are available for measuring urinary nitrogen losses. Generally, the patient requires 2–3g/day more than the daily loss [20]. If urinary nitrogen losses cannot be measured directly, a useful rule of thumb is to give approximately 0.2 g of nitrogen/day per kg of body weight. Standard commercial amino acid preparations are based on the aminogam of egg protein. They contain mixtures of synthetic L-amino acids, approximately 25% of which are the branched-chain amino acids (BCAA) leucine, isoleucine and valine. Recent work suggests that in stress the BCAAs are readily utilized as calorie sources by skeletal muscle. BCAAs are also known to exert an anabolic effect by decreasing protein catabolism and stimulating synthesis. BCAA-enriched amino acid solutions have been shown to have a greater effect on restoring nitrogen balance and immune competence than standard solutions. It must, however, be clearly stated that the role of BCAA-enriched solutions in clinical practice has yet to be clarified, for despite the apparent biochemical advantages described above they have not been shown to provide clinical benefit.

Both fat-soluble and water-soluble vitamins should be supplied. The stores of fat-soluble vitamins are greater and their half-life longer than those of the water-soluble vitamins. However, the water-soluble vitamins should be supplied daily, bearing in mind that injured and septic patients may have increased requirements, especially for the B group of vitamins. Supplements of the trace metals zinc, copper, etc. are unlikely to be required unless prolonged parenteral nutrition is needed, or the patient has abnormally high losses from fistulae, diarrhoea, etc. Certainly, even a modest oral intake in the form of drinks such as tea will supply these elements in sufficient quantities.

Parenteral nutrition: avoiding complications

Figures for catheter-related complications vary widely, depending on the experience of individual units. There is no doubt, however, that complications such as pneumothorax, misplacement of the catheter and sepsis can be kept at very low levels by observing a few simple rules. Feeding catheters should be inserted in the operating theatre, using full aseptic technique and with X-ray screening facilities available. Once inserted, the catheter must not be used for any purpose other than parenteral nutrition. There should be a strict protocol for dressing of the catheter and connecting and disconnecting it from the nutrient solutions. It is now well recognized that it is strict catheter-care protocol and not subcutaneous tunnelling of the catheter which leads to a low catheter sepsis rate.

Initially, feeding should be spread over 24 hours. Over a period of 4–5 days the infusion can be gradually speeded up until, ideally, the patient receives his entire daily requirements during an overnight 12 hour period. This is good for morale, as not only is there one less tube to worry about during the waking hours but also the patient can be more mobile. During the period that the catheter is not in use it is locked with 1000–1500 i.u. of heparin to prevent clotting. The rate of infusion must be slowed down towards the end of the feeding period to prevent reactive hypoglycaemia, which often follows abrupt cessation of the large carbohydrate load. Although the nutrient solution may be given in the form of 500 ml bottles, a 3 litre bag containing all the daily requirements is more convenient. The contents can be infused using a pump, a great advantage for overnight infusion because constant checks on the infusion rate are not necessary.

Monitoring

It is important to make frequent estimations of serum electrolytes, certainly until the patient is well stabilized on a particular feeding regimen. Knowledge of these, together with measurement of losses of body fluids will help in formulating the regimen. Haematological indices should be measured at regular intervals. In particular, the mean corpuscular volume, and prothrombin time will give a clue to deficiencies of folate, vitamin B12 and vitamin K.

Objective evidence of benefit from providing nutritional support is often difficult to obtain.

Body weight is a poor indicator of nutritional status because early changes are often due to water retention. In any case, it is not always possible to weigh patients who are confined to their beds and connected to traction, ventilators, etc. Thickness of the skin fold over the triceps is more useful, as is the trend in the serum albumin levels. Subjectively, however, it is usually rewarding simply to see a patient looking and feeling better.

Nutritional support is continued until the patient is able to meet his or her metabolic needs with a normal diet. It is important to remember that exercise is important for maintaining muscle bulk during feeding.

The decision to feed injured patients parenterally must be taken early and only if enteral feeding is thought to be contraindicated, inappropriate or inadequate. Attention to detail will keep the complication rate low. There is little doubt that the early institution of nutritional support in the severely injured patient reduces morbidity and, in some situations, even mortality.

References

1. Cuthbertson, D. P. (1942) Post shock metabolic response. *Lancet*, **1**, 433–437.
2. Stoner, H. B. (1981) Thermoregulation after trauma. In *Homeostasis in Injury and Shock* (eds Z. Biro *et al.*), Pergamon, New York, pp. 25–33.
3. Little, R. A. (1985) Heat production after injury. *Br. Med. Bull.*, **41**, 226–231.
4. Heath, D. F. (1985) Experimental studies on energy metabolism after injury and during sepsis. In *The Scientific Basis for the Care of the Critically Ill* (eds R. A. Little and K. N. Frayn), Manchester University Press, Manchester, pp. 75–101.
5. Gann, D. S. and Lilly, M. P. (1984) The endocrine response to injury. In *Progress in Critical Care Medicine Vol 1. Multiple Trauma* (ed. R. J. Wilder), Karger, Basel, pp. 15–47.
6. Stoner, H. B., Frayn, K. N., Barton, R. N. *et al.* (1979) The relationship between plasma substrates and hormones and the severity of injury in 277 recently injured patients. *Clin. Sci.*, **56**, 563–573.
7. Thoren, P. (1979) Role of cardiac vagal C. fibres in cardiovascular control. *Rev. Physiol. Biochem. Pharmacol.*, **86**, 1–94.
8. Chamberlin, W. H., Rice, C. L. and Moss, G. (1983) Pulmonary dysfunction in shock. In *Handbook of Shock and Trauma, Vol 1: Basic Science* (eds B. M. Altura *et al.*) Raven Press, New York, pp. 105–112.
9. Haglund, U. (1973) The small intestine in hypotension and haemorrhage. *Acta Physiol. Scand., Suppl.*, 387.
10. Sandor, P., Demchenko, I. T., Kovach, A. G. B. and Moskalenko, Y. E. (1976) Hypothalamic and thalamic blood flow during somatic efferent stimulation in dogs. *Am. J. Physiol.*, **231**, 270–274.
11. Yates, D. W. and Magill, P. J. (eds) (1978) Plasma volume replacement. *Arch. Emerg. Med.*, **1 (4)** (supplement), 1–58.
12. Dearden, N. M., Gibson, J. S., McDowall, D. G. *et al.* (1986) Effect of high-dose dexamethasone on outcome from severe head injury. *J. Neurosurg.*, **64**, 81–88.
13. Bone, R. C., Fisher, C. J., Clemmer, T. P., Slotman, G. J., Metz, C. A. and Balk, R. A. (1987) A controlled clinical trial of high-dose methylprednisolone in the treatment of severe sepsis and septic shock. *New Engl. J. Med.*, **317**, 653–658.
14. Mughal, M. M. (1987) Parenteral nutrition in injury. *Injury*, **18**, 82–86.
15. Kudsk, K. A., Stone, J. M. and Sheldon, G. F. (1982) Nutrition in trauma and burns. *Surg. Clin. North Am.*, **62**, 183–192.
16. Moore, F. A., Feliciano, D. V., Andrassy, R. J. *et al.* (1992) Early enteral feeding, compared with parenteral, reduces postoperative septic complications. *Ann. Surg.*, **216**, 172–183.
17. Frayn, K. N., Little, R. A., Stoner, H. B. and Galasko, C. S. B. (1984) Metabolic control in non-septic patients with musculoskeletal injuries. *Injury*, **16**, 73–79.
18. Bessey, P. Q., Walters, J. M., Acki, T. T. and Wilmore, D. W. (1984) Combined hormonal infusion simulates the metabolic response to injury. *Ann. Surg.*, **200**, 264–281.
19. Mullen, J. L., Buzby, G. P., Matthews, D. C. *et al.* (1980) Reduction of operative morbidity and mortality by combined preoperative and postoperation nutritional support. *Ann. Surg.*, **192**, 604–613.
20. Alexander-Williams, J. and Irving, M. (1982) *Intestinal Fistulas*. John Wright, Bristol.
21. Baker, S. P., O'Neill, B., Hadden, W. and Long, W. D. (1974) The injury severity score: a method for describing patients with multiple injuries and evaluating emergency care. *J. Trauma*, **14**, 187–196.
22. Stoner, H. B. (1984) The therapeutic implications of some recent research on trauma. *Arch. Emerg. Med.*, **1**, 5–16.

23. Rapp, R. P., Young, B., Twyman, D. *et al.* (1983) The favourable effect of early parenteral feeding on survival in head-injured patients. *J. Neurosurg.*, **58**, 906–912.

24. Dempsey, D. T., Guenter, P., Mullen, J. L. *et al.* (1985) Energy expenditure in acute trauma to the head with and without barbiturate therapy. *Surg. Gynecol. Obstet.*, **10**, 128–134.

25. Becker, D. P., Miller, J. D., Ward, J. D. *et al.* (1977) The outcome from severe head injury with early diagnosis and intensive management. *J. Neurosurg.*, **47**, 491–502.

26. Wilmore, D. W. (1977) *The Metabolic Management of the Critically Ill.* Plenum Press, New York.

27. Frayn, K. N. (1983) Calculation of substrate oxidation rates in vivo from gaseous exchange. *J. Appl. Physiol.*, **55**, 628–634.

28. Macfie, J. (1986) Towards cheaper intravenous nutrition. *Br. Med. J.*, **292**, 107–110.

29. Davies, J. W. L. (1982) *Physiological Responses to Burning Injury.* Academic Press, New York.

30. Askanazi, J., Rosenbaum, S. H., Hyman, A. I. *et al.* (1980) Respiratory changes induced by the large glucose loads of total parenteral nutrition. *JAMA*, **243**, 1444–1447.

11

Reconstructive orthopaedic surgery: skin cover following injury to a limb

P. L. G. Townsend

Acute injury

After debriding any injury, a decision has to be made whether the wound can, or should be closed. It the viability of skin is in doubt, closing a wound under tension is likely to lead to skin necrosis with infection complicating subsequent management.

A possible degloving injury should be looked for, especially in lower limb injuries. The history may be of help, for example if a limb is held against a rigid object such as a kerb, and a wheel passes over the limb, the effect may be to sheer the skin off the underlying structures, and with it its source of blood supply. Where the skin is completely degloved, the injury may be very obvious but where there are only small lacerations, the extent of the injury may not be immediately apparent. The wound should be explored, haematoma evacuated and if the degloving is extensive, circulation to the skin should be carefully assessed. If loss of an extensive area of skin is inevitable, removal of this skin should be carried out and the subcutaneous fat excised, leaving full thickness skin, which can then be stored in a skin bank or fridge at +4°C for secondary application.

Primary skin grafting of wounds is not often carried out except in facial injuries and in this situation it is important to remember the best subsequent cosmetic result is achieved by donor skin grafts taken as close as possible to the recipient site, so that a graft taken from the leg and placed on the face will be yellow in comparison with the adjacent skin.

Skin grafts will only take if there is a suitable vascular bed such as muscle or deep fascia; grafting onto fat is often unsatisfactory and it may be better to remove the fat, the viability of which may very well be in doubt, and graft onto fascia. Grafts will not take where there is no suitable vascular base, for example open joints, tendons without paratenon, bone without periosteum, or cartilage without perichondrium. These situations require some form of cover with its own blood supply and will be dealt with later.

Skin grafts may either be full thickness 'Wolfe' grafts or partial thickness 'Thiersch' grafts. Full thickness grafts require closure of the donor site after removal, which limits the size of the graft, although it is theoretically possible to put a partial thickness graft on the donor site. This is seldom done.

It is more difficult to get a good take of a full thickness graft, therefore their application requires more expertise. Their advantage is that if successful, the grafts do not produce as much fibrosis under them and therefore do not shrink. This is particularly important in, for example, finger contractures or syndactyly, where after release such a graft may be required.

The usual donor site for full thickness grafts is the groin, where quite a large ellipse of skin can be removed and the defect closed. The skin preferably should be taken from the left groin so there is no confusion subsequently about whether the appendix has been removed. An alternative site is the inner aspect of the upper arm, where quite large grafts can be taken and used, for example after release of recurrent Depuytren's contractures.

On the face small grafts can be taken from behind the ear, what is known as a post-auricular 'Wolfe' graft. In older people, similar grafts can be taken from in front of the ear. The defects can then again be closed directly.

Where a large graft is necessary, the supraclavicular fossa can be a suitable donor site. If even larger areas of skin graft are required, initial partial thickness grafts can be applied and after all the swelling has gone down, with shrinking of the graft, this may be excised and the area reconstructed with a better matching full thickness graft.

Partial thickness grafts in the acute situation often do not take well, due to difficulty in determining viability of tissues with wound contamination. As part of the initial management of a large wound at the time of debridement, skin grafts can be taken and stored. The wound site can then be dressed with an antiseptic dressing such as Flamazine or Betadine. After 24–48 hours the skin can be applied often without sedation directly onto the wound surface, the chance of haematoma under the graft is reduced and the prospects of infection diminished. Clinically, the percentage take of graft is enhanced and the wound can often be exposed.

It should not be forgotten that skin can act as a biological dressing reducing fluid loss and preventing infection; as a temporary expedient with exposed bone, it may provide cover until a suitable flap can be carried out as a delayed primary procedure.

In extensive wounds partial thickness grafts can be meshed using a suitable machine; this allows expansion up to three to five times the original size. Epithelium then grows into the gaps between the strands of skin usually within 2 weeks, depending on the amount of meshing and stretching. If the skin is meshed, but not expanded, this helps to allow skin grafts to drape over irregular wounds and at the same time allows blood and serous fluid to drain out through the slits.

Partial thickness grafts, if suitably stored, remain viable for up to 2 weeks; after this viability rapidly falls off. As indicated before, partial thickness grafts do heal with a larger amount of fibrosis underneath and therefore tend to contract.

Flap cover

As indicated, where there is no suitable bed for a graft, skin with its own blood supply must be used to cover exposed bone, cartilage, tendons or joints. To achieve acceptable results, there must be some understanding of the blood supply of the skin. Within skin, there are plexuses at dermal and subdermal levels; within the fat (often less well developed) and on the surface of the fascia, which itself is a relatively avascular structure. There is no longer felt to be an important plexus underneath the fascia. These plexuses all interconnect.

The arterial supply to the skin which vascularizes these plexuses can arise either be direct or indirect vessels. In the 'direct' cutaneous blood supply, there is an anatomically recognizable arteriovenous system, which supplies an area of skin which is the same on equivalent areas of the body. Unlike nerves, the blood supply of any particular area is not so fixed, so if one vessel is divided, alternative adjacent vessels may be able to open up and take over supply and drainage.

'Indirect' vascular supply occurs after blood vessels have supplied bone/muscle or fascia and then provide perforators to the skin.

When raising a flap, understanding the underlying anatomy is therefore vital.

Flaps can be described as:

1. Cutaneous – random;
   – axial;
2. Fascio-cutaneous;
3. Musculo-cutaneous;
4. Osteo-musculo-cutaneous.

Cutaneous random

For many years the concept of random pattern flaps was firmly adhered to, so that if a flap was raised, the breadth would correspond to the length on a one to one basis. Experimentally in pigs, this does seem to apply up to about 3 cm, but after that viability depends more on whether a large vessel is included in the flap.

An example of the use of a random pattern flap

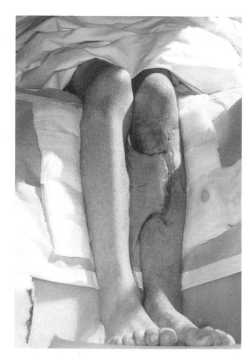

Fig. 11.1 Cross leg flap in position inset to cover exposed bone.

is (Fig. 11.1) the cross leg flap in the lower leg, for example, following skin loss with exposed bone, in the central third of the lower leg. The flap is raised from the inner aspect of the undamaged leg, leaving a graftable bed. The limbs are brought together and the skin of the flap is sutured to the edges of the wound. After about 3 weeks, the flap is divided across its base; by this time there has been extensive re-anastomosis of vessels between the edge and base of the flap and vessels on the damaged limb to maintain the blood supply of the transferred skin.

Axial pattern flaps

One of the great advances in plastic surgery was the discovery that a skin flap containing one of theses anatomically recognized direct cutaneous vessels can be made many times longer than its breadth. The first one described was the groin flap [1] in which skin from the lateral groin extending medially from the area of the anterior iliac spine, can be raised down to its supplying artery, the superficial circumflex iliac artery with accompanying vein.

The groin flap has been used especially on the hand where following injury or removal of malignant tumours; the flap can be raised and then inset onto the hand to cover the exposed tendons or bone. Usually after 3 weeks, often after initial delay by clamping the feeding vessels, the groin flap can be separated, the flap on the surface of the hand, having picked up an alternative supply via re-anastomosis with other vessels on its periphery and base.

Fascio-cutaneous flaps

In the lower limb, simple transposition of skin flaps, even with a ratio of 1:1, containing skin and subcutaneous tissue is fraught with difficulty and often unsuccessful.

Ponten [2], however, described flaps in the lower limb up to 22 cm long, incorporating skin and fascia. This incorporation of the fascia with its vascular plexus on the upper surface obviously increases the integrity and viability of the flap (Fig. 11.2).

Some flaps are difficult to categorize. An example is the valuable radial forearm flap, first described by Yang [3] in China and in the West-

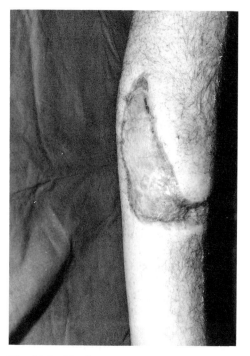

Fig. 11.2 Fascio-cutaneous flap in lower leg rotated to cover defect. Donor site grafted.

ern literature [4]. This flap, supplied by the radial artery, is composed of skin, subcutaneous tissue and fascia and can include segments of radius, or tendons such as palmaris longus or flexor carpi radialis.

The flap is nourished by vessels arising from the radial artery, which pass between the brachioradialis and pronator teres in the upper forearm and flexor carpi radialis and brachioradialis tendon distally. This flap can be based on the central or more distal parts of the radial artery. It has been used as a local flap, or a free flap, the latter to be discussed later. Subject to a satisfactory Allen test, the blood supply of the hand may be maintained via the ulnar artery and palmar arches, thus nourishing the radial artery retrogradely. This flap can be raised after division of the artery proximally and rotated distally. Of considerable interest is the fact that the venous return is then backwards via the vena comitans and the superficial draining veins. This flap can then be rotated to be used in reconstruction of hand injuries, either in the acute situation, where, for example, there has been loss of skin or tendons on the dorsum of the hand; or in later reconstruction, for example after a traumatic amputation where the skin is draped around a segment of radius it can be used in thumb reconstruction (Fig. 11.3).

The advantages of this flap over groin flaps are that only the damaged limb is involved and the patient does not have to be bed bound, the hand can be elevated and mobilization achieved earlier, with less morbidity. Where the flap has been raised, the defect is skin grafted.

Muscle and musculo-cutaneous flaps

Where there are muscles running under the skin, the blood supply to these muscles often give perforators to the overlying skin. If the muscle is raised with its blood supply, skin overlying the muscle can be taken with it, or alternatively, muscle can be raised as a flap and a skin graft applied on top, as muscle provides an excellent bed for grafting.

The lower leg can be divided into thirds, in the upper third and around the knee, injuries exposing the upper tibia or the knee joint may be covered by use of one or other bellies of the gastrocnemius muscle [5], still attached by its predominant blood supply from the popliteal fossa. Muscle drapes well, can be moulded into cavities and resists infection well. When more complicated reconstruction is likely on the underlying bone or joint, gastrocnemius with overlying skin is preferable (a musculo-cutaneous flap; Fig. 11.4) it can be more easily raised subsequently with skin-to-skin closure.

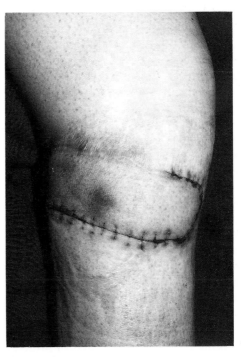

Fig. 11.4 Compound gastrocnemius–skin flap to cover defect below knee. Photo taken after thinning of flap.

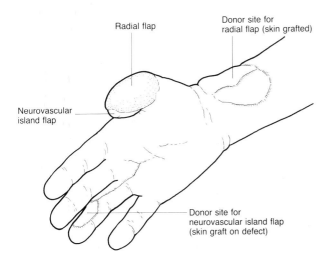

Radial flap

Donor site for radial flap (skin grafted)

Neurovascular island flap

Donor site for neurovascular island flap (skin graft on defect)

Fig. 11.3 Radial flap used to reconstruct thumb. Note neuro-vascular island flap from ring finger.

In the central tibial area the muscle flap used usually without overlying skin is soleus muscle. This can be separated from the gastrocnemius in a relatively avascular plane, divided off the Achilles tendon and rotated to cover the exposed tibia. Unlike the gastrocnemius, the blood supply is segmental from the posterior tibial vessels and the upper lateral part is also provided by the peroneal artery. In mobilization, some of these segmental vessels will have to be divided.

In the lower third, many muscles become tendons and muscle bulk available is small. If fascio-cutaneous flaps have either failed or are not possible, this is the area where free flaps are often indicated.

Free flaps

Local flap alternatives to covering ungraftable exposed structures should first be considered before use of microvascular 'free flaps'. Other injuries such as a fractured pelvis or injury to the other limb may make a cross-leg flap out of the question, or there may be so much local damage to exclude muscular, or fascio-cutaneous flaps, or else the site in the lower part of the leg may be such that no suitable muscle bellies can be used for cover.

The term 'free flap' is used where the donor flap is detached from its blood supply, transferred to the recipient area and revascularized. The first free flap was carried out by Daniel and Taylor [6] on the groin flap. It was found possible to maintain the viability of the groin flap on the predominant feeding artery, either superficial circumflex iliac artery, or superficial epigastric, together with the draining vein. Lymphatic re-anastomosis was therefore not essential.

Re-vascularization on the damaged leg depends on finding a suitable segment of un-damaged artery and draining vein. The vascular anastomoses are carried out under a microscope. Arterial anastomosis may be either end-to-end, or if possible, end-to-side, so that the peripheral run-off of the recipient vessel is still possible at the same time as nourishing the flap. Vein anastomosis is usually carried out by end-to-end anastomosis. In the situation where suitable recipient vessels are too far from the site for attachment of the flap, vein grafts may be required, reversed in the case of an arterial gap.

Microvascular surgery requires considerable training in the laboratory to achieve an acceptable level of clinical success and for this reason is best carried out in units where such surgery (including a replantation service) is a routine part of surgical practice.

The advantage of a 'free flap' is that it is usually a single stage procedure. While the surgery may take a long time, alternative techniques such as tube pedicles require a longer time in total and much longer in hospital. For this reason the latter technique is now seldom carried out. Another advantage of the free flap is that it brings an increased blood supply to the injured area which enhances healing of adjacent tissue such as an underlying fracture site.

Use of free flaps in an acute injury

Of considerable importance is the timing of the free flap. If bone is exposed and left to dry, it is likely to die off. Emergency free flaps have been carried out after debridement, but this is often an impractical situation. Often the best alternative, especially in a grossly contaminated wound, is initial debridement of the wound; exposed bone and tendons must then be kept moist, either by saturated dressings or using skin as a biological dressing. A delayed primary free flap can then be carried out, preferably within 48 hours, at which time a further debridement, if indicated, is carried out.

At the initial operation if there is an exposed fracture, or in a fractured limb where there are other non-graftable structures involved, some

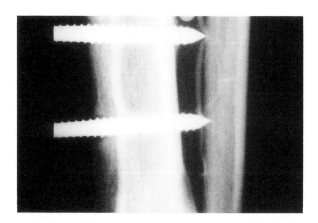

Fig. 11.5 Fixator pins compressing peroneal artery.

form of external fixation may be required. Obviously the pins must not be placed into the exposed bone as this will be the site of cover of the flap. Discussion should be made with the team responsible for the free flap, so the pins do not interfere with exploration or anastomosis of vessels (Fig. 11.5). Also, it should be borne in mind that if pins are passed from the medial side of the tibia, it is possible to damage the peroneal vessels (Fig. 11.5). Again, if pin sites have to be changed later, this undoubtedly reduces the viability of the bone and many produce annular sequestra.

Use of free flaps in chronic injury

Many cases are in this category, although any bone loss will be known from the time of the accident. Traumatized skin may die off under a plaster, a situation which is perhaps more likely to occur where internal fixation is carried out in an area of poor circulation which requires extra soft tissue mobilization to achieve.

Exposed bone and plates provide a difficult situation clinically. Gault and Quaba [7] found that in cases where there was an exposed fracture fixation device, or prosthetic joint, if preoperative wound cultures were negative, or only showed commensals, success rate of cover was high. If pathogenic bacteria were demonstrated preoperatively, then even covering the area with a well vascularized flap, allowing antibiotics to reach the affected area, success rate was low often resulting in chronic infection down to the metal.

In cases showing pathogenic bacteria, removal of the fixation device should be carried out and alternative fixation applied, preferably by external fixation, bearing in mind previous comments. The limb can be held out to length while all obvious dead bone is removed. Radical debridement is essential to prevent long term problems of osteomyelitis. This is preferably done in two stages. After initial debridement, daily antiseptic dressings can be carried out, such as Betadine. After a further week, further debridement can be carried out prior to reconstruction.

The choice of free flap depends on reconstructional requirements: skin, skin and tendons, or skin and bone.

Skin only

The first free flap, as indicated, was a groin flap (Fig. 11.6); its disadvantages are a short vascular pedicle, variability of vascular pattern and small vessels (range 0.8–3 mm). For this reason other

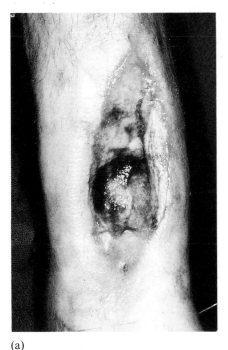

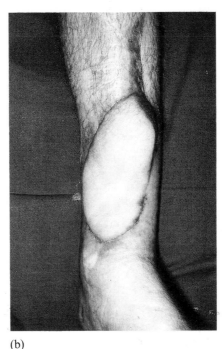

Fig. 11.6 (a) Skin loss and exposed bone lower leg. (b) Free groin flap. Note back cut to expose anterior tibial vessels away from site of trauma.

(a)   (b)

flaps have been developed; however, the groin area remains a good donor site as the wound can often be closed directly.

The radial forearm flap, mentioned earlier, may be used as a free, instead of transposition, flap, usually to resurface the other hand. The advantage of using it as a free flap is that the radial artery on the donor hand can be reconstituted using a vein graft.

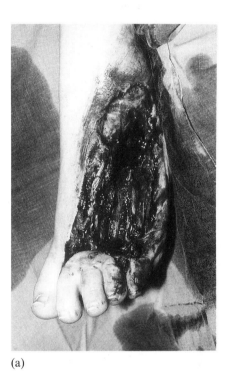

(a)

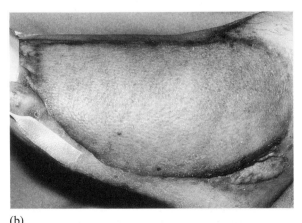

(b)

Fig. 11.7   (a) Degloving injury over foot prior to debridement with skin loss and tendon damage. (b) Free latissimus dorsi flap carried out as delayed primary procedure at 48 hours.

Latissimus dorsi flap

This is a musculo-cutaneous flap that can be used for local transposition or as a free flap (Fig. 11.7a, b). The flap can be used as 'free' muscle alone based on the thoraco-dorsal branch of the subscapular artery, whose origin lies in the axilla. After revascularization, skin grafts can be applied over the muscle. Postoperative management of continuing perfusion may be more difficult than if a cutaneous element is included. Muscle contraction in response to stimulation persists for a number of days after transfer if it remains viable.

The flap taken usually incorporates a skin 'paddle', being nourished by skin perforators coming through the muscle. In this situation, only a lateral strip of muscle need to be dissected with the skin flap, together with the perforating vessels.

The advantages of this flap are its long pedicle, about 10 cm, its versatility, incorporating skin/muscle, or even via its vascular branch to the serratus anterior. Segments of vascularized ribs can be mobilized with the flap. Depending on the size of the flap required the donor site can usually be closed. Disadvantages are a rather bulky flap and the necessity of dividing the nerve to the latissimus dorsi; however, it is sometimes possible to preserve one of the motor branches.

In cases of Volkmann's contracture, it is possible to get motor and therefore good functional recovery after micro-neuro-vascular anastomosis to the transferred latissimus dorsi muscle. The distal end of the thoraco-dorsal vessel can also be used to repair a defect in the radial or ulnar artery if present, producing a flow-through situation, as well as perfusion of the muscle.

Skin and tendon

The combined loss of skin and tendons, for example, over the dorsum of the hand or back of the heel, is a difficult problem, previously requiring firstly flap cover and secondary repair with tendon grafts. This may also require initial use of silastic rods.

Taylor and Townsend [8] showed it was possible to raise segments of tendons with a free flap maintaining their vascularity; for example, with the dorsalis pedis flap it is possible to use seg-

(b)

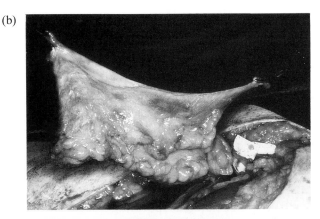

(c)

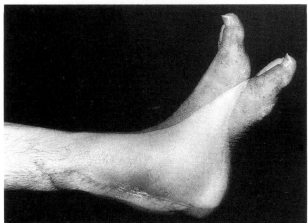

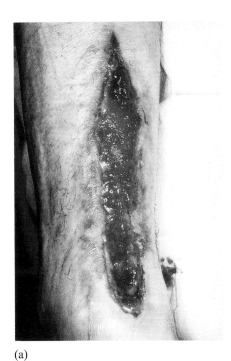

(a)

Fig. 11.8 (a) Skin and tendon loss on back of lower leg. (b) Composite groin flap containing skin, subcutaneous tissue and strip of external oblique aponeurosis. Background material placed behind superficial circumflex artery and vein. (c) Result following reconstruction. Note free flap inset on back of leg.

ments of foot extensor tendons to reconstruct the extensors of the fingers. For longer defects, segments of external oblique aponeurosis can be taken with the groin flap to reconstruct either a similar situation above, or for example the Achilles tendon under free flap cover (Fig. 11.8a–c).

As the tendons or tendon graft (external oblique aponeurosis) are still surrounded by normal vascularized connective tissue, gliding of these structures under the flap still occurs together with more rapid healing from the ends of the vascularized grafts.

More recently, it has been demonstrated that it is possible to take the radial forearm flap with palmaris longus and part of flexor carpi radialis tendons.

Innervated free flap transfer

Reconstruction, especially of a denuded thumb or over the heel, is best achieved if reinnervation is also carried out. Although some form of protective sensation occurs after a long time in the flaps already mentioned, it is possible to improve this by identifying the nerve supply to the skin being used in reconstruction and reanastomosing it to the divided nerves. For example, the terminal branches of the peroneal nerve can be identified while raising a dorsalis pedis flap, and after transfer to the thumb can be reanastomosed to the divided digital or other cutaneous nerves with much improved long term two point discrimination.

Skin and bone loss

The associated loss of skin and bone, especially in the lower leg, is perhaps one of the most difficult reconstruction problems. In the past, often a tube pedicle would be necessary to resurface the area and then subsequently bone grafts placed in position. The success rate was low and morbidity high.

Bone grafts placed as chips or pieces depend on revascularization to provide bony union and any infection diminishes the chance of success. Vascularized bone grafts, as part of a free flap, behave like a double fracture producing callus at both ends and if stressed undergo remodelling, there is therefore a very important fundamental difference between the types of graft. Vascularized bone also has a much greater resistence to infection.

In the hand, where often only a small segment of bone is required the radial forearm flap, either by pedicle or free flap incorporating a segment of radius, can be very useful in reconstruction, for example an amputated thumb [9].

The groin flap (superficial circumflex flap)

It was initially found possible to raise the crest of the ilium together with a groin flap, the bone remaining perfused via its periosteal supply. Although this was a considerable advance, there was a limit to the size of the bone graft which could be taken and would remain vascularized.

Deep circumflex iliac flap (DCIA) [8]

Perfusion studies of the DCIA vessel have shown that not only is skin perfused over the iliac crest, but that via the endosteal and periosteal circulation the whole of the ilium can be nourished by this vessel. For cases of bone loss between 6 and 12 cm this flap should now be considered.

The DCIA (1.5–3 mm in diameter) arises from the external iliac artery. The vena comitans draining the area usually join to form a single vessel draining into the external iliac vein.

The vessels can be identified posterior to the inguinal canal and be traced laterally behind the anterior superior iliac spine, allowing this to be left with the attachment of the inguinal ligament. Near this point, the vessels pierce the fascia transversalis and transversus abdominis and run close to the rim of the ilium between this latter muscle and the internal oblique. In this position, the artery gives off musculo-cutaneous branches. The flap can be raised, cutting a required segment of ilium together with a small cuff of muscles and skin flap according to need (Fig. 11.9).

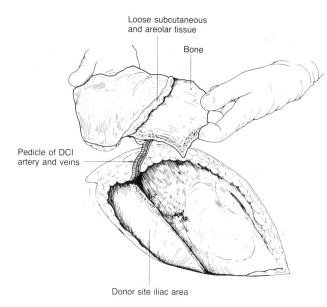

Loose subcutaneous and areolar tissue

Bone

Pedicle of DCI artery and veins

Donor site iliac area

Fig. 11.9   DCIA flap raised, showing skin and bone composite flap still attached by feeding vessels.

The typical case referred to earlier is a lower limb injury where bone loss has occurred either following the accident or subsequently (Fig. 11.10). The limb is held out to length by external fixators (Fig. 11.11) and all dead skin, bone and muscle extensively debrided.

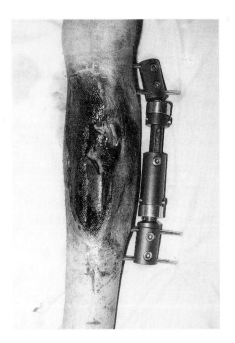

Fig. 11.10   Injury of lower leg with exposed dead bone and skin loss.

considered, the vessels being anastomosed to the posterior tibial vessels of the opposite leg. The legs are held together by rigid Hoffman fixation,

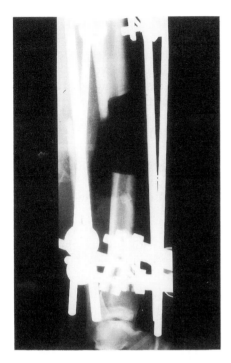

Fig. 11.11 After removal of dead bone, limb being held out to length by external fixators.

The pedicle of the DCIA flap is about 6 cm long, allowing anastomosis some distance away from the area of the bone loss. The bone graft is often stepped to allow locking into the ends of the tibia and then the anastomosis is carried out usually end-to-side to the anterior or posterior tibial artery, and end-to-end of the vena comitans to appropriate vena comitans, or to the long saphenous vein. The latter tends to go into spasm so the former is preferable.

If insufficient bony stability is provided by stepping the graft and tibia, a limited amount of fixation with wire may be required.

If the flap is successful (Fig. 11.12a, b) post-operative infection is usually not a problem unless bone chips or screws have been added.

In certain cases limb injuries are so severe, for example extensive skin loss with multiple fractures, or history of ischaemia within the limb, that anastomosis within the limb may add to the possible complications in view of the extra dissection required. There may be insufficient vascularized skin to cover either the pedicle, or long vein grafts which may be required to provide a blood supply from more proximal undamaged vessels.

In this situation a cross leg DCIA flap can be

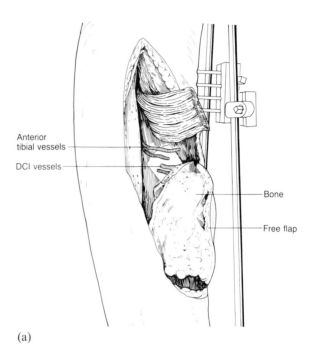

Anterior tibial vessels

DCI vessels

Bone

Free flap

(a)

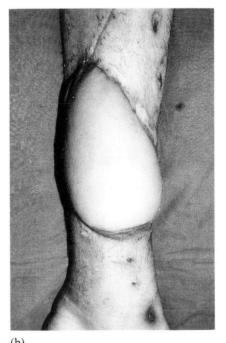

(b)

Fig. 11.12 (a) DCI vessels and flap placed adjacent to anterior tibial vessels prior to anastomosis. (b) Successful free DCIA flap in position over lower leg. Secondary skin thinning may be required later.

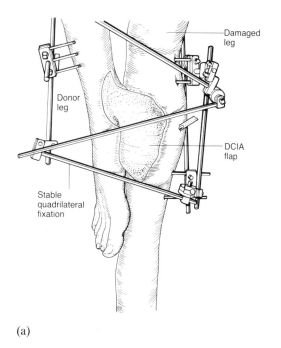

(a)

thus allowing elevation of the limb and mobilization of ankle, knee and hip joints (Fig. 11.13a, b).

The vessels and flaps are divided later than a traditional cross leg flap at 5 weeks, by which time anastomosis of vessels occurs between the cancellous bone to bone contact and skin to skin contact. Back bleeding from the damaged leg can usually be demonstrated from the DCIA after division.

That the flap and bone remain vascularized is confirmed by comparison between DCIA flaps with anastomosis based on the damaged leg and by the cross leg flap technique [10] of 23 cases, 13 based on the same leg and 10 cross leg cases. Time to clinical union with full weight bearing without external support in both groups was between 6 and 7 months. Following operation, the reconstructive situation is similar to a double fracture and in three of the former and one in the latter group, there was delayed or non-union. Further cancellous chips were added later after

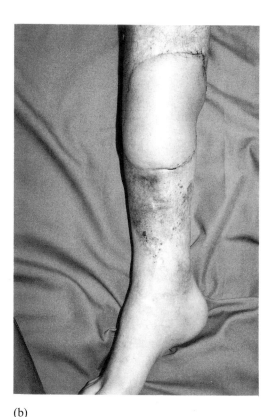

(b)

Fig. 11.13 (a) Cross leg free DCIA flap. Vessels anastomosed normal vessels right leg and flap inset into defect left leg. (b) Flap after division of DCIA vessels at 5 weeks.

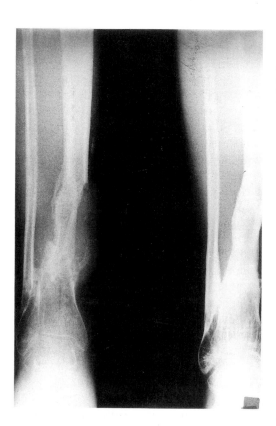

Fig. 11.14 Radiographs to illustrate remodelling of bone with vascularized bone graft. Left side at 6 months, right side at 18 months.

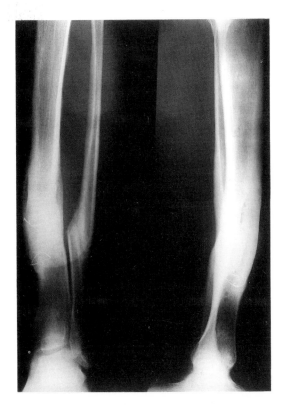

Fig. 11.15 Further case AP and lateral radiographs illustrating late remodelling. Bone graft area between wire loops.

freshening the ends. Extra time for this is taken into account in the overall figures quoted.

The normal postoperative treatment is to remove the Hoffman fixation when skin healing is achieved. The limb is then placed in a plaster of Paris cast and partial weight bearing started as soon as possible (Figs 11.14 and 11.15).

Vascularized fibula

Where there is a bony defect larger than 12 cm, the DCIA flap is unable to be used and in this situation the vascularized fibula based on the peroneal vessels can be considered. Provided about 6 cm are left at either end, the rest of the fibula can be taken as a free graft. To maintain stability in the ankle joint, a distal screw stabilizing the fibula remnant to the tibia is advised.

Even a small segment of fibula can be taken with a cuff of surrounding muscle. The nutrient artery lies in the middle third. In the case of congenital pseudoarthrosis of the tibia, this is probably the operation of choice. Vascularized fibula can, after removing the fibrous tissue between the tibial ends, be passed up and down the tibial medullary cavity ([11]).

Long term follow-up of a vascularized fibula indicates that with stress, the fibula hypertrophy remodels. This process may actually be enhanced if a greenstick or other fracture occurs. After about 2 years it may even be difficult to identify which is tibia and which fibula. Unlike the DCIA flap, the affected limb needs a lot longer external support, often over a year.

The vascularized fibula can be used in reconstruction of the forearm where there is loss of segments of both radius and ulna bones, converting it to a single bone forearm (Fig. 11.16a–d).

Although it is possible to take some skin with the fibula, it is quite small in comparison with a DCIA flap and it may be necessary to resurface the area of skin loss firstly by, for example, a cross leg flap prior to the microvascular procedure.

Replantation

The techniques used in replantation are of relevance to reconstructional problems; the indications are therefore worth briefly considering.

Amputation leading to ischaemia of part of a limb or digits may be partial or complete. In the former if revascularization is not carried out, necrosis of the end will occur.

Amputation may result from a clean cut, crushing, avulsion injury, or a combination of these.

The aim of any replantation should be not only to repair arteries, veins, but also tendons and nerves, as secondary surgery is more difficult to carry out.

The best results from revascularization occur if circulation is restored within 8 hours of injury, cooling the severed part increases this time.

Treatment of severed part

Without using any disinfectant for cleaning, the parts should be kept wrapped in a swab soaked in physiological saline and then placed within a plastic bag. Ice from a domestic refrigerator may

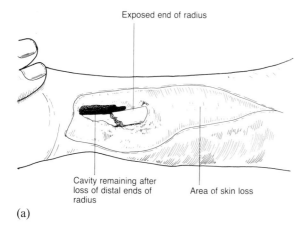

(a)

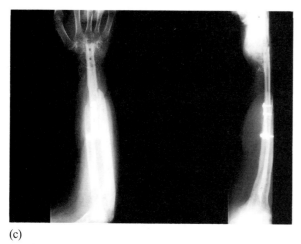

(c)

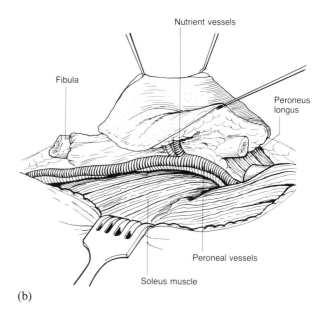

(b)

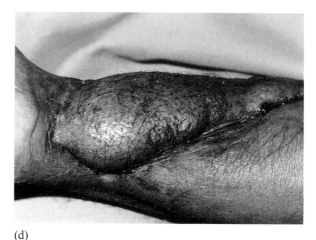

(d)

Fig. 11.16   (a) Compound injury left forearm, with skin loss and exposed dead bone. (b) Vascularized fibula being raised from leg with skin. Note feeding peroneal vessels (arrow). (c) Vascularized fibula in position forming single bone forearm. (d) Skin of flap inset on forearm.

be placed in an outer bag and an equal amount of water added.

On no account should a part be allowed to freeze, and the bag should not be placed in a thermos flask or an insulated container. The two bags can be sealed with one seal and placed in an open container. Cooling is especially important with larger amounts of muscle present in higher amputations, as they are more sensitive to anoxia.

Choice of cases suitable for replantation

Not every amputated digit is worth replanting, clean cut amputations do best. A narrow rim of crushing can be compensated for by adequate debridement and if necessary vein grafts. Avulsion injuries on the whole do badly.

Replantation of a single digit within no man's land is seldom indicated. Although successful replants should get metacarpo-phalangeal joint movement, there will be interphalangeal joint stiffness and if the other fingers are unaffected the patient will tend to exclude this digit and even demand amputation subsequently.

Indications for replantation are: thumb loss, multiple digit amputations, hand, and distal limb.

Other factors may have to be taken into account: age, sex, dominance of hand and social factors.

The centre which provides a replantation service should be notified, firstly to confirm indications and secondly to mobilize surgical teams and theatre, as time is obviously important. Two teams are preferable. One team debrides and identifies the structures on the amputated part and the other does the same on the stump.

Amputations at wrist level do well, as there are mainly tendons here. The more proximal the amputation, the more ischaemic muscle mass is involved and with it, an increasing risk to the patient's life from toxic breakdown products of anoxia being released into the general circulation after revascularization.

The results of proximal upper limb reimplantation can be unrewarding, mainly due to the poor nerve regeneration at this level. Motor and sensory modalities are more intermixed and accurate reapposition at axonal level is poor.

Incomplete lower limb amputations are usually well worth revascularizing. Replantation of complete amputation may not be so rewarding, as even if sensory return is achieved patients may complain of hyperaesthesia and this possibility has to be compared with the excellent functional results using a prosthesis after below knee amputation.

In multiple amputations where parts are not suitable for replantation, thought should be given to the possibility of providing spare tissue, such as vein or arterial grafts, or even a free flap. For example [12] in an arm and leg amputation where it was not possible to revascularize the arm, a radial forearm flap was raised from the amputated limb and transferred to cover the exposed tibia, allowing him to finish with a below, rather than above, knee amputation (Fig. 11.17a, b).

Reconstructional techniques used in replantation can be used in congenital or traumatic loss of a thumb or digits.

In trauma and in congenital loss due to amniotic bands, the anatomy proximal to the site of amputation is normal. In congenital hypoplasia, or aplasia, for example transverse arrest with loss of all fingers, this does not occur, so alternative tendons or nerves may have to be used, such as wrist flexors and extensors and a cutaneous nerve. The results are therefore very difficult to predict before exploration.

Thumb reconstruction was originally carried out using the big toe, although in many patients

this is too large. The wrap-around flap [13] is designed from the big toe, taking, the equivalent size of nail and skin to the remaining normal thumb, together with sensory and vascular supply on one side. The donor site is then skin

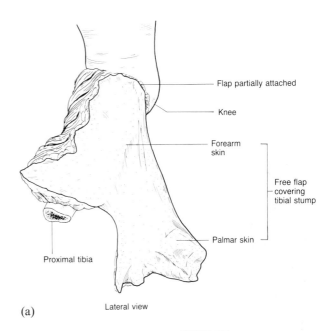

(a)   Lateral view

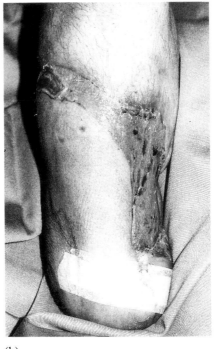

(b)

Fig. 11.17 (a) Free flap of forearm and hand. Skin draped over exposed upper tibia. (b) Amputation stump after healing. Palmar skin placed to cover end of stump.

grafted. The flap is then wrapped around an iliac bone graft and pegged into position into the site of the amputated thumb this flap is then revascularized. This technique provides a better match and reduces the morbidity of the donor big toe. To enhance bone graft take, a segment of distal phalanx is usually taken.

Digital reconstruction is usually from the second toe. This is based on the first dorsal metatarsal artery, a branch of the dorsalis pedis. If this toe is taken out together with the metatarso-phalangeal joint and a segment of the metatarsal, it is then possible to collapse in the donor deficit with a good cosmetic and functional result. Second toe transfer can produce a good sensory mobile digit, although not as powerful as the big toe.

In conclusion, the possibilities available of skin and composite reconstruction have considerably increased in recent years and it is important prior to making a decision on treatment to realize what these possibilities are, especially if local flaps or microvascular surgery are considered as this may affect the mode and placement of fixation. Also, by planning composite reconstruction of the various tissues lost the number of operations may be reduced with earlier rehabilitation of the patient.

References

1. McGregor, I. A. and Jackson, I. T. (1972) The groin flap. *Br. J. Plast. Surg.*, **25**, 3–16.
2. Ponten, B. (1981) The fasciocutaneous flap; its use in soft tissue defects of the lower leg. *Br. J. Plast. Surg.*, **34**, 215–220.
3. Yang, G., Chen, B., Gao, Y. *et al.* (1981) Forearm free skin flap transplantation. *Natl Med. J. China*, **61**, 139–141.
4. Song, R., Gao, Y., Song, Y. *et al.* (1982) The forearm flap. *Clin. Plast. Surg.*, **9(1)**, 21–26.
5. Ger, R. C. (1968) The management of pretibial skin loss. *Surgery*, **63**, 757.
6. Daniel, R. K. and Taylor, G. I. (1973) Distant transfer of an island flap by microvascular anastomosis. *Plast. Reconstr. Surg.*, **52**, 111–117.
7. Gault, D. T. and Quaba, A. (1986) Is free flap cases of exposed metalwork worthwhile? A review of 28 cases. *Br. J. Plast. Surg.*, **39**, 505–509.
8. Taylor, G. I. and Townsend, P. L. G. (1979) Composite free flaps and tendon transfer: an anatomical study and clinical technique. *Br. J. Plast. Surg.*, **32**, 170–183.
9. Biemer, E. and Stock, W. (1983) Total thumb reconstruction: one-stage reconstruction using an osteo-cutaneous forearm flap. *Br. J. Plast. Surg.*, **36**, 52–55.
10. Townsend, P. L. G. (1987) Indications and long term assessment of ten cases of cross leg free DCIA flaps. *Ann. Plast. Surg*, **19**.
11. Zhong-Wei, C., Dong Yue, Y. and Di-Sheng Chang, C. (1982) *Microsurgery*. Shanghai Scientific and Technical Publishers, Springer-Verlag Berlin, Heidelberg, New York, pp. 277–279.
12. Waterhouse, N., Moss, A. L. H and Townsend, P. L. G. (1984) Lower limb salvage using an extended free radial forearm flap. *Br. J. Plast. Surg.*, **38**, 394–397.
13. Morrison, W. A., O'Brien, B. M. and MacLeod, A. M. (1981) Thumb reconstruction with a free neurovascular wrap-around flap from the big toe. *J. Hand Surg.*, **5**, 575.

12

Arthroscopy of the knee

J. L. Pozo

Introduction

The advent of diagnostic arthroscopy and arthroscopic surgery in the last 10–15 years has greatly extended the accuracy of investigation, diagnosis, understanding and treatment of many of the common intra-articular pathologies of the knee.

Historical background

First reports of endoscopic practice date back to Philip Bozzini in Vienna around 1806 [1]. His 'lichtlieiter' or light conductor used candle light reflected down a bifid silver tube to visualize the interior of the nasopharynx, anal canal, vagina, urethra and orthopaedically the sinus of bones affected by osteomyelitis. In order to avoid burns to the surgeons' hands Herteloupe [2] resorted to *Lampyris noctiluca,* the female glow worm (the male only flashing intermittently) as an alternative source of illumination.

More conventional techniques of illumination were developed over the subsequent 50 years: Desormaux [3] used alcohol and turpentine, others experimented with camphor and petrol or burning magnesium filaments in the early cystoscope. The use of electricity to heat the platinum elements to white heat proved a more reliable and controllable source of illumination with David Newman in Glasgow in 1883 first using an incandescent lamp applied to an endoscope.

However, it was the development of the rod lens system by Professor Hopkins at Reading University which dramatically improved the clinical use of the endoscope.

Arthroscopy

In 1918 Professor Tagaki in Tokyo initially examined the inside of a knee in cadavers using a 7.3 mm cystoscope. Two years later he developed an instrument specifically for the examination of the knee: 'the arthroscope'. Although the first instruments did not have a lens system, rapid evolution led to the development of instruments which allowed still photography and cinematography [4] and colour photography by 1939.

In 1921 Bircher [5], working separately in Switzerland, presented the results of his knee examinations using the laparo-thoracoscope and nitrogen or oxygen to distend the joint.

In the USA, Burman, Finkelstein and Mayer [6], at the Hospital for Joint Diseases developed a 4 mm arthroscope which was used not only to examine the knee but also the elbow, ankle and shoulder. In 1934 they went on to describe their arthroscopic observations on 30 knees. There was little further advance in the subject until after the Second World War. Dr Watanabe [7], again in Japan, continued the technological development of the arthroscope, with publication of his water colour atlas of arthroscopy (1957) enhanced in 1969 with photographic material.

The first concrete report of arthroscopic surgery of the knee was the excision of posterior flap of the medial meniscus by Dr. Watanabe in 1962. However, it has been the enthusiastic work and teaching of Dr. R. Jackson on his return from Dr. Watanabe's unit, which led to the great interest and subsequent rapid development of arthroscopic surgery. In 1972 Jackson and Abe [8] reported 200 arthroscopic examinations of knee joints. It seems surprising that it was not until 1978 that the first clinical results of arthroscopic surgery were formally reported by Dandy [9]. By 1981 Johnson [10] was introducing the use of power instrumentation in the knee to trim menisci, excise synovium, shave articular cartilage and abrade articular surfaces.

Work is now being undertaken to investigate and develop the use of lasers in arthroscopic surgery. However, this remains largely restricted to specialist centres and the advantages of these techniques remain undefined.

Advantages and complications of arthroscopic surgery

Advantages

It is now universally agreed that arthroscopic surgery offers many major advantages, particularly when compared to similar procedures undertaken by open arthrotomy.

Diagnostic accuracy

Arthroscopy is reported to have a diagnostic accuracy of 97% in experienced hands [11]. It will often define multiple abnormalities where clinically only one pathology is evident. The findings may differ markedly from the clinical diagnosis, where accuracy ranges only from 60 to 75% [12]. Johnson [10] found that in 229 patients with a clinical diagnosis of a torn medial meniscus, only 21% had this isolated injury. Twenty-three percent had additional pathology and in 56% the diagnosis was completely different.

Access to all compartments and multiple pathologies

Arthroscopic surgery offers the facility to undertake multiple procedures, e.g. partial meni-

scectomy of torn medial and lateral menisci. It allows trimming of the torn posterior quadrant of the meniscus which is inaccessible through an arthrotomy. Drilling of osteochondral lesions can be undertaken with minimal postoperative morbidity. Debridement of joints with early degenerative disease, where more than one compartment may be affected, can produce excellent symptomatic improvement which would be impossible without multiple arthrotomy incisions.

Cost effectiveness

Patients undergoing arthroscopic surgery may be treated as day cases and the older population may require one overnight stay when the procedure is undertaken under general anaesthesia. By contrast after arthrotomy most patients require a minimum of 3–5 days as an inpatient.

Earlier mobilization and rehabilitation

Patients can readily mobilize with crutches or a walking stick and attain independent gait within a few days. Return to work of a sedentary nature is possible soon after, and to more strenuous activities, including driving, in one to two weeks. This contrasts with 10–14 days immobilization to allow sound healing of an arthrotomy incision and the invariable need for physiotherapy to regain full knee mobility over the subsequent 6–8 weeks. However, recent work suggests that incomplete motor control may persist for up to 8 weeks after arthroscopic meniscal surgery [13].

Cosmetic

Scars are minimum, often becoming virtually invisible over a few months. An arthrotomy scar can be unsightly and is not infrequently associated with an area of numbness or reduced sensation adjacent to the incision.

Low morbidity

Postoperative pain is minimal unless the procedure is complicated by a major haemarthrosis. The incidence of complications following arthroscopic procedures remains remarkably low. This allows for second procedures to be undertaken where necessary with little anticipated morbidity.

Complications

The complications of arthroscopic surgery are few and most are regarded as minor. A large study which scrutinized every single problem in a series of 2640 patients reported an overall complication rate of 8.2% [14]. The major complications amounted to 4.8% when cardiovascular episodes, paraesthesias, haemarthroses and effusions were excluded. Some surgeons would regard some of these minor and transient postoperative effusions and haemarthroses as almost inevitable in some procedures. The complication rate following open arthrotomy for meniscal procedures has been reported as 14.6% [15]. The major reduction has been in serious complications such as infection, neurological injury and venous thrombosis and embolism.

a) Any intra-articular structure can be damaged, but usually the anterior horn of the meniscus, the fat pad and the articular cartilage can be lacerated in making the portal incisions. The anterior cruciate ligament is most susceptible to injury during meniscal surgery in the intercondylar notch and during the use of motorized cutters.

b) Haemarthrosis, residual effusions, and fluid leakage from the posterior aspect of the knee represent some of the commoner complications.

c) Excessive or injudicious force in the use of the fine arthroscopic instruments in tight compartments can result in breakage within the knee joint; this is most often encountered in the course of lateral meniscectomies.

d) More serious complications include damage to the popliteal vessels from insertion of instruments via the posteromedial or posterolateral portals, or deep penetration of instruments through the intercondylar notch. The use of power instrumentation has also been associated with damage to the popliteal vessels. The blind passage of the meniscal suture needles has resulted in lacerations of these vessels and the peroneal nerves.

e) In general neurological complications are few. Delee's [16] review of 118 000 procedures revealed 65 neurological injuries, involving peroneal, saphenous, femoral, tibial and sciatic nerves. However, in a prospective study of 8791 procedures undertaken by experienced arthroscopists there was only one neurological complication–damage to the saphenous nerve during a medial meniscal suture. Tourniquet paresis seems uncommon, usually mild and undergoes early resolution [17].

f) The incidence of infection remains very low in all reported series, ranging from 0.04 to 0.08%:

> Johnson *et al.* [10]: 5 cases in 12 500 arthroscopies;
> Mullhollan [18]: 7 cases in 9000 arthroscopies;
> Delee [16]: 95 cases in 118 590 arthroscopies.

The possibility that intra-articular steroid injection following arthroscopy may increase the risk of infection has been raised by Montgomery and Campbell [19] following three cases of septic arthritis in their series of 15 500 patients, most of whom had such steroid injections.

g) As with all procedures involving general anaesthesia and tourniquet, there is a small incidence of deep vein thrombosis ranging from 0.1 to 3.2% [20].

Arthroscopic techniques

The low morbidity of arthroscopic examination has made the procedure justifiable as an adjunct to diagnosis, prognosis and treatment. However, these advantages must not allow arthroscopy to become a simple replacement for the clinical skills of a careful history and examination which so often provide an accurate diagnosis and assessment of the need for surgical intervention.

Anaesthesia

Arthroscopy can be undertaken under local, regional or general anaesthesia. The choice of anaesthesia is influenced by many factors including patient co-operation, the surgeon's expertise and the complexity of any surgical procedure.

Local anaesthesia

The use of local anaesthetic within the knee appears safe since blood levels have been shown to remain low during arthroscopic procedures [21]. Although local anaesthesia can be employed for routine diagnostic examination of the knee, the experience of the surgeon, the patient's tolerance and co-operation are of paramount importance. Furthermore, if a treatable lesion is encountered, it may not be possible to proceed, and a second operative procedure under general anaesthesia required at a second admission. In experienced hands, however, straightforward arthroscopic procedures can be undertaken safely and proficiently. It should be stressed that surgery under local anaesthesia requires well drilled, experienced nursing and theatre assistant staff and may nevertheless take longer than the same procedure undertaken under a general anaesthetic. A dose of 20–30 ml of 0.25% or 0.5% bupivacaine with 1:200 000 adrenaline can be used to infiltrate the skin, subcutaneous and capsular tissues and for anaesthetizing the joint [22]. The use of a tourniquet is optional but most patients find it too uncomfortable, and in its absence, intra-articular bleeding can make accurate visualization troublesome. Access for operative procedures can also prove difficult because of the lack of muscle relaxation. Local anaesthetic techniques tend to be time consuming and somewhat variable but eliminate the problems of general anaesthesia, including cardiopulmonary and thrombotic complications.

Regional anaesthesia

Spinal or regional anaesthesia with femoral nerve block [23] can be employed in patients where there are specific contraindications to general anaesthesia. However, this is rarely used as patients frequently complain of discomfort from the tourniquet despite adequate lower extremity anaesthesia. Femoral blocks fail to anaesthetize the posterior part of the knee and any manipulative procedures in this area can prove very painful. Quadriceps paralysis for 6–8 hours may delay patient discharge or require the use of rather cumbersome splints.

General anaesthesia

With these qualifications and the anticipation of an intra-articular surgical procedure, general anaesthesia is generally more widely employed. Overall, general anaesthesia appears to have a higher patient acceptance and is also more acceptable to the surgeon and the theatre staff as it seems much more efficient [21,23]. It has the further advantage that should the arthroscopic procedure fail, open arthrotomy can be promptly undertaken without the need for the patient to be readmitted for a second procedure.

Surgical techniques

The expertise, instrumentation and techniques necessary for arthroscopic diagnosis and surgery are now familiar and thoroughly covered in an extensive literature and in excellent hands-on courses. In this chapter these are not detailed and only specific points of interest are considered.

Tourniquet

A tourniquet is normally applied to the thigh but need not be inflated if only a diagnostic examination is undertaken. Tourniquet inflation tends to blanch the synovium and may impair the assessment of synovial disorders. If an intra-articular procedure is anticipated, then the use of a tourniquet following exsanguination of the limb is advantageous. In the presence of specific contraindications such as a history of thromboembolic disease it is preferable to proceed without inflating the tourniquet if possible. Impaired visualization due to bleeding can often be overcome by the assistance of low pressure suction through an outlet portal.

Patient position and leg holders

With the patient lying supine, one of three main techniques are employed for examination:

a) Using a leg holder: the patient lies with the legs hanging over the end of the operating table and the leg to be examined firmly held in a special leg holder. This allows the application of stress primarily to open the posteromedial compartment. However, leg holders restrict the range of positions the knee can be manoeuvred into and tend to disadvantage access to the patellofemoral and lateral compartments and interfere with instrumentation through superior portals. These supports incur further expenditure and are not without the potential hazard of damaging ligaments and even fracture to the femur in overforceful manoeuvres to open a tight joint.

b) Lateral post: other surgeons prefer to use a lateral post attached to the operating table, against which the femur can be levered to access the postero medial compartment. The post still allows the knee to be placed in almost any position, including the figure of four configuration to examine the lateral compartment.

c) Surgical assistant: some surgeons prefer to have the patient with the leg hanging over the side of the operating table and the foot supported and controlled on their lap. A varus or valgus stress, when necessary, can be applied by a surgical assistant. The technique tends to suffer from the inconsistent force applied to the knee as fatigue affects the assistant.

All these techniques have their strong proponents and essentially it is a question of trying out each technique before establishing a personal preference which the operator finds comfortable and efficient.

Arthroscopic equipment

Visualization of the intra-articular structures and operative field is now routinely undertaken via a television screen. This requires adequate illumination, with the use of a high intensity or xenon light source. Repeated direct viewing through the arthroscope with a xenon light source has been reputed to result in retinal burns. Video accessories allow the imaging of operations for record and teaching purposes. Efficient routine arthroscopic work requires a considerable financial outlay in specialized equipment, including a light source, camera unit and television monitor, a power unit to drive the motorized instruments and video recorder.

Arthroscopic instruments

The spectrum of manual instruments for intra-articular surgery is now extensive and very reliable. The advent of motorized power driven instruments has extended the arthroscopists'

armamentarium, not only facilitating existing techniques but improving and allowing the development of new procedures. These include, among others, meniscectomy, synovectomy, chondroplasty and abrader blades. It must be emphasized that these instruments are extremely powerful and although excellent in experienced hands they are capable of considerable damage not only to the intra-articular structures, particularly the anterior cruciate ligament, but also to the popliteal vessels, as reported in some studies. It is important to note that the negative pressure from the suction system used with these powered instruments can be sufficient to draw contaminated fluid back into the knee from a bucket at ground level collecting fluid from an accessory drainage tube in the knee.

Disposable cannula systems have also been developed to allow the repeated insertion of instruments through the same portal without repeatedly traumatizing the portal of entry.

Conventional entry portals

The success, safety and efficiency of arthroscopic surgery is highly dependent on the precise placement of the entry portals for adequate visualization and instrument access.

a) The anterolateral portal gives the most comprehensive view of all the compartments.

b) The anteromedial portal allows visualization of the lateral compartment.

c) The central transpatellar tendon portal: the entry point is approximately 1 cm distal to the inferior pole of the patella with the knee at 90° of flexion. The arthroscope is then introduced toward the superomedial quadrant with the knee in 90° of flexion to ensure the arthroscope passes above the fat pad. This central position can free the anteromedial and anterolateral portals for bimanual instrument manipulation. Proponents of this approach argue a better access to the posterior structures through the intercondylar notch, but usually only to best advantage if the 70° arthroscope is used. However, if the fat pad becomes swollen with irrigation fluid, visibility can become rapidly impaired.

d) The superolateral portal: this is the most valuable portal for assessing the patello-femoral articulation. This can also be used to visualize the anterior aspects of the medial compartment and conversely a superomedial portal used to view the anterior aspects of the lateral compartment.

e) The posteromedial portal can be safely accessed if the bony landmarks of the postero-medial edge of the femoral condyle and postero-medial border of the tibia are marked prior to distension, the joint is fully distended and the knee flexed to 90°. This portal allows visualization of the posterior horn of the medial meniscus and the posterior cruciate ligament.

f) The posterolateral portal: this lies approximately 2 cm above the posterolateral joint line at the posterior edge of the iliotibial band and the anterior margin of the biceps tendon. Entrance is along the posterior edge of the femoral condyle with the trocar directed slightly inferiorly.

Insertion of the arthroscope

Distension of the knee joint with normal saline is undertaken prior to insertion of the sharp trocar which is directed medially and superiorly through the skin towards the intercondylar notch with the knee in 30° of flexion. As soon as the synovium is penetrated, the sharp trocar is replaced with the blunt trocar. The knee is allowed to come slowly into full extension and the trocar, with a brisk push through the synovium, is negotiated under the patella towards the suprapatellar pouch. Distension of the knee joint can be adequately maintained using a 3 litre normal saline bag suspended about 2 metres above floor level. Whether delivered via the arthroscope or through the superolateral portal is a matter of the surgeon's preference.

Postoperative care

Portals may be closed with steristrip or nylon sutures removed 10–14 days after surgery. Except following specific procedures, most patients can fully weight bear immediately after surgery and most are walking freely by 48 hours. However, it is advisable to afford the patient the use of a walking stick or crutches for 1 or 2 days until they have regained their confidence following the general anaesthetic and their initial discomfort has settled.

Diversity of arthroscopic surgery

As expertise and confidence grew in the use of arthroscopy as a diagnostic tool, direct surgical intervention through arthroscopic visualization developed rapidly. This impetus was further promoted by the development of instruments and technology particularly adapted to arthroscopic surgery. The result has been an enormous expansion in the variety and complexity of surgical procedures which can now be safely undertaken arthroscopically, extending from relatively simple resection of synovial plicae, through resection and suturing of meniscal tears, to arthroscopically assisted anterior cruciate ligament reconstructions. The spectrum of arthroscopic operations is considered in further detail in the following sections.

Arthroscopy in the diagnosis of the acute haemarthrosis

It has become fashionable to arthroscope the knee presenting with an acute haemarthrosis [24–26].

Noyes *et al.* [21] found some damage to the anterior cruciate ligament in 72% of knees. Similarly Jones and Allum [27] found that 54% of their unselected group of patients had acute ACL tears. The incidence of meniscal tears was 22% compared to 62% by Noyes *et al.* [24] and 66% by Dehaven *et al.* [26], possibly reflecting the fact that these latter were studies exclusively on sports injured patients. Only 30% required definitive treatment at arthroscopy and no patient over 35 years required an operative procedure.

There are strong proponents of early arthroscopy since the diagnosis of an acute meniscal tear followed by immediate suture may increase the chances of successful healing. In athletes, early reconstruction of a torn anterior cruciate may be appropriate in order to return the patient to sporting activities with the minimum delay. It would seem preferable to be able to provide a definitive diagnosis and plan for rehabilitation based on arthroscopic examination. However, if primary reconstruction is not entertained at this point there is little to be lost by delay, since there may be resolution in 70% of patients without the necessity of an invasive surgical procedure and general anaesthetic.

Kannus and Jarvinen [28] have reported the outcome of 84 patients with an acute haemarthrosis after injury without instability as defined by clinical examination without anaesthesia. This group, which represented 25% of all knees attending with an acute haemarthrosis, underwent intensive rehabilitation. After an average 8-year follow-up, 86% were asymptomatic, suggesting that the stable knee with a haemarthrosis could sometimes be treated expectantly and was not always associated with an unstable prognosis.

Given the demands on the acute services, and the likelihood of resolution in 70% cases, it would seem appropriate to consider early arthroscopy largely in those patients in whom diagnosis of a major correctable injury would be followed by a definitive procedure at the same operation. It is important to emphasize that arthroscopy of the acutely injured knee is a difficult procedure.

If elective arthroscopy is difficult for the beginner, accurate identification of the sustained damage in the presence of continuous bleeding or when the synovium of the intercondylar notch is grossly swollen and haemorrhagic can present major difficulties of visualization. This type of surgery should only be undertaken by someone experienced in arthroscopic work. This is particularly so if identification of the damage then requires surgical intervention in the acute situation, where visualization can be so much more difficult than in the elective case. When persistent fresh bleeding is a problem, gentle continuous suction through a superolateral portal can clear the field of vision effectively to allow surgical procedures to be undertaken if a good flow of fluid can be achieved to maintain distension of the joint and flush the blood out the joint.

Meniscal surgery

It was as recent as the early 1980s that reports of large series of arthroscopic meniscectomies began to appear in the literature and hence establish the technique as a valuable tool in the orthopaedic armamentarium [29]. The very evident advantages of arthroscopic partial meniscectomy over open arthrotomy established the value of this type of surgery: in particular, the ability for surgery to be undertaken as a day case, the minimal requirement for postoperative analgesia,

and the early return to work and sports [30]. In a large series of 230 patients Simpson *et al.* [31] found that only 25% of patients following open meniscectomy had returned to sports by the 6th postoperative week compared with 86% of the patients who had undergone a similar procedure arthroscopically.

Though the basic techniques of partial meniscectomy will not be considered in this text it is essential to emphasize that accurate definition of the anatomy of the tear is crucial to an understanding and planning of successful arthroscopic meniscal surgery. O'Connor's classification [32] would appear to be eminently simple and valuable in this respect: a) longitudinal tears; b) horizontal tears; c) oblique tears; d) radial tears; e) variations or complex tears; e) degenerative tears. The use of a probe is therefore crucial to define the extent, type and configuration of the tear in the meniscal substance. A more detailed analysis has been presented by Dandy [33] in a report of 1000 symptomatic meniscal lesions. Eighty-one percent of the patients were male. The medial meniscus was involved in 70.5% and the lateral in 29.5%. Of the medial meniscal lesions 75% were vertical, 23% horizontal, the former occurring most frequently in the fourth and the latter in the fifth decade of life. Of the tears in the lateral meniscus, 54% were vertical, 15% oblique, 15% myxoid, 4% inverted and 5% discoid, the most common lesion being a vertical tear involving half the length and half the width of the meniscus. Each different morphological type of tear requires a particular technique to achieve the general objective of removing the unstable fragments whilst being as conservative as possible in retaining a stable rim.

The work of Cargill and Jackson [34], showing that patients with open partial meniscectomy for bucket handle tears did better than those who underwent open total meniscectomy, initiated a trend towards more conservative resection of only the damaged part of the meniscus. This was confirmed by McGinty *et al.* [15] in a study amply demonstrating that after 6 years the partial meniscectomy patients exhibited better functional results and 50% fewer radiological degenerative changes.

Arthroscopy has allowed clarification of the pathology of meniscal tears and has proved to be the ideal technique for further implementing the concept of a more conservative approach to meniscal surgery, allowing removal of only the damaged area of the meniscus. The objective is to remove the torn, mobile fragments and contour the peripheral edge, leaving a residual stable meniscal rim. The rim left after removal of a bucket handle can transmit up to 35% of the load across the joint [35]. Partial meniscectomy may not always be possible if the tear extends to the periphery and a subtotal excision would seem preferable to a total meniscectomy.

Developments in meniscal surgery are now being extended to the use of laser technology. The most commonly used are the Nd-Yag, CO_2 and argon lasers. All have limitations, but the development of a contact probe using a sapphire crystal for the Nd-Yag laser may have considerably advanced the application of the technique. O'Brien and Miller [36] have reported work on canine and rabbit samples which appears to indicate that the laser cuts meniscus tissue more effectively than articular cartilage. In their series of 15 patients there were no complications other than breakage of one contact tip which required retrieval from the joint. The advantages appeared to be mainly in the access to difficult areas of the joint. The system as a whole remains limited largely to research groups and the costs are not inconsiderable.

Meniscal suture

The important role which the meniscus plays in the function of the knee has become increasingly apparent over the last 10 years. It provides stability, transfers loads, lubricates and allows the nutrition of the articular cartilage. Biomechanical studies have demonstrated that in extension 50% of the compressive load of the knee joint is transmitted through the meniscus. In 90° of flexion this increases to approximately 85% of the load [37]. Complete meniscectomy reduces the contact area by 50% significantly increasing the load per unit area. The result is a marked incidence of early degenerative osteoarthritis in the subsequent 15–20 years [38,39]. There has therefore been great interest in the possibility of meniscal salvage by suture to encourage healing. The outer 10–20% of the meniscus is known to have reasonable blood supply provided by the perimeniscal capillary plexus [40].

Open meniscal suture was reported to be associated with a high incidence of healing in chronic peripheral tears and higher rates for acute tears [41]. The development of arthroscopic suture techniques has resulted in renewed interest and enthusiasm for the repair of the torn meniscus.

Reported results are impressive with healing rates of 78–100%. However, these results are not entirely based on second look arthroscopy but include arthrography and the absence of clinical symptoms. Keene and Paterson [42] reported healing in 10 of 11 re-arthroscoped knees out of a cohort of 20 patients with medial meniscal repairs. The most important factors contributing to successful resuture are a) acute tears, b) within 5 mm of the periphery of the meniscus (in the red-red or red-white area) c) in knees which do exhibit instability.

Two suture methods are generally in use: the inside-out technique uses long flexible needles passed into the knee through a curved cannula under arthroscopic vision and across the meniscal tear to emerge through the capsule. In the outside-in technique a needle is placed across the tear from the outside in. A suture is threaded through the needle, picked up in the joint and brought out of an anterior portal. A large knot is made in the end of the suture, which is then drawn back into the joint and against the meniscal surface. This is repeated and the free ends of the sutures tied on the capsular surface.

The potential for serious complications in terms of damage to the peroneal nerve and popliteal artery is considerable. The importance of ensuring that the needles emerge anterior to the semitendinosus tendon for medial repairs and anterior to the biceps tendon for lateral repairs cannot be sufficiently stressed. To ensure these problems are avoided a small incision down to the capsule allows retraction under direct vision of the structures at risk and permits access to emerging needles and suture ligation over the capsular tissues: so-called arthroscopically assisted meniscal repair.

Role of arthroscopy in the treatment of osteoarthritis

Debridement of osteoarthritic knees long precedes the development of arthroscopy. Magnuson [43] reported complete recovery of symptoms in a large number of knee joints following open debridement. Open removal of osteophytes and drilling of exposed subchondral bone became popular as the 'Pridie Procedure' following his reports of good results in 65% of his patients.

However, as far back as 1934, Burman *et al.* [6] noted a marked symptomatic improvement in two patients following diagnostic arthroscopy of their arthritic knees. Jackson and Rouse in 1982 reaffirmed this simple observation that lavage of the joint without any operative procedure resulted in persisting symptomatic benefit. This has now been confirmed by other workers. Attempts to further improve the outcome of simple arthroscopic lavage have led to the inclusion of added procedures to 'tidy up' the knee joint. These have included drilling of exposed bone areas, resection of unstable meniscal segments [44], removal of unstable chondral flaps, debridement of osteophytes and loose fragments of articular cartilage [45] and abrasion arthroplasty to permit capillary bleeding through to the joint surface.

Which of these procedures, or if all, contribute to symptomatic improvement remains largely unknown. However, some pointers are beginning to emerge. Jackson and Rouse [44] reported that excision of unstable, torn meniscal fragments proved beneficial. However, extensive partial meniscectomy of stable fragments appeared to be detrimental [45]. Salisbury *et al.* [46] report that normally aligned knees appear to do better than those with either varus or valgus deformities. Younger patients tended to do better than older patients and those with early degenerative disease again achieved more improvement than those with advanced changes [47]. Bird and Ring [48] confirmed these findings but felt that the procedure was of much less value in rheumatoid and seronegative knees.

In a prospective study of 276 knees with osteoarthritis followed for a mean of 44 months, Patel *et al.* [49] reported good beneficial results in 75% patients. Knees requiring meniscal debridement alone did better than those needing both meniscal and surface debridement and patients under the age of 60 years did better. Bert and Maschka [47] have found that abrasion arthroplasty offers no advantage over other procedures. In their series good results were maintained in 66% of their patients five years after arthroscopic debridement.

The indications for this type of surgery again require clearer definition. However, in certain groups the benefits appear to have been substantial. There seems to be an increasing impression that the older athlete with early degenerative changes can often benefit sufficiently to allow a return to some sporting activities. In some elderly patients conservative methods may fail, but their symptoms are not severe enough to warrant prosthetic replacement. This group may derive major symptomatic benefit from arthroscopic debridement and allow a considerable delay in major surgery.

The mechanism whereby significant symptomatic relief is achieved remains unknown. Whether it is the debridement or the simple act of distension followed by the washing out of debris that is responsible for the observed benefit is difficult to ascertain. However, it seems likely that removal of cartilage debris, crystals and inflammatory factors probably all play a contributary role. Similarly, the likely duration of the symptomatic improvement remains uncertain. Further detailed analyses are necessary before these answers emerge and more accurate indications for this type of treatment can be defined.

Arthroscopic synovectomy

Open synovectomy of the knee in rheumatoid arthritis is known to achieve a reduction in pain and severity of effusions, but only for a period of time due to recurrence of the synovitis [50]. Enthusiasm for this procedure waned because of the prolonged hospitalisation necessary to execute the painful rehabilitation required to regain the range of movement. Sometimes manipulation under anaesthesia became necessary and loss of the range of excursion was well documented [51].

The advent of arthroscopy and the introduction of motorized synovial resectors has led to renewed interest in the procedure particularly in the hope that some lasting benefits could be achieved without the marked drawbacks of open synovectomy.

Early studies were reported by Matsui *et al.* in 1989 [52] where they compared the long term results of arthroscopic (41 knees) versus open (26 knees) synovectomies using large punches. The outcome over ten years was similar in both groups, with 80% of the knees being rated as good at 3 years but deteriorating to 57% good at 8 years. However, the authors found that the radiological changes of deterioration were less marked after arthroscopic synovectomy. Their findings at 2–3 years have been confirmed by Klein and Jensen [53] in a series of 45 patients using a powered synovectomy system. All the patients showed a reduction in pain and swelling and an improvement in the activities of daily living. The majority maintained an increase in the range of movement achieved postoperatively. Where articular damage was established the benefits were less substantial.

Although there are few large studies, and in some series, patients with different inflammatory conditions were included, the general impression appears to be that arthroscopic synovectomy offers many major early advantages.

There was little postoperative pain and both knees could be operated at the same admission. Hospitalization was only over a few days and return to work was rapid. One major advantage was that the majority of patients gained and maintained an improved range of movement. Because of the low morbidity repeat operations were felt to be acceptable in the longer term management. In patients with marked disease and grade IV articular damage, total knee replacement was postponed by more than 2 years.

It must be emphasized that arthroscopic synovectomy is an incomplete synovectomy. It may retard synovial growth. Regrowth is inevitable but then rheumatoid synovium recurs even in complete synovectomy performed by open arthrotomy [54].

Further large detailed studies are necessary in this field before an accurate assessment of the value of this procedure, not only in rheumatoid arthritis but also in other synovial proliferative diseases, can be ascertained.

Synovial plicae

Synovial plicae represent unresolved partition remnants of the three synovial compartments which fuse to form the single knee cavity during embryological development:

a) The infrapatellar plica or ligamentum mucosum is usually a thin band of synovium running from the fat pad to the superior aspect of the intercondylar notch. It can sometimes interfere with the passage of the arthroscope to other compartments. It should not be mistaken for the anterior cruciate ligament, in front of which it lies, initially obscuring the ligament.

b) The suprapatellar plica can divide the suprapatellar pouch into two separate compartments. As with the ligamentum mucosum, it is not thought to be responsible for any symptomatic complaints.

c) The lateral patellar plica is very rare, though described.

d) The medial patellar plica arises superior to the patella and runs down the medial side of the joint over the medial femoral condyle to insert into the fat pad. It is thought that trauma, usually a direct blow, to the overlying part of the knee can result in chronic inflammation and thickening of the plica which can then become symptomatic. The patient complains of pain in the anteromedial aspect of the knee, worse on activity, and sometimes of a clicking sensation and pain on flexion of the knee, often in the arc of 45–60° of the range. This represents the thickened plica flicking across the medial femoral condyle on flexion. Tenderness can be elicited about 1 cm above the medial condyle and the plica can sometimes be palpated or rolled under the finger.

In the absence of other pathology which might account for symptoms in this part of the knee, the presence of a thickened inelastic tough plica on arthroscopic examination, may account for the patient's symptoms.

Initially simple division of the plica was thought to be sufficient treatment. However, in view of the recurrence of symptoms in some patients, probably due to the development of dense fibrous tissue at the site of the previous incision, resection or saucerization of the plica down to the side wall is preferable. This can usually be undertaken with relative ease by introducing the cutting instruments or a powered synovial resector through the superomedial portal or superolateral portal. The patients often report an immediate improvement or resolution of their symptoms.

Loose bodies

The majority of loose bodies are either a) cartilagenous or b) osteochondral in nature. The former usually arise as the result of trauma to the hyaline cartilage of the articular surfaces. The radio-opaque osteochondral loose bodies usually arise from osteochondritis dissecans, osteochondral fractures, osteophytic processes, or synovial chondromatosis. 'Rice bodies' represent multiple fibrinous lesions secondary to chronic inflammatory conditions, such as rheumatoid arthritis and sometimes tuberculosis.

The removal of the loose bodies must be allied to identification and treatment of the underlying pathology causing the formation of these fragments. A recent radiograph prior to surgery may be of considerable value in identifying the location and number of radio-opaque loose bodies. A thorough systematic examination of the knee is essential to locate all the fragments. Sometimes difficulty may be encountered when a loose body is obscured behind a large plica or small fragments may come to lie under the meniscus. Once located, the fragment can be pierced with a needle or 'incarcerated' between two needles if it cannot be effectively pierced. A strong grasper is essential to secure a hold on larger loose bodies. On removal, it is best to ensure an adequately sized exit portal than to risk losing the fragment back into the joint.

Small loose bodies in the posterior compartment of the knee may be completely asymptomatic and do not always require removal. Where appropriate, visualization can be undertaken through posteromedial or posterolateral portals. Visualization through the intercondylar notch may then allow instrument access via posteromedial or posterolateral portals. These techniques can however present considerable difficulties.

Multiple loose bodies can be removed without difficulty by repeated washouts and suction of the joint cavity. The removal of small foreign bodies follows the same basic principles. However, when instrument breakage occurs, it is essential to keep the piece on vision until it can be grasped and removed. Small fragments can be held at the tip of a small bore sucker until they can be grasped with an appropriate instrument. Magnetic instruments are now available to immobilize metal foreign bodies until they can be secured and removed.

Lateral release of the patella

Arthroscopic lateral release or perhaps percutaneous arthroscopically assisted lateral release of the patella offers more rapid recovery, less pain, and easier rehabilitation than the equivalent open procedure. The knee is always fully examined before the release is undertaken in order to identify any coincidental pathology, and to assess the congruency of the patello-femoral articulation and the condition of the articular cartilage. The lateral portal can be slightly enlarged and the skin undermined from the margin of the lateral tibial plateau, along the lateral border of the patella tendon and patella to beyond the superior pole border of the patella into the fibres of vastus lateralis, 4 cm above the patella being recommended by Dandy and Griffiths [55]. An incision is made through the capsular retinaculum and into the joint, although some surgeons prefer to maintain the integrity of the synovium. Either using scissors or a special lateral release knife the structures are then split longitudinally from tibial margin to vastus lateralis. It is suggested that unless the patella can be tilted through 90° from the femoral articulation the release is incomplete and further dissection is necessary to ensure the likelihood of an effective procedure. A drain may be left in the line of the release. A compression pad is applied to contain the haemarthrosis when the tourniquet is released. After 48 hours knee flexion and static quadriceps exercises are initiated.

The main difficulties however, have been not so much with the technique of the procedure as to the selection of appropriate cases for this operation. Dandy and Griffiths [55] reporting on their series of 41 knees recommended the procedure as highly successful in patients with recurrent dislocation of the patella in flexion but not for those with subluxation in extension. The procedure again seemed less satisfactory in patients with ligamentous laxity. Although many studies have been reported, difficulties of interpretation arise because few define the type of patellar instability being addressed, and a miscellaneous group of patella subluxation and dislocation often forms the basis of such studies [56]. The problem is further compounded by the fact that the lateral release may have been undertaken specifically for pain in association with instability. Reported success rates vary widely from 44% [57] to 75% [58].

In cases where there is a tight lateral retinaculum with patella tilting or in the lateral facet compression syndrome an isolated lateral release can be considered justifiable when properly supervised conservative treatment has failed to improve symptoms over three to six months.

Arthroscopy in children

The accurate diagnosis of knee problems, particularly acute presentations, in children can be extremely difficult. Arthroscopy provides a minimally invasive technique to reach a diagnosis and afford definitive treatment where appropriate. A clinical diagnostic accuracy ranging from 42% [59] to 55% [60, 61] in the under 13 years-old age-group appears consistent in the literature.

a) Acute injuries: The presentation of a significant haemarthrosis and a very painful knee invariably requires arthroscopic examination. The importance and prevalence of injuries to the anterior cruciate ligament in children is becoming increasingly appreciated. Bergstrom [62] reported damage to the ACL in 43% and Eiskjaer and Larsen [63] in 45% of older children arthroscoped because of an acute haemarthrosis. The injury may be partial or full mid-substance tear and overall represents the single most common diagnosis in these patients with a haemarthrosis. When there is avulsion of the tibial insertion of the ACL with a bone attachment, it may be possible to relocate the fragment accurately either arthroscopically or by open arthrotomy. Tears of the meniscus can be particularly difficult to diagnose. Meniscal injuries, including medial bucket handle tears, occur more frequently than originally expected and are commoner than injuries to the lateral meniscus [60, 63]. Early diagnosis of an osteochondral fracture, usually of the femoral condyle, will allow easier relocation of the fragment for pinning or Herbert screw fixation depending on the size of the lesion.

b) Discoid lateral meniscus: Although initially thought to represent an arrested stage of development of the lateral meniscus, Kaplan [64] did not find any stage at which the meniscus had the discoid configuration. It is rather postulated that as the result of the abnormal posterior ligamentous attachments, the meniscus cannot move back with the femur and with time is pushed into the joint, so that the central concavity becomes obliterated and a discoid shape develops. In the past, the symptomatic discoid meniscus was

treated by open resection of the whole meniscus. The advent of arthroscopy has allowed a more accurate diagnosis and a more conservative partial meniscectomy leaving a residual rim in cases of midsubstance tears. Watanabe *et al.* [65] have classified the discoid meniscus as i) complete, ii) incomplete and iii) Wrisberg ligament type. The discoid meniscus, because of its relative immobility, poor vascularization and posterior attachment, is more susceptible to injury. The majority of patients are aged 10–15 years on presentation and complain of pain clicking, snapping, locking and giving way. Lack of extension and a positive McMurray's test may be found in a proportion of these patients. The decision to operate on a suspected discoid meniscus can be difficult, particularly when the history is only of clicking and there is little pain or giving way and with few objective signs. However, Hayashi *et al.* [66] propose that the symptomatic discoid lateral meniscus indicates a tear in the substance of the meniscus or a peripheral detachment. Identification of tears in the midsubstance may be difficult even at arthroscopy. Excision of the meniscus in one piece is the only way to confirm a tear postoperatively. Hayashi *et al.* [66] argue that all discoid menisci have a posterior attachment which then ruptures as part of the mechanism of the posterior tear or peripheral detachment and indicate that in their series of 46 children they did not identify any Wrisberg ligament type of lesions. They recommend complete excision of the meniscus if the lesion is near the periphery, or if the fascicle in the popliteal area is torn, i.e. the Wrisberg ligament type. For a midsubstance tear, about 4 mm–6 mm rim can be left in situ. Surgery can be technically difficult and sometimes a combination of arthroscopic and open techniques becomes necessary to remove the discoid fragment effectively. Long-term data is lacking on whether meniscectomy, partial or total, in these children results in early osteoarthritis of the lateral compartment.

c) Chondromalacia patella: The diagnosis of chondromalacia patella is based on clinical examination and findings, and the absence of any radiological abnormalities. The role and value of arthroscopy in the management of adolescent knee pain remains a matter of vigorous contention. However, there seems to be little to be gained by submitting patients, particularly those with a classical history, clinical findings, the absence of an effusion and normal radiograph, to an intrusive and invasive procedure when the chance of discovering any abnormal findings remains small, the significance of these uncertain and the likelihood of symptomatic improvement little if any. Furthermore the natural history of the condition suggests that spontaneous improvement would occur without surgical interference in at least 50% of the cases and there is no evidence that arthroscopy has improved on this natural outcome [68].

d) Osteochondritis dissecans: The diagnosis of osteochondritis dissecans is generally straightforward and based on radiological examination. Its management is considered in a separate section.

e) Septic arthritis: Arthroscopic techniques of drainage and lavage have been found to be very successful in the treatment of septic arthritis of the knee in children [60, 68, 69]. It allows for thorough débridement and lavage, and may be repeated if necessary. Treatment must include the appropriate antibiotics in adequate doses. The use of passive continuous motion techniques may be used as an adjunct to help maintain the range of movement during the recovery phase of treatment.

Osteochondritis dissecans

The exact aetiology of osteochondritis dissecans remains unknown. The generally accepted view is that a localized area of subchondral bone undergoes infarction, probably against a background of a traumatic event, allowing separation of the overlying articular cartilage.

Arthroscopy has allowed ready access and visualization of the osteochondritis dissecans fragment and an understanding of the natural history of the disease. The locations of the lesions are described as classical (69%), extended classical (6%) and inferocentral (10%) on the medial condyle and inferocentral (13%) and anterior (2%) the lateral condyle [70].

Undisplaced lesions in young children may heal if further trauma is avoided particularly if located in the non-weightbearing area. No treatment is usually necessary other than careful follow-up until the lesion is noted to be incorporated radiologically. In the older age groups, where surgical treatment is indicated, arthro-

scopy is becoming the commonest approach to surgical intervention.

Guhl [71] recommends arthroscopic examination and treatment of children over the age of 12 with lesions larger than 1 cm in diameter.

a) In patients with no overt loosening of the fragment, careful probing is necessary to define its location as there is often no obvious break in the continuity of the articular surface. The preferred treatment is multiple drilling with a small diameter K wire through the fragment into the underlying subchondral bone to stimulate vascularity and healing [72].

b) If the fragment is not completely loose but still attached by a tissue hinge, it can be turned back to expose the base which is then curetted. The fragment is secured with two slightly divergent K wires which are drilled through the fragment and condyle to emerge through the condyle in the area of the femoral epicondyle. Once the wires appear under the skin they can be withdrawn retrogradely whilst the intra-articular end is viewed directly via the arthroscope until it is just below the articular surface. The K wires are cut off under the skin to allow for easy removal 6–8 weeks later. The patient can be maintained in a partial or non-weightbearing status for 6–8 weeks.

Care should be taken not to damage the epiphysis by drilling the K wire through epiphyseal plates which are still open.

c) In the older patient with a well established hinged fragment, the latter may be excised and the underlying crater curetted or drilled as above to stimulate the development of fibrous or fibrocartilaginous growth. If the fragment is free as a loose body, it should be removed and the crater treated as above. If the lesion is fragmented, multiple fixation is unlikely to achieve healing and the fragments are best removed and the crater treated appropriately.

Osteochondral fractures

In the adult, articular cartilage shears at the junction between the calcified and uncalcified zones. The adolescent cartilage does not have a calcified zone and the shear forces are transmitted directly to the subchondral bone resulting in an osteochondral fracture [73]. In these cases, diagnosis is usually early because of the acute presentation following the injury. The patient invariably has a significant haemarthrosis and the knee may be locked. The fresh detached fragment can usually be reattached into the crater with stability, and secured by the pinning technique described above.

Arthroscopically assisted anterior cruciate reconstruction

Numerous methods are available for augmentation or reconstruction of the torn anterior cruciate ligament, using prosthetics, allografts or autografts. The development of interference screw fixation allowing early mobilization, together with the early success of the bone–patella tendon–bone graft technique, accurate drill guides and reproducible isometry techniques, has resulted in an enormous interest and work in ACL reconstruction. The results of open arthrotomy techniques appear to be reproducible and reliable with Clancy *et al.* [74] and O'Brien *et al.* [75] reporting 90% good results in the short to medium term. However, many of these cases were protected with an extra-articular reinforcement.

One of the technical problems in reconstruction has been the placement of the graft material at the exact anatomic location of the anterior cruciate ligament on the distal femur. The advances in arthroscopic techniques and technological equipment, has encouraged arthroscopic or arthroscopically assisted ACL reconstruction to try and overcome some of the problems presented by conventional arthrotomy.

Arthroscopically assisted reconstruction is said to offer superior visualization of the anatomic cruciate attachments and site for graft placement. The notchplasty can be undertaken with greater ease. There is improved cosmesis for the patient because of the smaller scars. There are no major incisions through the extensor retinaculum or joint capsule which theoretically should result in less quadriceps inhibition and easier rehabilitation [76].

In a comparison of arthroscopically assisted reconstruction versus a miniarthrotomy using dacron grafts, Gilquist and Oldesten [77] reported the operation time was significantly longer in the former but the Lysholm scores and activity levels were the same in both groups. No benefit was defined in terms of rehabilitation and they found the access for the notchplasty was easier through a miniarthrotomy. In the series reported by Buss *et al.* [78] the average operating time for arthroscopic reconstruction was 173 minutes (range 109–254 minutes). Short term reviews of miniarthrotomy or arthroscopic reconstruction using bone-patellar tendon–bone autografts have shown no statistically significant differences [79]. The short term success rate of 87% for the arthroscopic assisted procedure [78] appears no different from that achieved by open techniques. In a study with a 4-year average follow-up, Aglietti and co-workers [80] reported an 81% satisfactory outcome, but 23% of the group had undergone a lateral tenodesis. The need for an extra-articular reinforcement, particularly when arthroscopic techniques are used remains undefined. No long-term prospective study of the arthroscopic and open techniques is available as yet and therefore the final verdict remains to be established.

Role of magnetic resonance imaging

In experienced hands arthroscopy can reach a diagnostic accuracy of 98%, with correspondingly high levels of specificity and sensitivity [81]. Magnetic resonance imaging now provides a non-invasive method of assessing injury particularly to the soft tissues of the knee. This may significantly reduce the number of patients undergoing arthroscopy with normal findings and without the need for definitive surgical treatment.

Recent MRI studies followed by arthroscopic examinations have confirmed the high diagnostic accuracy of MRI. An accuracy of 78 to 97% for lesions of the anterior cruciate ligament and 99% for the posterior cruciate tears have been reported by Fischer *et al.* [82] from their multi-centre study of 1014 patients. Diagnostic accuracy for medial meniscal tears at 89–91% – sensitivity 96% and specificity of 91% – is lower than for lateral meniscal injuries where the diagnostic accuracy is rated at 88–97% – sensitivity 96% and specificity 98% [82,83]. The main contentious area remains the over-diagnosis of tears in the posterior horn of the medial meniscus.

Some of these may be inferior incomplete tears not identified at arthroscopy or simple degenerative myxoid change within this area of the meniscus not extending to the surface. The false positive group is of considerable concern and emphasizes the need to match clinical to MRI findings.

With increasing experience and rapidly advancing technology producing higher quality imaging, the diagnostic reliability of the technique will undoubtedly improve. As yet, it remains a very expensive and time-consuming diagnostic modality. The indications for its use must as always be considered as an aid to diagnosis and not simply supplant the clinical skills and management of the physician. Boden *et al.* [84] showed that in 74 asymptomatic volunteers who underwent MRI, 13% under, and 36% over, the age of 45 years were diagnosed as having meniscal tears.

The commonsense and pragmatic approach as defined by Richard Senghas [85] cannot be more simply and succinctly expressed: 'If an arthroscopy is indicated by the severity or duration of the patient's symptoms, what is the point in doing an MRI. If a negative result would mean the continuation of non-operative treatment, whilst a positive result would mean arthroscopy is indicated, then an MRI might save the patient an invasive procedure under anaesthesia.' Nevertheless, MRI will undoubtedly contribute enormously to the pre-operative management of difficult cases and help clarify the need for arthroscopy where the significance of clinical history and findings are uncertain.

References

1. Bozzini, P. (1806) Lichtleiter, eine Erfindung zur Anschauung innerer Thiele und Krakenheiten nebst der Abbildung. In *Journal der practishen Arzneykunde und Wundarzneykunst Berlin* (ed. C. W. Hufenland), **24**, 107–124.
2. Herteloupe, C. L. S. (1827) *La Lithotritie.* Academie des Sciences, Paris.
3. Desormaux, A. J. (1853) De L'Endoscope. *Bull. Acad. Med. Academie des Sciences.*
4. Tagaki, K. (1933) Practical experience using Tagaki's arthroscope. *J. Jpn Orthop. Assoc.*, **8**, 132.
5. Bircher, E. (1921) Die arthroendoskopie. *Zentralbl. Chir.*, **48**, 1460.
6. Burman, M. S., Finkelstein, H. and Mayer, L. (1934) Arthroscopy of the knee joint. *J. Bone Joint Surg.*, **16**, 225–268.
7. Watanabe, M., Takeda, S. and Ikeuchi, H. (1957) *Atlas of Arthroscopy.* Igaku Shoin, Tokyo.
8. Jackson, R. and Abe, I. (1972) The role of arthroscopy in the management of the knee: an analysis of two hundred cases. *J. Bone Joint Surg.*, **54-B**, 310.
9. Dandy, D. J. (1978) Early results of closed partial meniscectomy. *Br. Med. J.*, **1**, 1099–1100.
10. Johnson, L. L. (1981) *Diagnostic Surgical Arthroscopy: the Knee and Other Joints.* Mosby, New York.
11. Dandy, D. J. and Jackson, R. W. (1975) The impact of arthroscopy in the management of disorders of the knee. *J. Bone Joint Surg.*, **57B**, 346.
12. Curran, W. P. and Woodward, E. P. (1980) Arthroscopy: its role in diagnosis and treatment of athletic knee injuries. *Am. J. Sports Med.*, **8**, 415.
13. Durand, A., Richards, C. L., Moulin, F. and Bravo, G. (1993) Motor recovery after arthroscopic partial meniscectomy. *J. Bone Joint Surg.*, **75A**, 202–213.
14. Sherman, O. H., Fox, J. M., Synder, S. J. *et al.* (1986) Arthroscopy – 'no problem surgery'. *J. Bone Joint Surg.*, **68A**, 256–265.
15. McGinty, J. B., Guess, L. F. and Marvin, R. A. (1977) Partial or total meniscectomy. A comparative analysis. *J. Bone Joint Surg.*, **59A**, 763–766.
16. Delee, J. C. (1983) Complications of arthroscopy and arthroscopic surgery. Results of a national survey. *J. Arthroscopic Rel. Res.*, **1**, 214–220.
17. Small, N. C. (1988) Complications in arthroscopic surgery performed by experienced arthroscopists. *Arthroscopy*, **2**, 253–252.
18. Mulhollan, J. S. (1982) Swedish arthroscopic system. *Orthop. Clin. North Am.*, **13**, 349.
19. Montgomery, S. C. and Campbell, J. (1989) Septic arthritis following arthroscopy and intra-articular steroids. *J. Bone Joint Surg.*, **71B**, 540.
20. Walker, R. H. and Illingham, M. (1983) Thrombophlebitis following arthroscopic surgery. *Contemp. Orthop.*, **6**, 29–33.
21. Eriksson, E., Haggmark, T., Saartok, T. *et al.* (1986) Knee arthroscopy with local anesthesia in ambulatory patients. *Orthopaedics*, **8**, 186–188.
22. Fairclough, J. A., Graham, G. P. and Pemberton, D. (1990) Local or general anaesthesia in day case arthroscopy. *Ann. R. Coll. Surg. Eng.*, **72**, 104–107.
23. Fairclough, J. A., Graham, G. P. and Pemberton, D. (1990) Local or general anaesthesia in day case arthroscopy. *Ann. R. Coll. Surg. Eng.*, **72**, 104–107.
24. Noyes, F. R., Bassett, R. W., Grood, E. S. and

Butler, D. L. (1980) Arthroscopy in acute traumatic haemarthosis of the knee. *J. Bone Joint Surg.*, **62A**, 687–697.

25. Gilquist, J., Hagberg, G. and Oretorp, N. (1977) Arthroscopy in acute injuries of the knee joint. *Acta Orthop. Scand.*, **48**, 190–196.

26. Dehaven, K. E. (1983) Arthroscopy in the diagnosis and management of the anterior cruciate ligament deficient knee. *Clin. Orthop.*, **172**, 52–56.

27. Jones, J. and Allum, R. (1977) Acute traumatic Haemarthrosis of the knee, expectant treatment or arthroscopy. *Ann. R. Coll. Surg. Eng.*, **48**, 190–196.

28. Kannus, P. and Jarvinen, M. (1987) Long term prognosis of nonoperatively treated acute knee distortions having primary haemarthrosis without clinical instability. *Am. J. Sports Med.*, **15**, 138–143.

29. Hamburg, P., Gilquist, J. and Lysholm, J. (1983) Suture of new and old peripheral meniscus tear. *J. Bone Joint Surg.*, **65A**, 193–197.

30. Firer, P. (1985) Arthroscopic meniscectomy. South African experience. *J. Bone Joint Surg.*, **67B**, 507.

31. Simpson, D. A., Thomas, N. P. and Aichcroth, P. M. (1986) Open and closed meniscectomy, a comparative study. *J. Bone Joint Surg.*, **68B**, 301–304.

32. O'Connor, R. L. (1977) Arthroscopy of the knee. *Surg. Ann.*, **9**, 265.

33. Dandy, D. J. (1990) The arthroscopic anatomy of symptomatic meniscal lesions. *J. Bone Joint Surg.*, **72B**, 628–633.

34. Cargill, A. O. and Jackson, J. O. (1976) Bucket handle tear of the medial meniscus. *J. Bone Joint Surg.*, **58A**, 248.

35. Hargreaves, D. J. and Seedhom, B. B. (1979) On the 'bucket handle tear': Partial or total meniscectomy? a quantitative study. *J. Bone Joint Surg.*, **61B**, 381.

36. O'Brien, S. J. and Miller, D. V. (1990) The contact Nd-yttrium-aluminium garnet laser – a new approach to arthroscopic laser surgery. *Clin. Orthop. Rel. Res.*, **252**, 95–100.

37. Seedholm, B. B., Dowson, D. and Wright, V. (1974) Functions of the menisci – a preliminary report. *J. Bone Joint Surg.*, **56B**, 381.

38. Fairbank, T. J. (1948) Knee joint changes after meniscectomy. *J. Bone Joint Surg.*, **30**, 664.

39. Jackson, J. P. (1968) Degenerative changes in the knee after meniscectomy. *Br. Med. J.*, **2**, 525–527.

40. Arnoczky, S. P. and Warren, R. F. (1982) Microvasculature of the human meniscus. *Am. J. Sports Med.*, **10**, 90–95.

41. Hamburg, P., Gilquist, J. and Lysholm, J. (1983) Suture of new and old peripheral meniscus tear. *J. Bone Joint Surg.*, **65A**, 193–197.

42. Keene, G. C. R. and Paterson, R. S. (1987) Arthroscopic meniscal suture. *J. Bone Joint Surg.*, **69B**, 162.

43. Magnuson, P. B. (1941) Joint debridement: a surgical treatment of degenerative arthritis. *Surg. Gynecol. Obstet.*, **73**, 1–9.

44. Jackson, R. W. and Rouse, D. W. (1982) The results of partial arthroscopic meniscectomy in patients over 40 years of age. *J. Bone Joint Surg.*, **64B**, 481–485.

45. Salisbury, R. B., Nottage, W. M. and Gardner, V. (1985) The effect of alignment on results in arthroscopic debridement of the degenerative knee. *Clin. Orthop.*, **198**, 268–272.

46. Jones, R. E., Smith, E. C. and Reisch, J. S. (1978) The effects of medial meiscectomy in patients older than 40 years. *J. Bone Joint Surg.*, **60A**, 783–786.

47. Bert, J. M. and Maschka, K. (1989) The arthroscopic treatment of unicompartmental gonarthrosis: a five year follow-up study of abrasion arthroplasty plus arthroscopic debridement and arthroscopic debridement alone. *Arthroscopy*, **5**, 25–32.

48. Bird, H. A. and Ring, E. F. (1978) Therapeutic value of arthroscopy. *Ann. Rheum. Dis.*, **37**, 78–79.

49. Patel, D. V., Aichroth, P. M. and Mayes, S. T. (1990) Arthroplastic debridement for degenerative arthritis of the knee. *J. Bone Joint Surg.*, **72B**, 1091.

50. Taylor, A. R. (1973) Synovectomy of the knee: long term results. *J. Bone Joint Surg.*, **61B**, 121.

51. Laurin, C. A., Desmarchais, J., Daziano, L. et al. (1974) Long term results of synovectomy of the knee in rheumatoid patients. *J. Bone Joint Surg.*, **56A**, 521–531.

52. Matsui, M., Taneda, Y., Ohta., S., Itoh, T. and Tsuboguchi, S. (1989) Arthroscopic versus open synovectomy in the rheumatoid knee. *Int. Orthop.*, **13**, 17–20.

53. Klein, W. and Jensen, K. U. (1988) Arthroscopic synovectomy of the knee joint: indication, technique and follow-up results. *J. Arthrosc. Rel. Surg.*, **4**, 63–71.

54. Gschwend, N. (1981) Synovectomy. In *Textbook of Rheumatology*. Saunders, Philadelphia, p. 1874.

55. Dandy, D. and Griffiths, D. (1989) Lateral release for recurrent dislocation of the patella. *J. Bone Joint Surg.*, **71B**, 121–125.

56. Aglietti, P., Pisaneschi, A., Buzzi, R. et al. (1989) Arthroscopic lateral release for pateller pain or instability. *Arthroscopy*, **5**, 176–183.

57. Ogilvie-Harris, D. J. and Jackson, R. W. (1984) The arthroscopic treatment of chondromalacia patellae. *J. Bone Joint Surg.*, **66B**, 660–665.

58. Sherman, O. H., Fox, J. M., Sperling, H. et al.

(1987) Patellar instability treatment by arthroscopic electrosurgical lateral release. *Arthroscopy*, **3**, 152–160.

59. Suman, R., Stother, I. G. and Illingworth, G. (1985) Diagnostic arthroscopy of the knee in children. *J. Bone Joint Surg.*, **67B**, 675.

60. Angel, K. A. and Hall, D. J. (1989) The role of arthroscopy in children and adolescents. *J. Arthr. Rel. Surg.*, **5**, 192–196.

61. Harvell, J. C., Fu, F. H. and Stanistsk, C. L. (1989) Diagnostic arthroscopy of the knee in children and adolescents. *Orthopaedics*, **12**, 1555–1560.

62. Bergstrom, R., Gilquist, J., Lysholm, J. and Hamburg, P. (1984) Arthroscopy of the knee in Children. *J. Paed. Orthop.*, **4**, 542–545.

63. Eiskjar, S. and Larsen, S. T. (1987) Arthroscopy of the knee in children. *Acta Orthop. Scand.*, **58**, 273–276.

64. Kaplan, E. B. (1957) Discoid lateral meniscus of the knee joint: nature, mechanism and operative treatment. *J. Bone Joint Surg.*, **39A**, 77.

65. Watanabe, M., Takeda, S. and Ikeuchi, H. (1978) *Atlas of Arthroscopy*. 3rd edn, Igaku-Shoin, Tokyo, p. 88.

66. Hayashi, L. K., Yamaga, H., Ida, K. and Miura, T. (1988) Arthroscopic meniscectomy for discoid lateral meniscus in children. *J. Bone Joint Surg.*, **70A**, 1495–1500.

67. Goodfellow, J. W. and Sandow, M. J. (1985) The natural history of anterior knee pain in adolescents. *J. Bone Joint Surg.*, **67B**, 36–38.

68. Nade, S. (1983) Acute septic arthritis in infancy and childhood. *J. Bone Joint Surg.*, **65B**, 234–241.

69. Smith, M. J. (1986) Arthoscopic treatment of the septic knee. *Arthroscopy*, **2**, 30–34.

70. Aichroth, P. M. (1971) Osteochondritis dissecans of the knee. *J. Bone Joint Surg.*, **53B**, 440–447.

71. Guhl, J. F. (1982) Arthroscopic treatment of osteochondritis dissecans. *Clin. Orthop.*, **65**, 167.

72. Bradley, J. and Dandy, D. J. (1989) Results of drilling osteochondritis dissecans before skeletal maturity. *J. Bone Joint Surg.*, **71B**, 642–644.

73. Rosenberg, N. J. (1964) Osteochondral fractures of the lateral femoral condyle. *J. Bone Joint Surg.*, **62A**, 2.

74. Clancy, W. G., Nelson, D. S., Reider, B. and Narchania, R. G. (1982) Anterior cruciate ligament reconstruction using one-third patellar ligament, augmented by extra-articular tendon transfers. *J. Bone Joint Surg.*, **64A**, 353–359.

75. O'Brien, S. J., Warren, R. E., Pavlov, H., Panariello, R. and Wickiewicz, T. L. (1991) Reconstruction of the chronically insufficient anterior cruciate ligament with the central third of the patellar ligament. *J. Bone Joint Surg.*, **73A**, 278–286.

76. Rosenberg, T. D., Paulos, L. E., Victoroff, B. N. and Abbott, P. J. (1988) Arthroscopic cruciate repair and reconstruction. In *The Crucial Ligaments* (ed. J. A. Feagin), Churchill Livingstone, New York, Edinburgh.

77. Gilquist, J. and Odensten, M. (1988) Arthroscopic reconstruction of the anterior cruciate ligament. *Arthroscopy*, **4**, 5–9.

78. Buss, D. D., Warren, R. F., Wickiewicz, T. L., Galinat, B. J. and Panariello, R. (1993) Arthroscopically assisted reconstruction of the anterior cruciate ligament with use of autogenous Patella-Ligament grafts. Results after twenty-four to forty-two months. *J. Bone Joint Surg.*, **75-A**, 1346–1355.

79. Shelbourne, K. D., Rettig, A. C., Hardin, G. and Williams, R. I. (1993) Miniarthrotomy versus arthroscopic assisted ACL reconstruction with autogenous patellar tendon graft. *Arthroscopy*, **9**, 72–75.

80. Aglietti, P., Buzzi, R. and D'Andria, S. (1991) Arthoscopic anterior cruciate ligament reconstruction with patella tendon. *Arthroscopy*, **8**, 5–10.

81. Jackson, R. W. and Dehaven, K. E. (1975) Arthroscopy of the knee. *Clin. Orthop.*, **107**, 87–92.

82. Fischer, S. P., Fox, J. M., Del Pizzo, W. *et al.* (1991) Accuracy of diagnosis from magnetic resonance imaging of the knee. *J. Bone Joint Surg.*, **73A**, 2–10.

83. Boree, N. R., Watkinson, A. F., Ackroyd, C. E. and Johnson, C. (1991) Magnetic resonance imaging of meniscal and cruciate injuries of the knee. *J. Bone Joint Surg.*, **73B**, 452–457.

84. Boden, A. D., Davis, D. O., Dina, T. S. *et al.* (1992) A prospective and blinded investigation of magnetic resonance imaging of the knee. Abnormal findings in asymptomatic patients. *Clin. Orth.*, **282**, 177–185.

85. Senghas, R. E. (1991) Indications for magnetic resonance imaging. *J. Bone Joint Surg.*, **73A**, 1.

13

Flexor tendon surgery

C. Semple

Flexor tendon surgery continues to present considerable problems to the surgeon, despite numerous advances in scientific knowledge, and applied surgical techniques over the past two decades. Most population centres now have two or three surgeons who specialize in hand surgery and are capable of carrying out effective primary tendon repair and this has now supplanted the previous enthusiasm for tendon grafting, carried out at a later stage once the original wound had healed.

Applied anatomy and physiology

The basic topographical anatomy of the flexor tendons has been understood for many years, but recently the precise anatomy of the tendon sheaths, their vincula, associated blood supply and synovial fluid nourishment of the tendon has been explained in considerable detail. Bunnell coined the phrase 'no man's land' for the area of the flexor tendon sheath between the distal palmar crease and up to the proximal interphalangeal joint including both tendons; and he felt that repair of tendons in this region was extremely complex and advocated delayed repair rather than attempting surgery in such a difficult area. Doyle has described the fibrous flexor sheath of the flexor tendon in a way which has now become standard (Fig. 13.1), and this should be understood by all surgeons carrying out operations on flexor tendons. From the point of view of damaged flexor tendons and their repair

the A2 and A4 annular pulleys are the most important, and significant problems will occur postoperatively, with bow-stringing of tendons and other difficulties if the A2 pulley is com-

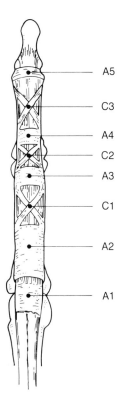

Fig. 13.1 Fibrous flexor sheath. A2 and A4 are the most important. Bow stringing will occur if A2 is removed; A3 and C pulleys can be removed if absolutely necessary to gain access.

pletely removed or divided. The A3 pulley is a very short one and does not contribute significantly to the overall integrity of the sheath, and the cruciate, or C pulleys can also be divided if necessary to obtain access to tendons.

Inside the fibrous flexor sheaths the synovial sheath maintains a valuable fluid environment, and there is good evidence that this fluid environment provides at least as much nourishment to the tendon as the intratendinous vascular network. Indeed in some it may even supply the majority of such nutrition. Removal of portions of the synovial sheaths at the end of a surgical repair, as advocated by some surgeons, is bound to affect the synovial fluid environment of the tendon and disturb the healing process.

The vascular network of flexor tendons is now well understood, although some debate still exists regarding the exact movement of nutrients in and out of the tendon in the natural human situation. The majority of the blood supply to the tendon comes from the vincular vessels. Some of it comes from the proximal portion of the musculo-tendonous junction, and probably very little comes from the distal portion of the tendon at its osseous insertion. The vincula to the tendons vary considerably in their position and length, particularly in the ring and little finger. Armenta and Lehrman have described these vincula as arising from four levels of the volar aspect of the phalanges and define them as Vl, V2, V3 and V4; these small vascular reflexions have some relevance, particularly in the region of the superficialis decussation, as fairly short strong vincula may prevent tendons from retracting, and on the other hand a long thin vinculum may be torn resulting in bleeding in the sheath and some damage to a tendon, particularly the profundus tendon.

For many years it was considered that flexor tendons were incapable of healing from their own intrinsic cellular tissues and that adhesions of one type or another were necessary in order to bring fibrocytes in from external areas to unite the two tendon ends. It now appears clear, however, that given appropriate circumstances flexor tendons are capable of healing satisfactorily from their own tissues, and this is particularly so when they lie in a natural synovial fluid environment. Lundborg's careful studies have shown that isolated small portions of tendon can commence healing when totally isolated in the knee joint of a rabbit,

devoid of any blood supply or external cellular factors. In practice, many factors are involved, including damage to the tendon sheath, and vascular elements of the vincula.

The overall message appears clear; tendon repair must be carried out as carefully as possible, preserving all potential blood supply to the tendon and respecting the synovial sheath at all levels.

Surgical repair of flexor tendons

The diagnosis of a divided flexor tendon might appear straight forward to someone experienced in hand surgery, but a disturbing number of damaged flexor tendons remain undiagnosed until the patient turns up some weeks later with a healed wound and an inability to flex a finger. At this stage the treatment options are restricted, as the flexor tendon may well have shortened into the palm, the fibrous sheath may have collapsed particularly at the level of the proximal phalanx, and considerable skill will be required to obtain a satisfactory result.

Assuming, however, that the divided flexor tendon is diagnosed shortly after the injury it is now standard practice to recommend *primary repair* of that tendon or tendons, providing an experienced hand surgeon and appropriate surgical facilities are available. It is also vitally important to have good quality follow-up facilities, including physiotherapy and occupational therapy. Given good quality facilities, and a co-operative patient, it should be possible to obtain 70% good or excellent results following primary flexor tendon repair, and these are the sort of results which have been published over the last decade, generally coming from good quality hand surgery units. A number of technical aspects of flexor tendon surgery are common to all surgical units, while in other fields there is some difference in approach or technique. All surgeons carry out such surgery under an exsanguinating tourniquet, a bloodless field, and there is an increasing use of brachial block anaesthesia, rather than general anaesthesia for such surgery. Brachial block anaesthesia has a number of advantages, particularly that one can instruct the patient on how to take care of his hand in the immediate postoperative period and obtain his immediate cooperation. With an increased knowledge of anatomy, and good quality surgical instruments it is possible to make a neat approach to the damaged tendon and its sheath without harming the neighbouring structures such as vessels or nerves, generally making use of the original wound which is usually transverse in the finger. The great majority of flexor tendon injuries occur in young males, between the ages of 10 and 30, and the vast majority of wounds are caused by glass or knife and occasionally by sharp machinery. The type of tendon suture used very much dictates the type of exposure of the finger and tendon sheath. If a long Bunnell type zig zag suture is to be used then a considerable amount of tendon will have to be exposed in order to place the suture, whereas a shorter H-shaped suture (such as a Kessler or its variants) enables a much smaller exposure of the tendon to be used. The general trend now is to use a short core suture to hold the two ends of the tendon together and supplement this by some fine circumferential sutures to tidy up and closely approximate the epitenon, or synovial surface of the tendon to reduce any rough areas which might cause adhesions. Most core sutures which have been described recently are variations on the Kessler/Mason/Allan suture (Fig. 13.2), although other methods such as Tsuge (Fig. 13.3) and Becker (Fig. 13.4) have been described.

Some surgeons prefer to release the tourniquet and achieve haemostasis before suturing the skin, whereas others are prepared to suture the skin and completely close the wound before releasing the tourniquet. There is general agreement that some form of protected motion is necessary after flexor tendon surgery, and the method popularized by Kleinert is widely used. This involves

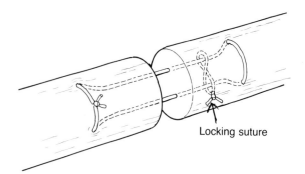

Fig. 13.3   Tsuge suture.

attaching an elastic band to the relevant finger or fingers and thereby preventing the patient from producing an active pull on their repaired tendon, yet allowing active extension of the finger and passive flexion so that the flexor tendon can move passively in its sheath without undue tension being applied to it. Various refinements of this type of controlled motion have been described; most surgeons and therapists allow a

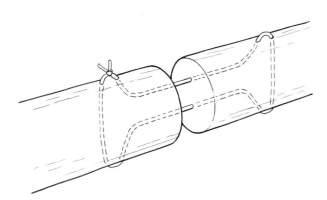

Fig. 13.2   Kessler/Mason Allen suture.

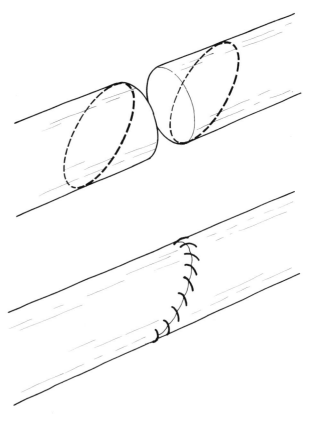

Fig. 13.4   Becker suture.

graduated release from this type of controlled movement over a period of 4–6 weeks. Careful control of such movements is necessary by the hand therapist, together with a considerable degree of patient cooperation.

After repair of the tendon, debate continues about the need for formal repair of the tendon sheath over the tendon repair. It appears clear from physiological evidence that the synovial lining of the sheath is extremely important in providing an appropriate nutritional milieu for the healing tendon, but it is often difficult or impossible to formally close the sheath. In some situations where a considerable amount of damage has occurred to the finger, the tendon sheath may be deficient over a significant length and reconstruction of tendon sheaths/annular pulleys may be necessary. This is always difficult and a number of substitutes have been suggested such as palmaris longus, as a weave between the remnants of the original tendon sheath, or a piece of fascia lata or palmaris longus taken right round the proximal phalanx of the finger to reconstruct an A2 pulley. Lister has described a neat method using a portion of the extensor retinaculum, which has the advantage of including a portion of synovial lining which can be used to cover the tendon at the A2 level.

Author's preferred technique

The fact that a tendon division has occurred does not automatically mean that a tendon requires repair, and certainly when the patient presents late, after the original wound has healed, the actual deficit of function following loss of one tendon only in the finger is often remarkably small. The matter should be carefully discussed with the patient before proceeding to tendon repair. A number of papers have been published which recommend repair of both superficial and profundus tendons in no mans land, that is at the level of the distal palm/proximal phalanx, and have shown that statistically these are likely to produce better results than repair of one tendon only and excision of the other tendons. The reasons for this are not entirely clear, but are almost certainly related to the better preservation of the vascular circulation and the pulley system when both tendons are carefully repaired at that level.

Primary tendon repair is carried out in a bloodless field under a pneumatic tourniquet, and brachial block anaesthesia. If the wound in the finger is a transverse one then it is open via a bayonet extension, or alternatively a Bruner type of incision may be used, particularly in the central two fingers. Exposure of the tendon is by careful trap door extension of the original wound in the tendon sheath, and the two tendon ends are delivered into the wound by flexing the finger at the relevant joints, although occasionally the proximal end of the profundus tendon may require to be retrieved by means of a separate incision in the distal palm. The tendon surfaces are not handled at all with any forceps or instruments, although once the tendon has been retrieved it can be held in the wound by means of fine hypodermic needles passed through the tendon sheath. A core suture of the Kessler type is placed using 4/0 braided polyester suture (Ethibond), with the knot generally placed in the gap between the tendon ends. If the tendon ends lie easily together with no irregularities then no further sutures are placed, but generally a few further sutures, and sometimes a complete circumferential suture of fine 8/0 nylon is required to tidy up the tendon ends and encourage them to lie easily flush with each other. Both flexor tendons are repaired at all levels unless there is significant tearing or crushing of the tendon ends which make the prospect of a successful outcome remote, in which case one tendon only will be repaired and the other one removed. If the trap door in the sheath can be easily repaired this is done, but this may produce excessive tightness over the repaired tendon and the trap door may simply be laid across the tendon with one or two very slack sutures. Care is taken to ensure that the A2 pulley system is at least 50% intact. Digital nerves are repaired at this stage if they were also damaged in the original wound. A suture of 4/0 nylon or prolene is inserted into the finger nail, avoiding the nailbed so that elastic traction can be applied to the finger postoperatively. If the finger nail is badly bitten or otherwise damaged, traction on the finger can be achieved by a button hook glued onto the nail postoperatively. The wound is closed and a complete hand dressing applied with careful compression, using a crepe bandage and small dressings to each individual finger and plaster support applied on volar and dorsal aspects before the tourniquet is released. All hand surgeons have their own particular way of applying bandages and dressings, and it is important to gain experience and confidence in a particular style of applying a bandage so that the circulation to the hand is not impeded but also that effective support of the soft tissues and prevention of haematoma formation occurs.

On the day following surgery the patient is seen by the hand therapist, who carefully instructs the patient in the degree of movement that he/she may use, involving elastic band traction to encourage gentle movement of the repaired tendon in its sheath, yet avoid excessive tension at the repair. Plaster protection of the wrist and hand is used, with the wrist moderately flexed, about 30°, and with a dorsal hood to prevent full extension of the finger yet allowing an almost full range of flexion. Considerable care has to be taken over this type of postoperative splintage and elastic traction, and the therapist has to carefully control the patient so that the proper joints, particularly the proximal interphalangeal joint, are flexing adequately; it is all too easy for the metacarpophalangeal joint to do all the movement and leave the interphalangeal joints stiff. Routine antibiotics are not used and the patient is followed up in the dressings clinic until the wound has healed and sutures have been removed. Regular hand therapy sessions continue initially two or three times a week, decreasing as the patient gains more confidence and use in the finger. The patient is generally fit for discharge from follow-up at the 2- or 3-month stage.

The above comments relate essentially to damage to the flexor tendons at the level of the proximal phalanx, but similar techniques are used at all levels, although one generally expects a better result in patients with divisions of the flexor tendons in the distal forearm or wrist: divisions of the flexor profundus tendon only, in the distal portion of the finger, may be more easily dealt with by simple advancement of the flexor tendon by 1.5 cm, which can generally be managed without difficulty. As implied above, a number of authors have described good or excellent results in 75% of patients undergoing primary tendon repair, but we have found this level of success difficult to achieve. We feel that at least part of this difficulty may lie in the unselected nature of patients dealt with in an NHS hospital in the UK and the varied level of patient co-operation and drive which exists.

Delayed repair

Primary tendon repair, as described above is generally taken to mean repair within 24 hours of the original injury, but the patient may not present for a day or two, and other factors may make such prompt repair impossible. Delayed primary repair up to a week is perfectly possible, although much depends on the state of the wound and if there is any suggestion of infection then the wound must be cleaned and left to heal naturally before contemplating any tendon surgery. When the wound has healed tendon repair may still be possible, although much will depend on the position of the proximal end of the tendon: if this has contracted back to the palm, and the superficialis decussation has closed, or the fibrous flexor sheath has collapsed, particularly at the level of the A2 pulley, then the prospect of achieving a good result is diminished. When discussing flexor tendon surgery with the patient it is extremely important to explain the potential risks and disadvantages of such surgery. While some series describe success rates of 75%, it must be stressed that these are generally private clinics in the United States run by very experienced hand surgeons and the general results of flexor tendon surgery in public hospitals in the United States, and the NHS in the UK are generally much poorer. It must be remembered that patients are likely to strongly resent a lot of time, surgery and rehabilitation spent on a finger which ends up stiff and useless, and indeed they occasionally take this resentment to Court. For the patient with a healed wound and a divided tendon or tendons it is important to clearly define the advantages and disadvantages of prospective flexor tendon surgery, and the patient may well be better off with his hand as it is, rather than embarking on a long and complex period of surgery and rehabilitation, with only a possibility of improving matters.

Tendon grafting

When direct tendon repair is impossible, either due to the long delay which has occurred since the original injury, or to the degree of damage to the tendon, its sheath or the finger as a whole, then some form of tendon replacement may be appropriate. Free tendon grafting, as described by Pulvertaft, requires considerable care with regard to surgical technique and postoperative rehabilitation, and furthermore the finger should have a good or excellent range of passive movement preoperatively. It must be stressed that no form of tendon grafting can ever improve on the preoperative passive range of movement. All too often flexor tendon reconstructive surgery fails because the patient does not start off with a good passive range of movements. The essential techniques of free tendon grafting have not changed since Pulvertaft's original descriptions, and the reader is referred to his article for a description of that surgery. The concept of a staged tendon reconstruction, using a silicone spacer rod to form a pseudosheath has gained popularity since Hunter's original description and this is the method of choice in situations where the tendon sheath is badly damaged by scarring, previous burns, etc. It must be stressed, however, that this technique which is time-consuming and difficult to carry out, is no substitute for standard free tendon grafting which is still the appropriate method if the tissues of the finger are satisfactory. With the staged tendon reconstruction technique the initial surgery involves removing all scarred and unsatisfactory tissue from the region of the tendon and its sheath, repairing or reconstructing tendon pulleys, particularly the A2 pulley, and inserting a silicon rod to run from the distal phalanx to the palm or wrist. The proximal portion of the rod is left free, and it simply moves in and out in a pistoning fashion with passive movements of the finger and thereby forms a sheath around itself. It is important to appreciate that the sheath which is formed is not a true synovial sheath, as Lundborg has shown, but is simply a sheath lined by granulation tissue and this is one of the factors which can complicate the second stage of the procedure when the formal tendon graft is inserted. Significant scarring and adhesions may form between the granulation tissue and the new tendon. The time between the first and second stages is generally 3 or 4 months, as long as the skin and subcutaneous tissues of the finger have healed satisfactorily and the finger has regained a full passive range of movements at all joints. The second stage operation should be a very much less traumatic one than the first stage, with simple retrieval of both ends of the tendon and insertion of a free tendon graft, generally palmaris longus or plantaris. An appropriate suture will secure the graft firmly into the distal phalanx and an 'in and out weave' and/or 'fish mouth suture' is made proximally in the palm or wrist. Controlled gentle active movement is commenced once the wounds have healed, generally at the 10 day stage and remains under the care of the hand therapist for at least 3 months. In all types of tendon surgery, but particularly following tendon grafting, some adhesions are always likely to form and they are most likely to resolve following repeated small active movements of the tendon rather than by any attempts at passive manipulation. La Salle and Strickland found that in their series of 43 patients with two stage tendon grafting, different types of rod designs made no particular difference to the results, nor did placement of the proximal end of the rod in the palm or wrist, or the degree of immobilization/mobilization used postoperatively. They also found that it made no significant difference whether the profundus or superficialis was used as the motor for the tendon graft, although most surgeons consider that the most appropriate motor muscle is that which has the easiest excursion at the time of the grafting procedure.

Further reading

Armenta, E. and Lehrman, A. (1980) The vincula to the flexor tendons of the hand. *J. Hand Surg.*, **5**, 127–134.

Doyle, J. R. and Blyth, W. (1975) The finger flexor sheath. *AAOS, Symposium on Tendon Surgery in the Hand*, pp. 81–87.

Hunter, J. M. and Schneider, L. H. (1977) *Staged Flexor Tendon Reconstruction*, AAOS Instructional Course Lecture, 26, Mosby, St Louis.

La Salle, W. B. and Strickland, J. W. (1983) An evaluation of digital performance following two-stage flexor tendon reconstruction. *J. Hand Surg.*, **8**, 263–267.

Lister, G. D. (1979) Reconstruction of pulleys employing extensor retinaculum. *J. Hand Surg.*, **4**, 461.

Lundborg, G. and Rank, F. (1978) Experimental healing of flexor tendons based on synovial fluid nutrition. *J. Hand Surg.*, **3**, 21–31.

Lundborg, G. *et al.* (1980) Superficial repair of

severed flexor tendons in synovial environment. *J. Hand Surg.*, **5**, 451–461.

Manske, P. R. and Lesker, P. A. (1982) Nutrient pathways of flexor tendons in primates. *J. Hand Surg.*, **7**, 436-444.

Neilsen, A. B. and Jensen, P. O. (1985) Methods of evaluation of flexor tendon results. *J. Hand Surg.*, **10B**, 60–61.

Pulvertaft, R. G. (1959) Experience in flexor tendon grafting. *J. Bone Joint Surg.*, **41B**, 629.

14

Musculoskeletal trauma: nerve

D. Marsh and N. J. Barton

Division of a peripheral nerve is a unique injury. In laceration of any other tissue, one group of cells is separated from another group of cells. Even when a hollow tube is cut, such as a blood vessel or ureter, the two ends consist of independent masses of viable cells, with the potential for the divided structure to *repair* itself by formation of scar tissue. A peripheral nerve injury is different; the nerve cells themselves are cut into two pieces. The distal portion of the neuron, amputated from the cell body, must die. Repair, in the sense of a join between tissues, is therefore impossible. The only hope for restoration of communication lies in a totally different process – *regeneration*.

Surgeons must therefore understand something of the unique and fascinating nature of nerve cells and their response to injury. They must approach the divided nerve in the full knowledge that they cannot truly repair it; they can only give it the best environment in which to regenerate.

Structure and function of normal nerve

Each peripheral nerve (Fig. 14.1) consists of thousands of axons, whose cell bodies lie either in the dorsal root ganglion (for sensory fibres) or in the anterior horn of the spinal cord (for motor fibres), held together by connective tissue elements. The latter are of fundamental impor-

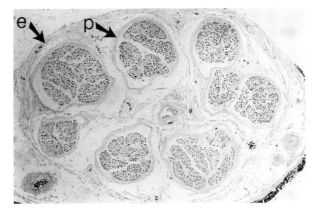

Fig. 14.1 Transverse section of sural nerve, showing epineurium (e) and perineurium (p). Haematoxylin and eosin × 50.

tance in the processes of recovery from peripheral nerve injury and in our attempts to help.

Axons may be a metre or more in length, but even the thicker myelinated fibres are only 20 microns wide; this is equivalent to a 5/0 nylon suture 5 m long. Such a formidable arrangement is sustained by virtue of a highly efficient axoplasmic transport system, capable of moving chemicals and cellular organelles in both directions at rates up to 400 mm/day. The Nissl granules in the cell body (Fig. 14.2) are the enzyme manufacturing endoplasmic reticulum; their profusion is evidence of the Herculean metabolic task of sustaining a total volume of axoplasm which may be 200 times that of the cell body.

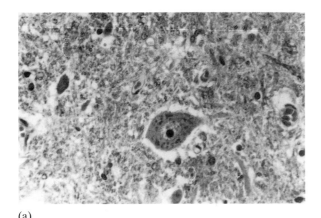

(a)

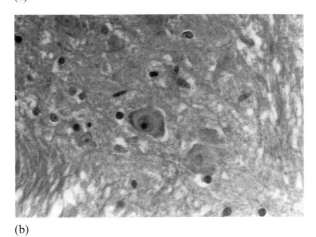

(b)

Fig. 14.2   (a) Anterior horn neuron with Nissl substance in clumps in the cytoplasm (haematoxylin and eosin × 650). (b) Anterior horn cell showing chromatolysis (× 800).

Every nerve fibre has associated Schwann cells; in a minority, these produce a myelin sheath. This allows up to a 100-fold increase in conduction velocity for a relatively small increase in diameter. Equally important, it allows many more action potentials to be transmitted per second. The Schwann cells are also gifted in other ways and their versatility is given full play after injury, as we shall see. They sit on a basement membrane, which forms the inner lining of the endoneurial tube, whose great significance is that it forms a conduit, specific to each fibre, leading directly to the correct target organ.

Nerve fibres are grouped together in fascicles which are ensheathed in perineurium. This membrane is mainly responsible for the biochemical environment in which the nerve fibres lie and has been described as the blood–nerve barrier due to its highly selective permeability. Fascicular grouping varies greatly from nerve to nerve, ranging from a few large to many small fascicles. The pattern of fascicles also varies along the length of a given nerve, as Sunderland [1] showed, although towards the periphery it is more constant [2].

The membrane surrounding the whole nerve trunk is the epineurium, whose chief characteristic is its physical strength. It normally lies in some longitudinal tension, so that the two ends of a divided nerve spring apart. Considerable longitudinal traction on the nerve can be sustained by the epineurium without the nerve fibres suffering rupture. However, this is *not* true at the points of emergence of the nerves from the spinal cord, where the epineurium is relatively deficient and small tensile forces can cause enormous damage.

Degeneration and regeneration

Damage to axons, severe enough to lead to their death distal to the lesion, may be due to stretch, crush, or a cut. The outcome of these different types of injury is vastly different, but all produce one constant feature: an apparently preprogrammed response to injury by the parent cell body proximally and the Schwann cells below the lesion. This response can be divided into degenerative and regenerative phases, though these overlap in time and are both highly constructive in what they achieve.

Degenerative phase

This consists of changes in the cell body and Wallerian degeneration in the distal axons. The former is called chromatolysis, because of the observed dissolution of the deeply staining Nissl granules, signalling a change in the synthetic machinery of the cell, like a factory re-tooling. Ribosomes which were designed for production of transmitter substances are replaced by new ones, dedicated to the production of cellular building material. Energy production, previously geared to transmission of action potentials, is switched to the pentose phosphate pathway, more suited to the work of chemical synthesis. Glial cells proliferate over the surface of the injured cell and prise loose the synaptic endings from other CNS cells, as if taking the cell out of service to concentrate on the business of regeneration. These changes begin within hours of injury and the signal initiating them is presumably brought from the site of injury in the axoplasmic transport system.

Wallerian degeneration is the work primarily of the Schwann cells. It does not necessarily start at once; transmission of action potentials below a complete transection has been observed for up to a week. Myelin surrounding the axons is rapidly broken down followed by the axons themselves, the Schwann cells acting as phagocytes. The basement membrane remains intact and the Schwann cells, increased in number, form solid columns (the bands of Büngner) within the endoneurial tubes. These extend from both cut ends of the nerve toward each other and unite, forming an attractive surface down which the regenerating axon sprouts can grow. Evidence is accumulating that the Schwann cells also create gradients of neurotropic substances which draw axon sprouts in their direction.

Augustus Waller (1816–1870) was a busy general practitioner at St Mary Abbott's Terrace in Kensington, London where he carried out the research on degeneration of nerves in frogs with which his name is associated and for which he was elected a Fellow of the Royal Society at the age of 35. This shows that one need not be prevented from doing research by shortage of time or facilities; the real impediment is the lack of will to do it. Waller was also interested in the ability of white blood corpuscles to escape from capillaries and such was his dedication that he courageously attempted to study the microcirculation in his own prepuce, though after a few attempts he changed to the frog's tongue and was able to demonstrate that pus contained extravasated leucocytes. In the same period he also published papers on the physiology of vision, the microscopy of hailstones, and the formation of coloured films by the action of halogens on metals. After 10 years in practice, he moved first to Bonn and then to Paris to obtain more favourable opportunities for carrying out his scientific work, and returned to England in 1858 as Professor of Physiology in Queens College, Birmingham (which has since become the University) and Consultant Physician to the Queen's Hospital in Bath Row (whose buildings now house the Birmingham Accident Hospital).

Regenerative phase

The 'degenerative' process creates the conditions under which regeneration proper can proceed. The first stage is a sprouting of new axons at the level of the lesion; several fine filaments of axoplasm reach out from each axon. This is not a passive process, like toothpaste being squeezed from a tube; the tip of the advancing axon sprout has a specialized structure, known as the growth cone and containing actin and myosin, which burrows actively through the tissues and drags the axon after it. If the endoneurial tubes are intact (as in axonotmesis due to crush) the axon sprouts have an easy job and can progress to their correct target organs at a rate of about 1 mm per day.

However, in the case of a cut, the sprouts must first find their way through granulation tissue into the endoneurial tubes of the distal stump and this is a powerful factor working against the re-establishment of useful connections. Some sprouts will never find the distal stump and will only contribute to a tender neuroma at the suture site. Whatever chemotactic signals are being produced by the ever-resourceful Schwann cells, the chances of any axon finding its old, correct, conduit are remote. Even if a sensory axon finds a sensory tube, it is likely to lead to the wrong species of touch receptor, located in the wrong area of skin. An enormous degree of topographic disorganization is inevitable.

The new axons must then undergo a process of maturation, including remyelination. Finally, the quality of sensibility regained will depend crucially on the re-establishment of useful connections with the specialized sensory receptors [3].

Much effort is being directed towards unravelling the mechanisms by which these processes are initiated and controlled. There is certainly room for improvement: experimental studies involving ideal sutures in primates have shown that about half of the axons fail to regenerate. A few adjuvant treatments, apparently effective in laboratory animals, have been shown to enhance the vigour of the regenerative response after suture. However, at the time of writing, no safe and reliable method for enhancing regeneration in the clinical context exists.

The above gloomy facts underly the poor results obtained after peripheral nerve repair, at least on the sensory side. They suggest two cardinal principles which should guide the surgical approach:

- Do nothing to interfere with the process of axonal regeneration. In particular, *minimize fibrosis.*
- Minimize the spatial disorganization by trying to appose fascicles correctly to one another.

Different surgeons apply these two principles with different emphasis. To some it is a transgression of the first to suture individual fascicles; to others it is necessary to do precisely that in order to satisfy the second. There is no reliable evidence which indicates that either point of view has more to commend it.

Factors influencing results

The most powerful factors determining the outcome of peripheral nerve injuries are not under the control of the surgeon. These are the age of the patient and the level and nature of the lesion. Young patients with lesions in continuity or clean cuts, sustained at a distal level, do well.

We all hope that in future years we will be able to do more to determine the quality of the outcome, whether by improved surgery or adjuvant chemical therapy, but at present, the single most effective step in improving results overall would be the elimination of delay in diagnosis and treatment.

Avoidable delay in diagnosis

From the moment of injury, patients begin to learn how to cope without the function that they have lost. Skills for which the injured hand may previously have been preferred begin to be transferred. Evidence is accumulating that structural changes occur in the CNS due to the loss of afferent input from the denervated part. These processes will continue until reinnervation takes place and the longer that is, the less complete will be the eventual recovery of function. The end organs, whether motor or sensory, also deteriorate; therefore suture of a divided nerve should be carried out with minimal delay. The most frequent cause of delay is missed diagnosis at the time of injury.

There are six reasons why it may not be realized that a nerve has been cut:

1. The relevant nerve is not examined. Sometimes the patient does not consult a doctor, but if he does then *failure to examine* the function of any nerves which may be divided is *negligence* and will be so judged in the Courts. The diagnosis is made by testing the motor and sensory function of the nerve distal to the cut, not by looking at or poking around in the wound. This includes all nerves which could conceivably be cut, remembering that a long thin blade or sliver of glass may pass deeply and obliquely into the tissues and divide structures far from the cut in the skin: we have seen an injury with an entry wound on the lateral side of the upper arm which divided the *ulnar* nerve only, just falling short of coming out again through the skin on the medial side of the arm.

2. Sensory testing may be inadequate. Remember that a patient may take some time to realize that part of the body has become anaesthetic. It is totally inadequate to test sensibility by touching the part and asking 'can you feel that?'; an affirmative reply cannot be trusted even from the scrupulously honest. Also dangerous is 'tell me when I touch you'; a falsely reassuring picture may be obtained due to tiny movements or vibrations caused by the touch which are picked up by highly sensitive receptors in adjacent nerve territories.

Better is to ask the patient 'does this feel different from normal?' (or 'different from this?' – comparing it with an area of skin supplied by a different nerve). If it does feel different, you must assume that the nerve is divided until proved otherwise. Best is to set some sort of discrimination task ('am I touching you with the sharp end or the blunt end?' – Fig. 14.3). In applying such a test, take care to eliminate vision and *repeat* the test a few times in random sequence; with only one application, the patient with a divided nerve will get it right 50% of the time.

These sorts of tests are hard to perform in young children. Here it is best to follow Dellon's [4] advice and use the innocuous tuning fork (the pronged end), the feeling is one of tickling and they laugh; with sharp pins they cry. Again, do not be misled by the ability to *detect* the buzz;

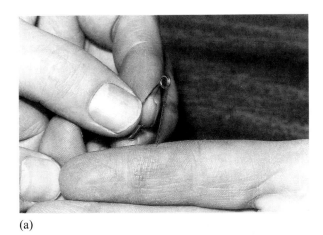

(a)

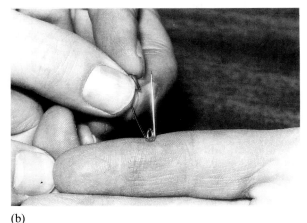

(b)

Fig. 14.3 Testing the ability to distinguish (a) sharp from (b) blunt.

vibrations travel far across the skin. Ask for a difference in quality of sensation between two sides or two nerve territories. Another innocuous test suitable for children is to immerse the digits in warm water for 30 minutes and check for wrinkling of the pulp skin [5].

3. Important clues, provided by the consequences of autonomic denervation, are ignored. Affected digits are warm, due to vasodilatation, and dry, due to cessation of sweat production. The skin dries within a few minutes of division of sudomotor fibres and a simple means of assessing this is to feel the frictional drag in moving a plastic pen across the skin – dry skin shows low friction. A more precise (and documentable) measure is obtainable with a cheap skin resistance meter [6]. In either case it is obviously necessary to avoid confusion by blood or cleansing agents on the skin.

4. A partial division may lead to error: there may be a cut in the median nerve but the patient may have normal sensibility in, say, the thumb. There are ten digital nerves and with any cut on the front of the palm, wrist or arm the territories of all ten must be examined.

5. There may be unexpected anatomical variation. For example, every fifth patient with complete division of the median nerve can still oppose the thumb because the opponens pollicis is ulnar-innervated. It is important to record this, because after repair of the nerve, a functioning opponens may be wrongly interpreted as evidence of recovery. Similarly, one patient in five has a sensory frontier between the median and ulnar nerves which does *not* run down the centre of the ring finger.

6. Even after the most rigorous testing, suspicion must be maintained whenever a penetrating injury *could* have damaged a nerve. At the time of writing two authors have provided evidence that divided nerves, lying in contact, can transmit action potentials across the gap in the first few hours after injury, albeit unphysiologically evoked synchronized action potentials [7,8]. This ceases, of course, after Wallerian degeneration begins.

There is only one sensible response to all these pitfalls: have a low threshold for exploring the wound, or at the very least arrange an immediate review by an experienced surgeon.

Timing of repair

Seddon and his co-workers [9] favoured secondary repair of nerve lacerations. However, their main experience was with nerves injured in war, where both the nature of the wounds and the circumstances of early surgery are very different from those usually occurring in civilian practice. It should be possible in the 1990s to get the patient to a surgeon experienced in this type of work with a fully equipped operating theatre and plenty of time, within a short time after the injury.

If, as is generally the case, the wound is a clean-cut and tidy one, and direct apposition of the cut ends is possible, then current opinion is that the best chance for regeneration is given by primary repair [10]. Primary repair is now preferred, because the cut fascicles can be directly matched (not possible after a scarred section has been resected), the nerve can be repaired under no more tension than it normally has, and regeneration can start straight away.

Suture should be done immediately whenever possible, within the limits of common sense. A patient not available for surgery until late at night will probably gain more than he or she loses if the surgeon sleeps and then performs the operation the following morning, *provided* the limb is elevated in the meantime to minimize oedema. A wait of up to 24 hours does no harm (unless arterial repair is also necessary, in which case there must be no delay at all).

The desire for primary repair must be tempered by basic surgical principles and there are three main reasons why delayed repair may be indicated. The first is that the wound is too contaminated (including an initially clean wound in which diagnosis has been delayed beyond 24 hours). The second is that the nerve injury involves an element of crush or traction and it is not possible to judge how much of the proximal stump needs to be resected to find viable axons. The third is that there is a skeletal injury which for some reason cannot be stabilized immediately, so that a nerve repair is at risk of subsequent disruption.

If delay is appropriate, then a preliminary operation must be performed, during which the wound is cleaned and the cut ends of the nerve are *apposed*, not just marked. This is to prevent retraction of the nerve ends, which would necessitate a graft rather than direct suture subsequently.

Principles of wound care

Remember that a cardinal aim of treatment is avoidance of fibrosis:

- prevent oedema formation. Insist on elevation of the injured hand above the level of the patient's head at all times both while waiting for surgery and for several days afterwards. A sling is not enough;
- prevent ischaemia. The main blood supply to a peripheral nerve is via longitudinal internal plexuses and these are compromised by stretch; therefore tension is a very bad

thing. This argues for generous mobilization of nerve to avoid tension, but this must be tempered by awareness of the risk of damaging feeder vessels, particularly in the distal stump; dissect outside the adventitia. In the case of the ulnar nerve, divided at the wrist, use the ulnar artery. If it is also divided, repair it (or at least suture together the tied-off ends); this takes most of the tension off the nerve as well as improving arterial supply;

- prevent haematoma. Expose the nerve under tourniquet; insist on having a fine bipolar diathermy and use it, after removal of the tourniquet but before suture of the nerve, to prevent intraneural haematoma. This is particularly important when dealing with the median nerve, which may have a large artery within it;
- prevent drying out of the tissues. Keep the nerve moist with saline at all times;
- avoid unnecessary interfascicular dissection and suture. If you suture fascicles, then use a monofilament synthetic suture of 10/0 grade or finer. Do not excise epineurium.

Use of microsurgical technique

Twenty-five years ago the argument was about *when* the nerve should be sutured; since then the area of debate has shifted and the main question now is how the nerve should be repaired. Many experts believe that results are better when the

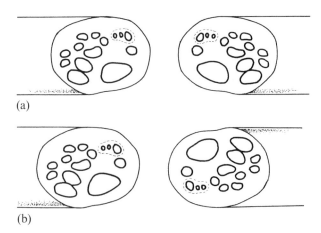

Fig. 14.4 (a) Correct and (b) incorrect alignment of fascicles.

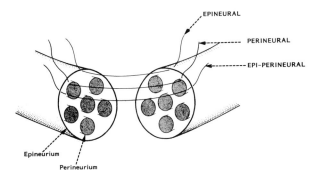

Fig. 14.5 Epineural, perineural and epi-perineural sutures.

operating microscope, microsurgical instruments and microsurgical techniques are used for nerve repair [11].

Microsurgical repair does not necessarily mean fascicular suture; with the microscope it is possible to orient the nerve ends better (Fig. 14.4) and insert the sutures more accurately, whether they are epineural, perineural or epi-perineural (Fig. 14.5). However, although the naked eye can discern the fascicles as well as the epineurium, it is only with the microscope that one can see and therefore suture the perineurium. Advocates of immediate fascicular suture argue that the formal coaptation of matching fasciculi must reduce misdirection of regenerating axons.

Although one would expect this gentler and more precise surgery to produce a better result, the place of microsurgery is not so firmly established for nerves as it is for small blood vessels. It is important to remember that it is not axons, but large groups of axons which are being coapted; the evidence for significant benefit from improved topographic accuracy is inconsistent:

Animal experiments have the advantage that at a later date the repaired nerve can be removed and studied in various ways; in particular they allow histological assessment of axon regeneration. Dog peroneal, cat sciatic and, rarely, primate median nerve have been used as models.

Approximately half of the published studies report improved histological appearances and electrophysiological function after perineural repair performed under the microscope. However, the other half (by and large the more recent studies) reported that epineural repair, sometimes performed with the aid of the microscope, sometimes not, was just as good.

Clinical studies have the advantage that humans can cooperate with much more sophisticated tests of function of the sutured nerves, particularly sensory function. This ought to allow measurement of the ability to transmit information accurately, and thus demonstrate the advantage of better fascicular orientation and coaptation, if there is any.

However, this is not as easy as it sounds and there has been a remarkable dearth of comparative clinical trials of different suture techniques. Series reported by Salvi [12] and Donoso *et al.* [13] suggested there might be some advantage to microscopic perineural repair. Neither Young *et al.* [14] nor Marsh and Barton [15] could demonstrate any benefit.

What, therefore, should you do?

If you work in a hospital which possesses a suitable operating microscope (one with pedals controlling focus and magnification and binocular eyepieces for an assistant) together with microsurgical instruments and sutures, and you have learned how to use all these, we would recommend that you do so. However, be careful that you do not in the process contaminate your field or prolong tourniquet time beyond acceptable limits. Consider also that, if there is a choice between an early operation with magnifying spectacles versus a late one with the microscope, the former is preferable. You may say this choice should never have to be made, but under pressure of many cases waiting for theatre time, it can happen. It is more likely to happen if you get a reputation among nurses and anaesthetists for making a prolonged circus out of nerve repair, so if you use the microscope be quiet and efficient about it.

Make sure in advance that *you* know how to set it up and operate all its features. Adjust it for the intended field before you scrub, then roll it back and expose the nerve under tourniquet using ordinary instruments. Then release the tourniquet, use the diathermy (bipolar near the nerve) and pack the wound with swabs while you bring the microscope in again. It is a good idea for your assistant to let the scrub nurse have a look every now and then to relieve boredom.

Fascicular suture is not something you should embark upon without expert instruction. You are likely to do more harm (by production of intraneural fibrosis) than good (by accurate co-

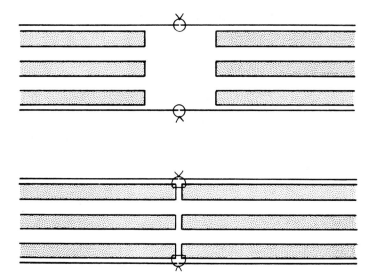

Fig. 14.6 Improved fascicular coaptation with epi-perineural sutures.

aptation). If you need to read this before operating on a nerve, then do an epineural repair – with or without the microscope – but as carefully and accurately as you can, and with the finest possible non-absorbable and non-reactive suture material.

Our own preference is for an epi-perineural suture because an epineural suture may drag the epineurium forwards (Fig. 14.6), like a sleeve pulled down over the end of the fingers, leaving the cut fascicles separated. The suture must pass through connective tissue (epineurium or perineurium), not nerve tissue.

Rehabilitation

After the nerve has regenerated, the information passing along it to and from the patient's brain will be scrambled. No electronic device could function after such an insult, but people can, due to the plasticity which is a feature of the CNS. Almquist *et al.* [16] suggest that it is because childrens' brains are more adaptable that they do better following nerve repair, not because the nerve actually regenerates better.

In order to make the most of their potential, patients need help in two respects. First, they need to know the time-course of regeneration. If they know what to expect they will not become dismayed or demoralized by the prolonged and imperfect recovery and will make the best of what they have. Warn them that:

- the affected part will remain numb for some months after the operation; they must be very careful not to burn themselves during this time;
- the first sensation to return will be 'protopathic': unpleasant and abnormal, but usefully protective;
- discriminatory touch sensibility will come more slowly and may continue to improve for 4 or 5 years;
- sensibility will never return to normal (in adults);
- they will experience many and varied paraesthesiae during regeneration.

Second, they need hand therapy. For the first few weeks, the nerve repair must be protected from tension by suitable splintage. Following this, they need to be helped to regain full mobility. In addition, they may be helped at a later stage by formal sensory re-education: graded sensory exercises under supervision. This depends on there being an enthusiast in your physiotherapy or occupational therapy departments. For many patients, their normal work constitutes much the best form of re-education.

Surgical methods

If it is possible to appose the two cut ends without undue tension, then direct suture is the method of choice.

Early direct suture

Having made a prompt diagnosis of nerve division, cover the wound with a betadine-soaked swab and start antibiotics. Admit the patient and organize theatre and the most experienced surgeon available. We have already discussed the use of magnification and the principles of wound care.

Expose the cut ends and study the pattern of the fascicles, with the aim of matching them accurately. Even without the microscope, one can get some idea by matching up the small blood vessels on the surface of the nerve, and if the cut is oblique then there is no difficulty in getting the rotation correct.

In our opinion, it is unwise to try to trim the ends of the nerve. If it was a clean sharp cut, you will probably only make it worse, as it is very difficult to hold the nerve still while you cut it whereas, when the patient cut it, it was held steady by surrounding tissues. Moreover, if you resect the bulging endoneurium, it only forms another bulge quite quickly. If the cut was not a clean sharp one, you should not be doing primary repair.

The essential point in technique is that the nerve ends must not be dragged together under tension. That is one reason for using fine suture material (not larger than 6/0); if there is tension, the suture breaks. However, the elasticity in the nerve does make the ends retract from each other, and to help yourself get in the first two stitches you may flex the adjacent joint through about half its range. You should not stick needles across the nerve as this may cause further injury, but we find it helpful to use a strong sub-epineural stay suture to take the tension while the finer sutures are put in.

The initial stay suture is the one which determines the rotation and the nerve ends must be carefully aligned before it is inserted. The main sutures are then inserted and, as we have said, a fine accurately placed epineural stitch is perfectly acceptable. A few epi-perineural sutures are preferable, after which the gaps are filled in by simple epineural sutures, and the stay suture is removed.

After completion of the repair, it should be possible to relax the adjacent joint into an almost neutral position, though it is wise to splint it in slight flexion for 2 weeks and in a neutral position for another 2 weeks.

Late direct suture

If it was not possible or desirable to repair the nerve within 24, or at most 48 hours, it is better to wait for about 8 weeks and then do a secondary procedure. The argument for this used to be that the epineurium thickened up and made it easier to suture, but with modern techniques we do not need this extra assistance. What is more important is to ensure that the initial phase of healing and deposition of scar has taken place.

In a secondary procedure it is necessary, even if the nerve ends have been apposed, to resect both ends back to healthy unscarred nerve tissue. This can be the most difficult part of the operation. You need a very sharp straight cutting edge: half of a razor blade (cut longitudinally) held in a strong needle holder is best. You also need something to hold the nerve still; special instruments are made, but if you have not got them you can sterilize one of the plastic bracelets used to identify patients, wrap it around the nerve, and then cut through bracelet and nerve together on to a wooden or metal spatula. It is better to press than to saw.

Then inspect the cut surface and see whether you have got back to healthy white bundles or can still see homogeneous grey scar tissue, in which case further resection is necessary. For this, the microscope is very helpful. In practice, any visible neuroma swelling is full of scar so you must cut back to where the nerve is of normal diameter.

Now is the time of decision. Can the cut ends be brought together easily or not? You are allowed some, but not full, flexion of adjacent joints, but mobilization of the nerve for several inches on either side is discouraged because of damage to its blood supply. A gap of 1 cm can usually be closed using the same technique as for primary repair; with a gap of more than 2 cm, this will produce unacceptable tension.

Grafting

The alternative is a nerve graft. Although this means two suture lines instead of one and an intervening segment of initially avascular connective tissue elements, it is better than suture under tension [17]. The absence of need for prolonged splintage with flexed joints also allows earlier hand therapy and use of the hand.

The usual donor site is the sural nerve and it is possible to obtain 35 cm from each leg. Three or four strands are used and the epineurium of the graft is sutured to the epineurium or perineurium of the main nerve. It is wise to use two stitches at each end to prevent rotation and thus loss of apposition of the cut ends at the junction. The most extensive use of nerve grafts is in reconstruction of the brachial plexus and, to save time, various sorts of nerve 'glue' have been used. These are not new, and nerve grafting used to be done by gluing together several parallel strands of sural nerve and then suturing them, as one, into the defect; this was called a cable graft. Nowadays it is preferred to spread the strands of graft apart so that each can acquire a blood supply as soon as possible.

Better still, the blood supply can be brought with the nerve, a vascularized nerve graft, with microvascular suture of the vessels from which the blood supply of the nerve is derived. The problem is in finding a suitable donor and at present the method is largely confined to brachial plexus injuries in which the prognosis for recovery of the ulnar nerve is considered hopeless; this nerve is then used as a vascularized graft to the trunks and cords which lead to the median and radial nerves. The long-term results are not yet known.

The future: adjunctive therapy

Many surgeons now believe that there is a limit, a low limit, to the quality of reinnervation following nerve transection which can be achieved by prompt diagnosis and optimal surgical technique. This is set by the regenerative power of the nerves themselves and by the problem of topographic disorganization (regenerating axons failing to find their correct end-organs). It would seem that any further improvement in results, and any progress in treatment of more central lesions which show no, or hardly any, regeneration, requires a leap in understanding of the process at the level of neurobiology.

We may speculate that new knowledge may enable us to intervene biochemically, as an adjunct to physical coaptation of the divided nerve. We may one day be able to switch back on the growth potential of the embryonic neurones, perhaps even utilize mechanisms by which axons find their correct target organs in the first place.

At present, we have only a few animal studies to encourage us, showing some enhancement of regeneration by a variety of agents, none of which is yet ready for clinical application. Physical agents showing some effect include pulsed electromagnetic fields and low-dose lasers. Biochemical agents include gangliosides, leupeptin, laminin and triamcinolone.

Assessment of results

There are two completely separate reasons for assessing the results of nerve repair. The first is clinical: to check, in the individual case, that regeneration is proceeding at a reasonable pace and that re-suture or grafting is not required. The second is in a research context, to compare two different methods of treatment. These two objectives require different methods.

Checking regeneration

Here there is little point in trying to express quantitatively the regeneration which has taken place. One is interested primarily in the *rate* at which things are happening; simple, qualitative tests suffice, but must be carried out regularly. As far as motor fibres are concerned, the matter is simple, pick a muscle which is recorded as having been completely paralysed at the time of the nerve injury, and whose function can be unambiguously detected without confusion from trick movements.

The return of function in sensory fibres can be detected by application of stimuli either to the nerve trunk or to the skin innervated by it. The former includes Tinel's sign – an 'electric' sensation in the territory of the nerve produced by percussion over the nerve trunk. The most distal point at which this is elicited is the level the regenerating axon tips have reached and should progress at about 1 mm per day. It is important to start distally and work proximally, or you flood the hand with paraesthesiae and cannot continue the examination. Another approach is to keep the site of stimulation constant and vary the power of the (electrical) stimulus. This is the idea of sensory threshold measurement [8].

In applying stimuli to the skin in the territory of the nerve, one is seeking answers to two questions. When does protective sensibility recover? When does the sense of light touch recover (if at all)? Protective sensibility can be tested by asking the patient to discriminate between the sharp and blunt ends of a pin. Touch sense implies tactile gnosis: the ability to discriminate different textures, shapes of coins or other objects and so on. For those who like to describe events in terms of grades and numbers, the return of skin sensibility is more easily recorded by use of the Medical Research Council sensory scale of S0 to S4 [18]. However, the numbers should not obscure the fact that this is a qualitative, descriptive grading only.

The decision to re-suture because of failure of regeneration is very difficult. The cost (in lost time) of starting again from scratch is high and there is no guarantee of better luck next time. Much would depend on what the patient's wishes are and the level of experience of the surgeon who did the first operation. Rarely is such a decision taken because of dissatisfaction with the quality of tactile gnosis, when protective sensibility and some motor function have returned.

Comparing different treatments

Injuries to neural tissue throughout the body remain the source of massive morbidity. As already stated, much basic neurobiological work is in progress, aimed at finding ways to reawaken or enhance the ability of nerve cells to regenerate. Transections of peripheral nerves in the upper limb are the most likely human test bed for such new treatments because they are common and do show at least some regenerative ability. Comparative trials between different treatments could be very helpful.

Qualitative measures, such as the MRC S 0–4 scale, are of little use in this context. For these purposes, a quantitative expression of the end result is exactly what is needed.

This has proved very elusive, so much so that it is impossible to compare the results of one author with those of another. Again the problem is

mainly on the sensory side; unlike muscle function, which an outside observer can measure, sensation is known only to the subject. Although psychologists have many elaborate methods for investigating mechanisms underlying sensation, few have addressed themselves to the problems of applying them to people whose sensations are abnormal, as they are after peripheral nerve suture. Their methods are apt to be misleading, since patients do not recover a certain proportion of normal sensation, rather a new kind of sensation.

For example, a test such as two-point discrimination is very difficult to apply reliably in people with disordered sensation. False positives are common unless a rigorous testing technique is employed and most values obtained in outpatient clinics or occupational therapy departments are probably worthless [19]. Particularly misleading is the habit of using two-point discrimination as a summary measure of sensibility; there is no evidence that performance of any one sensory task adequately sums up sensory function in the normal hand, let alone the highly abnormal.

Overall function is probably best assessed by tests which involve the performance of integrated tasks with a high sensory component, such, as picking up small objects (Fig. 14.7), discriminating shapes or textures and so on [20]. These can be so arranged to give a quantitative result by scoring speed and accuracy. The score must be expressed as a ratio to performance by the patient's normal hand, not by reference to population norms: variation between people is far

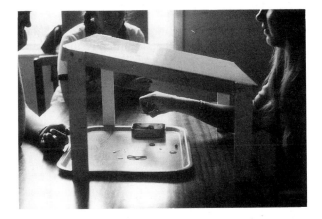

Fig. 14.7 The picking-up test, performed against the clock, developed from Moberg [20].

higher than variation between dominant and non-dominant hands.

More detailed assessment of sensory function is a specialist topic; ideally one would like to estimate both the numbers of the various populations of touch receptors reinnervated and the degree of topographic disorganization, but that is beyond the scope of this chapter.

Summary

The present situation is that results of nerve suture in adults are at best poor, because of the limited regenerative power of nerve cells and the topographic disorganization caused by transection of the endoneurial tubes. This will not change until huge strides have been made in understanding the neurobiology of regeneration.

In practice, even worse results often occur because of delay in diagnosis; this is avoidable by application of known principles. Immediate careful direct suture is the best treatment for the clean cut nerve. One should strive to

- appose the fascicles accurately;
- avoid intraneural fibrosis by gentle tissue handling.

References

1. Sunderland, S. (1945) The intraneural topography of the radial, median and ulnar nerves. *Brain*, **68**, 243–298.
2. Jabaley, M. E., Wallace, W. H. and Heckler, F. R. (1980) Internal topography of major nerves of the forearm and hand: a current view. *J. Hand Surg.*, **5**, 1–18
3. Mackel, R. (1985) Human cutaneous mechanoreceptors during regeneration: physiology and interpretation. *Ann. Neurol.*, **18**, 165–172.
4. Dellon, A. L. (1981) *Evaluation of Sensibility and Re-education of Sensation in the Hand*. Williams & Wilkins, Baltimore.
5. O'Riain, S. (1973) New and simple test of nerve function in the hand. *Br. Med. J.*, **3**, 615–616.
6. Wilson, G. R. (1985) A simple device for the objective evaluation of peripheral nerve injuries. *J. Hand Surg.*, **10B**, 324–330.
7. Lynch, G. and Quinlan, D. (1986). Jump function following nerve division. *Br. J. Plast. Surg.*, **39**, 364–366.
8. Smith, P. J. and Mott, G. (1986) Sensory threshold and conductance testing in nerve injuries. *J. Hand Surg.*, **11B**, 157–162.
9. Seddon, H. (1975) *Surgical Disorders of the Peripheral Nerves*, Churchill Livingstone, London, p. 275.
10. Birch, R. (1986) Lesions of peripheral nerves: the present position. *J. Bone Joint Surg.*, **68B**, 2–8.
11. Narakas, A. (1986) Editorial. *Peripheral Nerve. Repair and Regeneration*, **1**, 3–4.
12. Salvi, V. (1973) Problems connected with the repair of nerve sections. *Hand*, **5**, 25–32.
13. Donoso, R. S., Ballantyne, J. P. and Hansen, S. (1979) Regeneration of sutured human peripheral nerves: an electrophysiological study. *J. Neurol. Neurosurg. Psychiatry*, **42**, 97–106.
14. Young, L., Wray, C. and Weeks, P. M. (1981) A randomised prospective comparison of fascicular and epineural digital nerve repairs. *Plast. Reconstr. Surg.*, **68**, 89–93.
15. Marsh, D. and Barton, N. (1987) Does the use of the operating microscope improve the results of peripheral nerve suture? *J. Bone Joint Surg.*, **69B**, 625–630.
16. Almquist, E. E., Smith, O. A. and Fry, L. (1983) Nerve conduction velocity, microscopic, and electron microscopy studies comparing repaired adult and baby monkey median nerves. *J. Hand Surg.*, **8**, 406–410.
17. Millesi, H., Meissl, G. and Berger, A. (1972) The interfascicular grafting of the median and ulnar nerves. *J. Bone Joint Surg.*, **54A**, 727–750.
18. Medical Research Council (1954) Special Report Series no. 282. *Peripheral Nerve Injuries*. HMSO, London.
19. Moberg, E. (1987) Personal Communication.
20. Moberg, E. (1958) Objective methods for determining the functional value of sensibility in the hand. *J. Bone Joint Surg.*, **40B**, 454–476.

15

External skeletal fixation for the treatment of fractures

J. Kenwright

Introduction

External skeletal fixation was used in the last century and developed extensively by Hoffmann in 1938, who employed fixation for various types of fracture including fractures of the facial bones. Enthusiasm for the treatment method has waxed and waned, but since 1980 there has been a surge of increased use for many different types of fracture and it is interesting to define why this has occurred.

There have been major advances in plastic surgical techniques for replacing lost or severely damaged soft tissue, and these treatments rely on effective skeletal stabilization. Modern external skeletal fixation systems can always supply this need. Similarly, operations are available for reconstruction of large segmental bone defects, and an increased use of such methods has led to a greater need for external skeletal fixation. Infected fractures still present some of the most difficult problems in orthopaedic surgery and lead to prolonged morbidity. Although improved wound care has decreased the incidence of such disasters, the widespread use of internal fixation and the salvage of many limbs which might previously have been amputated has resulted in many infected pseudarthroses. External skeletal fixation is one of the mainstays of treatment for such problems. There have also been major advances in frame technology, so that complex fractures can be effectively stabilized.

These include fractures of the pelvis and juxta-articular regions as well as those of short bones.

More confident management of screw tracks has led to reduced fear of complications associated with infected tracks. Finally, the transfer of experiences through international communication has led to a widened use of external skeletal fixation in many countries over the last 10 years.

In the following sections the main indications for the use of external skeletal fixation in the treatment of the injured will be discussed. External fixator frame technology and application, the principles of treatment and the problems created will also be presented.

Indications

Fractures associated with severe soft tissue injury

External skeletal fixation has become the method of choice for stabilization of fractures associated with severe open or closed soft tissue injury (Fig. 15.1). Dramatic results have now been described from many sources, demonstrating that early stabilization of severe injuries can lead regularly to sound healing with a painless and functioning limb. Most of the studies are retrospective analyses of large numbers of patients but they do show clearly that effective stabilization by whatever means leads to lower rates of infection than seen for injuries of equivalent severity treated in casts. Hicks [1] first demonstrated this influence of stability using internal fixation; primary and secondary amputation rates were decreased for

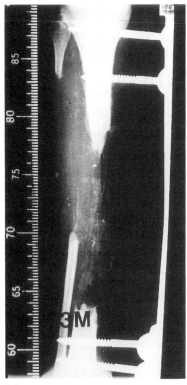

(a)

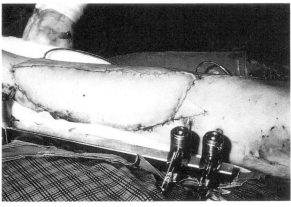

(b)

Fig. 15.1 Frames may need to meet considerable mechanical demands as seen here in (a) where there has been major bone loss. The patient could mobilize freely (b) following free vascularized grafting with skin, muscle and bone.

open tibial diaphyseal fractures if early stabilization with plates was used. In general, external skeletal fixation is now used for stabilizing such fractures, though internal fixation should still be considered first in the forearm and in femoral fractures. Internal fixation usually means increas-

ing local soft tissue damage in order to apply the implant, and such dissection is unnecessary with external skeletal fixation. Many of these injuries can now be treated by reamed or unreamed intramedullary nailing. For most open diaphyseal fractures there is little difference seen in the results from either nailing or treatment by external fixture.

With the use of effective stabilization, fracture infection rates for tibial diaphyseal fractures can be reduced to approximately 2% for grade I and II open fractures [2]. Infection rates of between 20% and 40% are still recorded for grade III open wounds even when employing modern methods of stabilization. In order to maintain these low rates of infection for lesser wounds and to try and reduce the infection rates for major wounds, it would seem important to stabilize fractures effectively very early after injury. The importance of obtaining vascularized soft tissue closure within 72 hours of injury has now also been demonstrated. There is little place for the use of skeletal traction or fracture stabilization with casts in the primary treatment of grade II or III open fractures, as neither offers sufficient stability for wound healing.

Less severe soft tissue injuries with skin of doubtful viability

Apparent simple skin contusion is often unmasked as necrosis several days from injury. This necrosis will then need excision, and fracture stabilization with external skeletal fixation will be required if the bone is subcutaneous. Such contusion with suspect skin is often treated best by stabilization of the fracture using external skeletal fixation as the primary treatment on the first day. This allows stable healing conditions for the damaged skin and may limit the extent of the subsequent necrosis. The serious and often unrecognized nature of many closed soft tissue injuries has been stressed by Tscherne and incorporated in his most useful system of classification of fractures in which closed fractures are classified into four types according to the scale CO–CIII [3].

Neurovascular injuries

If surgical repair of a major vascular or neurological structure is to be made, stabilization of the skeleton is needed. External skeletal fixation as a preliminary to vessel repair is usually the method of choice in such circumstances.

Compartment syndrome

If this crisis arises in the leg or forearm, the wide decompression needed invariably destabilizes the fracture completely and external skeletal fixation should be applied.

Multiple injuries

It has been shown recently that stabilization of multiple fractures within the first 24 hours of injury reduces the incidence and severity of adult respiratory distress syndrome (ARDS) [4]. External skeletal fixation can usually be applied to one or more fractures and be built into the operative programme so that several fractures are stabilized simultaneously. Such a plan of combined surgery is needed for multiple fractures to reduce the time of the initial emergency surgical programme.

Early application of external skeletal frames may even be needed in the receiving area of the Accident Department in order to reduce haemorrhage associated with severe pelvic fractures. The application of anterior frames under such circumstances may reduce pelvic volume and add just sufficient stability to reduce blood loss even if there is incomplete stabilization of the posterior elements of a fracture dislocation; this can be a life saving procedure.

The use of early external skeletal fixation of the tibia combined with closed nailing of a femoral fracture sustained in the same leg is especially indicated in order to facilitate early rehabilitation of the knee joint, and of muscle function in the leg.

Acute bone loss

Such loss is usually associated with severe soft tissue wounds and external skeletal fixation is the method usually chosen for fracture stabilization (Fig. 15.1). The defect can be treated by grafting, or acute shortening and remote distraction osteogenesis.

Fracture instability

External skeletal fixation is indicated frequently for treatment of unstable juxta-articular fractures of the radius and for fractures of the pelvis, where the main objective is to control fracture position, and where the degree of comminution or displacement may make internal fixation difficult. The use of external skeletal fixation for treatment of unstable closed fractures of the tibia or femur is advocated by some surgeons [5,6]; though fracture control is very effective the method is not universally popular, however, due to the significant incidence of screw track infections, and the prolonged healing times often seen with this method of treatment. Closed intramedullary nailing with locking screws is now the most effective treatment for such unstable fractures. The combination of external fixation and limited internal fixation is very safe and useful for pilon fractures.

Fracture infection

External skeletal fixation has revolutionized the treatment of fracture infection. The main principle of such treatment is the uncompromising excision of dead bone and creation of a healthy wound. Once this is accomplished, one of the following procedures for reconstruction of soft tissue or bony defect is selected.

i. Pappineau method with massive cancellous graft.
ii. Fibular transposition for tibial fractures.
iii. Free vascularized transfer of bone and soft tissue.
iv. Bone transport by the Ilizarov technique.

Each of these methods depends upon stabilization of the bony fragments in the presence of bone loss, this stabilization to be maintained for 6–12 months in many instances. This is a demanding situation for fixation which can now be treated effectively by external skeletal fixation.

Non-union

Stabilization is usually needed for the treatment of any atrophic, hypertrophic or infected non-union and external skeletal fixation should be considered for each problem. External fixation allows wound care, stabilization of fragments and mobilization of adjacent joints, and this often in patients in whom there are stiff joints due to previous prolonged conservative treatment. Bone graft can be applied through incisions remote from damaged skin.

External skeletal fixation may also be indicated for the treatment of many short bone fractures in the hand or wrist, for dislocations, for the correction of post-fracture deformity, or for arthrodesis performed early after devastating joint injuries.

Frames, screws and the bone screw interface

The ideal system

Many different external fixation frames are available, each designed to try to meet the specifications for an ideal fixation system. These are that frames should be (i) simple to apply by relatively inexperienced operators; (ii) convenient for the patient allowing overall mobility as well as muscle and joint rehabilitation; (iii) adjustable so that fracture position can be corrected after application and so that the mechanical conditions at the fracture site can be adjusted i.e., dynamization should be possible; (iv) versatile so that fractures in long and short bones as well as in the pelvis can be treated; (v) inexpensive and re-usable; and (vi) have standardized instruments designed for their application. Each available system has attempted to embrace many of the features that would make it 'ideal' but each has limitations because several of these specifications for the perfect frame are mutually exclusive.

In clinical practice it is probably necessary to have two types of frame available in an accident unit, including a simple unilateral system for diaphyseal fractures which represent the vast majority of fractures requiring treatment; a versatile complex system for pelvic, short bone, and complicated fractures is also essential. Circular frames are rarely needed for acute treatment of injuries.

Frame stability

Knowledge of frame stability has accumulated from clinical experience and from investigations made on material testing machines. The scientific literature and the manuals accompanying the frames describe the geometrical configurations which will give adequate stability and prevent loss of fracture position during rehabilitation for most fracture patterns [7,8].

The weakest link in all systems is the screw clamp junction, and loss of fracture position is usually due to failure at this point. When stiffness of the frame/fracture system is considered as opposed to failure strength all unilateral frames are considerably less stiff in antero-posterior bending than in other axes [7] Stiffness of the frame system depends on the material properties of the frame and on the geometry of the frame and screws as applied. Simple measures which give predictable increases in stability include decreasing the offset of the frame from the bone, increasing the number of screws, increasing the distance between screws and changing the angle of the screws so that they are not all in one plane. In the lower leg the bending moments are principally sagittal: if mechanical conditions alone were the most important ones then one set of screws should be inserted in the antero-posterior plane so as to resist effectively this

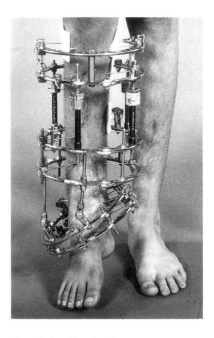

Fig. 15.2 Circular frames with tensioned thin wires give high degrees of bending stiffness but allow axial flexibility on weight bearing. Their main use is for correcting fracture deformity and for bone transport.

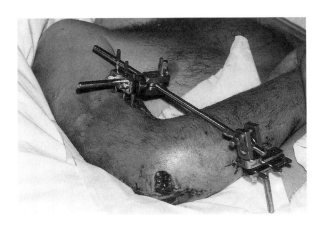

Fig. 15.3 Frames bridging joints should be removed as soon as possible; the wrist and inferior radio-ulnar joints will tolerate frames for approximately 4 weeks. The elbow joint is less tolerant.

bending moment. For very unstable fractures major modifications may be needed such as triangulation of the frame, the use of a dual frame configuration or change to a circular frame (Fig. 15.2).

A lot of emphasis has been placed upon the results obtained from tests upon simulated fractures fixed by frames and loaded in material testing machines. The conditions within these tests are often ideal with perfectly applied bone screws, a situation which is not always possible to achieve in clinical practice. In patients there may be very unstable or comminuted fractures, and the bone itself may be osteoporotic. Hence in clinical practice allowance needs to be made for these factors when planning application of a frame and when planning postoperative weight-bearing.

There is a considerable body of opinion now which advocates decreasing the stability of frames in one or more axis during the early or later stages of fracture healing to improve the mechanical environment for the healing fracture. Progressive dismantling of frames can be performed [9] or frames selected with features which allow dynamization [5,10]. It should, however, be noted that decreasing rigidity (and hence stiffness) in one axis may lead to a decrease in stiffness in another axis. For example, torsional stiffness may be reduced unevenly by such manoeuvres and this may lead to an inappropriate shear at the fracture on loading [8].

Choice of frame

In general unilateral frames are satisfactory for most diaphyseal fractures. Juxta-articular fractures may cause special problems as will any need to create fixation across a joint (Fig. 15.3), and for such circumstances a more complex frame will be needed. If progressive correction of deformity is required or bone transport is planned, circular frames are the most appropriate.

Bone pins and screws

The geometry of an external fixator results in large bending loads being carried by the screw in addition to some tensile and compressive loads. In experimental cadaveric studies, the application of a moderate value of cyclically applied load has been shown to result in an increased incidence of screw loosening over unloaded or statically loaded screws [11].

The likely mechanism causing this loosening would appear to be related to the amount of relative movement which occurs between the screw and the bone [12,13]. Hence, if the movement between the screw and the bone can be reduced, for example by using a larger stiffer screw, then the incidence of screw loosening may be expected to reduce. Large diameter screws also greatly enhance the stiffness of the fixator system.

Various types of screw threads have been tested, although there is insufficient evidence that one particular type is more effective than another. Most external fixators offer a specific screw for use with the fixator and some offer specific screws for both cancellous and cortical bone.

The concept of inserting crossed thin wires under tension with circular frames is an interesting alternative to the use of conventional screws. With these wires there can be considerable rigidity of a fracture and bone fragments in bending, yet flexibility in axial loading. This mechanical combination is claimed to give the most appropriate environment for fracture healing.

Fatigue failure of screws and pins is uncommon and is not considered to be a practical problem.

On fixator removal, the refracture rate through either small or large diameter screw holes is low. Remodelling occurs rapidly around screw holes which enhances local bone strength unless there is gross and continuing infection.

Application of frames

Planning

Preoperative planning is needed, making allowance for the nature of both the bone and soft tissue injury, as well as the mechanical demands that will be placed upon the fixation system. An overall plan for the type of frame to be used and its configuration should be made before entering the operating theatre so that necessary equipment can be available.

Detailed planning is needed for siting of the screws. Draping should show the whole contour of both limbs so that accurate alignment can be achieved. For many injuries, including fractures of the pelvis and in the distal forearm, certain standard positions for screw insertion have been well tested and are nearly always selected. For tibial and femoral fractures screw positions have to be chosen carefully for individual situations. Screws should be inserted at least 2 cm from the fracture itself, but this rule may have to be broken if there is severe comminution or if there are longitudinal splits through the bone. Under these circumstances fracture fragments may be penetrated and despite occasional infection of such screw tracks infection of fractures does not occur. Sites for screw insertion are chosen, other factors being equal, where there is thin soft tissue coverage between the skin surface and the bone, and where skin moves little during joint function. For tibial fractures the medial surface of the tibia is the most appropriate from this point of view and should be chosen, though the anterior crest is the most sound mechanically when using a unilateral frame. Other factors may predominate when choosing screw sites. These include planning for future plastic or other soft tissue surgery when adequate access to wounds may be a critical factor.

The normal anatomical siting of neurovascular structures will influence the placement of screws and this is a particularly important factor when inserting screws through the femur, tibia or humerus especially with the use of circular frames. The exact site of neurovascular structures should be checked in an atlas preoperatively: safe corridors for insertion for each bone have been defined by both Green [14] and Behrens [9].

Finally, when planning, the mechanical demands on the fixator should be considered carefully. The fracture may be very unstable and a plan must be made to use the appropriate frame and an adequate number of screws, these placed with optimum geometry. Postoperative demands on the fixator are affected by the patient's weight, the weight-bearing programme to be prescribed, and the overall activity related to the personality of the patient will also require consideration.

If there is a strong possibility that subsequent internal fixation may be needed, and exchange nailing is now frequently needed, the screw holes should be placed allowing for future skin incisions.

Insertion of screws

Having planned the sites of insertion for screws, an incision is made approximately 1 cm long so that tenting of the skin is not seen around the screw when joints function: this avoids skin necrosis which is accompanied by inevitable infection. Screw holes should be pre-drilled using a sharp drill bit to reduce thermal necrosis, and the surrounding skin needs protection during drilling. It is very easy to over-penetrate the distal cortex and injure nerves or vessels, this being a particular risk in the central half of the tibia. Screws can be placed accurately using image intensification and should be inserted through the centre of the bone for maximum mechanical effect. The screws should be inserted in a meticulous manner applying similar mechanical principles to those used with internal fixation.

Fracture reduction

Before tightening the clamps upon the screws major efforts should be made to reduce the fracture using any open wound for accurate reduction.

After care

At the end of the procedure, and whilst still within the operating theatre, the screw holes should be assessed in different positions of function to make sure there is no tenting of the skin. The frame should be offset from the limb sufficiently to allow for the considerable oedema which frequently follows serious injury. Reduction is checked on radiographs.

Postoperatively screw-hole management can be performed effectively by many means. Screw holes should be dressed each day and can be left wet with dressings or dry. If there are scabs, these should be removed to allow drainage.

Problem areas and complications

Major complications are rare as a direct result of the use of external skeletal fixation, but there are many minor problems and it is these which sway the surgeon away from the universal use of external skeletal fixation for the treatment of all unstable fractures.

Screw track problems (Fig. 15.4)

Screw track complications rarely cause permanent disability but their high incidence is one of the major objections to the use of external skeletal fixation. Well placed screw tracks, maintained in a meticulous manner can remain trouble free for approximately one month after insertion. There then follows an increasing in-

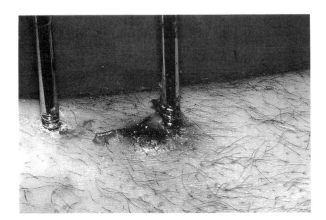

Fig. 15.4 Screw track problems are very common. The screw has to be replaced in infections like this. Skin tenting always leads to necrosis and secondary infection. Despite large residual screw holes in the bone late fracture through these is rare.

cidence of infection with or without loosening associated with increased patient activity. Reddening around the screw hole is seen frequently during excess use and responds well to immobilization for 24 hours, which both reduces the loading of the bone screw interface and the fretting of the screw on the soft tissues. Positive signs of infection require antibiotic therapy as well as rest. If infection continues with discharge, and lysis is seen on radiographs the screw needs replacing at a site at least 1.5 cm from the initial placement. Despite many problems seen with screw tracks, it is unusual to have to abandon the treatment method prematurely because of these complications. When treating complex conditions such as infected non-unions, frames can be maintained for over 1 year.

After removal of screws infection nearly always resolves. Ugly pitted scars may remain but are amenable to minor surgical procedures. Osteomyelitis may persist following screw removal and radiographs including tomograms may show a small ring sequestrum. In this situation the track needs full curettage under general anaesthetic when the condition nearly always resolves. Refracture through screw holes is very unusual even when using 6.0 mm screws.

Loss of fracture position

This complication should be guarded against and usually follows incorrect insertion of screws or gross overloading of the system.

Joint function

Loss of function can be associated with any fracture but is encountered commonly in both the ankle joint after tibial fractures and in the knee joint after stabilization of femoral fractures. When treating tibial fractures equinus deformity develops very readily due mainly to postoperative discomfort with inhibited muscle action: the equinus remains and is often impossible to correct at a later stage; however, this problem is avoidable. An intensive physiotherapy programme is needed with this type of injury, starting immediately after frame application, and it is advisable to apply a plastic or plaster of Paris splint with the foot in the plantargrade position

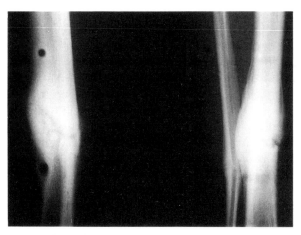

Fig. 15.5 Healing with external callus formation is 'ideal'. There is often a gap at the fracture site, and also rapid healing is needed so that frames can be removed as early as possible.

at the time of initial frame application. If the frame has to be applied on the lateral side of the leg because of soft tissue damage the screws passing through the anterior compartment will increase the risk of equinus deformity and vigorous steps need to be taken to prevent permanent deformity.

When stabilizing femoral fractures through the lower third of the femur the screws pass through the fascia lata: it is crucial that longitudinal division of this fascia is made at the time of frame application and that the knee is put through its normal range of movement in the operating theatre. If this is not done, extensive knee stiffness will follow. Patients need to be encouraged firmly to use the knee during the early days after femoral fixation and adequate sedation and supervision of movement is needed in the first week.

If a joint has to be bridged by a frame the joint will nearly always have permanent substandard function, although bridging the wrist joint during the treatment of lower radial fractures does not appear to lead to major stiffness so long as the frames are removed within 4 weeks.

Problems with fracture healing

Fixation systems and the fracture healing process

Experimental and clinical experiences have shown that the fracture healing process is acutely sensitive to the mechanical environment at the fracture site. It is also claimed that external skeletal fixation inhibits healing of diaphyseal fractures, and that most frames offer too much rigidity. This latter point is difficult to prove, as external skeletal fixation is used in general for the most severe types of fracture which have very long and varied healing times whatever treatment method is employed.

The pattern of healing when using external skeletal fixation for diaphyseal fractures is that of secondary fracture healing, or healing by external callus formation (Fig. 15.5). Even with meticulous reduction of such fractures at the time of frame application, there is always a significant gap or incongruity at the fracture site so that primary bone healing or 'gap healing' cannot occur. It is now known that under such fracture healing conditions functional stimulation is required, and this at an early stage during the treatment. With serious long bone fractures treated by external skeletal fixation using rigid frames such stimulation is unlikely to occur. This has been confirmed in patients being treated by unilateral external skeletal fixation by measuring the amount of movement that does occur at the fracture site during weightbearing in the early weeks after fracture. It was shown that very little movement occurs at the fracture site in the first 6 weeks after injury [15]. Burny [6] has shown that many fractures of the tibia heal rapidly if treated with external skeletal fixation using 'minimum fixation' with a non-rigid unilateral Hoffmann frame configuration.

Similarly De Bastiani [5] and Behrens [9] have proposed that fractures of the tibia should be dynamized after an interval of 6 weeks, either by adjusting the frame to allow dynamic loading during weightbearing or by progressive dismantling of the frame.

There is also evidence that strain should be applied to fractures within the early weeks after injury, though the timing must vary with the severity of soft tissue injury [10,16].

With the types of programme described in these studies frames were applied as early as possible after injury and maintained at least until clinical union had been reached. There is a school of thought which proposes that frames be removed as soon as the initial soft tissue injury has healed; subsequent treatment would be by a cast. In this way the advantages of external skeletal fixation and functional cast treatment can be embraced so that the most appropriate mechanical environment exists throughout treatment. In our experience removing frames at early stages has nearly always led to unsatisfactory bone healing and if this method is to be used it is suggested that bone grafting is applied at the time of frame removal.

Combinations of internal and external fixation can be employed and accurate reduction be maintained by minimal internal fixation (Fig. 15.6), the external skeletal fixation system supplying the majority of stability. The mechanical environment associated with this type of combined fixation inhibits external callus formation. Healing of the fracture will occur eventually after many months but if the frame is removed before such healing has occurred very careful protection of the fracture will be needed and it is recommended that bone graft should also be applied, with the frame *in situ*.

Failure of healing

Delayed or non-union is common in diaphyseal fractures treated by external skeletal fixation. External fixation is used for the most severe types of injury and long healing times of over 20 weeks are common for tibial fractures. With these types of injury there must be a strong case for adding bone graft if there is any bone loss, or significant comminution. The graft is applied at the initial operation or within the first 6 weeks of injury.

Despite a low threshold for the use of bone graft, non-union may still develop. This can then be treated by further bone grafting of the fracture whilst maintaining the frame *in situ*, but other methods should be considered in this situation. If the soft tissues have healed soundly it may be appropriate to change to internal fixation, preferably with the use of a locked intra-medullary nail for diaphyseal fractures. If this change in treatment method is to be used the limb should be

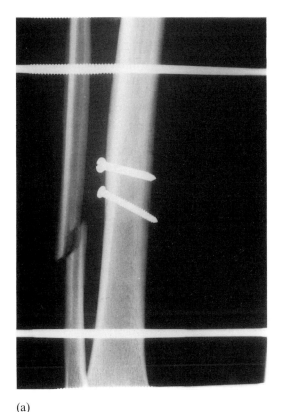 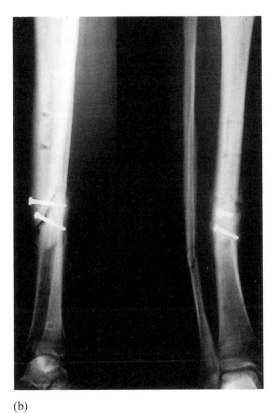

(a)   (b)

Fig. 15.6 Combinations of internal and external fixation enable accurate reductions to be maintained as seen in radiograph (a). Such stabilization inhibits external callus formation and predisposes to mechanical failure when the frame is removed (b).

immobilized in a cast for at least 1 month after frame removal before embarking on the internal fixation. This interval allows local screw tracks to heal soundly and reduces the risk of fracture through the screw holes. If internal fixation is planned the screw tracks should be curetted formally at the time of frame removal.

The treatment of infected non-union is a complex subject which cannot be covered within the scope of this chapter. All the principles of external skeletal fixation apply to these difficult problems.

Patient tolerance

Frames are well tolerated by patients despite intermittent screw-track infections and the need for multiple hospital attendances. A few patients have an unfavourable psychological response to external skeletal fixation and develop a strong rejection response to the presence of the appliance on the limb; if this occurs the frame must be removed.

Conclusions

The recent developments in external skeletal fixation have changed the management of many types of fracture and particularly severe open fractures, fractures with bone loss and fracture infection; the method offers safe, atraumatic, and effective stabilization of complex fractures.

Planning is required even in the emergency situation; it is important for subsequent care for the frames to be applied with meticulous attention to mechanical details in the same way as employed with internal fixation. Planning should also take into account the mechanical demands that will be placed upon the leg and the subsequent surgery that might be needed both to bone and soft tissue.

This type of stabilization when used for open fractures is associated with very low rates of fracture infection if there has also been correct wound care. It is, however, becoming clear that certain types of devastating fracture below the knee might still best be treated by primary amputation [17]. Careful review of the long-term results of type III C tibial fractures, with associated vascular damage and soft tissue loss, shows that most patients in this group still require a secondary amputation; this end result is seen despite technically satisfactory primary fixation and rescue of a viable limb. If this group is excluded it is probable that external skeletal fixation is the method of choice for stabilization of most diaphyseal fractures with grade 2 or 3 open wounds.

The future for external skeletal fixation for fracture control for severe injuries is clear, but the place of the treatment method for treatment of simple fracture instability is still in doubt.

There is still room for development of frame technology perhaps incorporating new materials, and for further studies of the influence of adjustment of flexibility to enable the most appropriate mechanical environment to be applied at the different stages of fracture healing for an individual fracture.

References

1. Hicks, J. H. (1964) Amputation in fractures of the tibia. *J. Bone Joint Surg.*, **46B**, 388–392.
2. Gustilo, R. B. and Anderson, J. T. (1976) Prevention of infection in the treatment of one thousand and twenty-five open fractures of long bones. *J. Bone Joint Surg.*, **58A**, 453–458.
3. Tscherne, H. and Oestern, H. J. (1982) Quoted in Szyszkowitz, R. (1988) *Curr. Orthop.*, **2**, 14–17.
4. Johnson, K. D., Cadambi, A. and Burton, S. (1985) Incidence of adult respiratory distress syndrome in patients with multiple skeletal injuries. Effects of early operative stabilisation of fractures. *J. Trauma*, **25**, 375–384.
5. De Bastiani, G., Aldegheri, R. and Brivio, L. R. (1984) The treatment of fractures with a dynamic axial fixator. *J. Bone Joint Surg.*, **66B**, 538–545.
6. Burny, F. (1979) Elastic external fixation of tibial fractures: study of 1421 cases. In: *External Fixation: the Current State of the Art* (eds H. F. Brooker and C. C. Edwards), Williams & Wilkins, Baltimore.
7. McCoy, M. T., Kasman, R. A. and Chao, E. Y. (1983) Comparison of mechanical performance in four types of external fixators. *Clin. Orthop. Rel. Res.*, **180**, 23–33.
8. Finlay, J. B., Moroz, T. K., Rorabeck, C. H., Davey, J. R. and Bourne, R. B. (1985) Stability of ten configurations of the Hoffman external fixation frame. *J. Bone Joint Surg.*, **67B**, 734–744.

9. Behrens, F. and Searls, K. (1986) External fixation of the tibia. Basic concepts and prospective evaluation. *J. Bone Joint Surg.*, **68B**, 246–254.

10. Kenwright, J., Goodship, A. E., Kelly, D. J., Newman, J. H., Harris, J. D., Richardson, J. B., Evans, M., Spriggins, A. J., Burrough, S. J. and Rowley, D. I. (1986) Effect of controlled axial micromovement on healing of tibial fractures. *Lancet*, **ii**, 1185–1187.

11. Pettine, K. A., Kelly, P. J., Chao, E. Y. S. and Huiskes, R. (1986) Histologic and biomechanical analysis of external fixator pin-bone interface. *Orthop. Transac.*, **10**, 337.

12. Scatzker, J., Horne, J. G. and Sumner-Smith, G. (1975) The effect of movement on the holding power of screws in bone. *Clin. Orthop. Rel. Res.*, **111**, 257–262.

13. Uthoff, H. K. (1973) Mechanical factors influencing the holding power of screws in compact bone. *J. Bone Joint Surg.*, **55B**, 633–639.

14. Green, S. A. (1981) *Complications of External Skeletal Fixation: Causes, Prevention, Treatment.* C. Thomas, Springfield, Illinois.

15. Cunningham, J. L., Evans, M. and Kenwright, J. (1989) The measurement of fracture movement in patients treated with unilateral external skeletal fixation. *J. Biom. Eng.*, **11(2)**, 118–122.

16. Goodship, A. E. and Kenwright, J. (1985) The influence of induced micromovement upon the healing of experimental tibial fractures. *J. Bone Joint Surg.*, **66B**, 650–655.

17. Hansen, S. T. (1987) Editorial. The type III C tibial fracture, salvage or amputation. *J. Bone Joint Surg.*, **69A**, 799–780.

16

Brachial plexus injuries

A. O. Narakas†, P. M. Yeoman and C. B. Wynn Parry

Part 1 Surgical Reconstruction

A. O. Narakas

Introduction

During the last 22 years the author has been confronted with over 1200 various plexopathies (Tables 16.1 and 16.2), 864 patients being victims of accidents in their postnatal life. It is this latter group which will be presented.

At first sight these 864 patients with traumatic brachial plexus injury (BPI) are numerous enough to yield valuable statistics. In reality, this is hardly the case because we do not see all cases of BPI, but only the severe ones, and many come from neighbouring countries. In the first 500 patients seen only 360 were living in Switzerland, in the last 300 seen only 246. Therefore it is difficult to establish the frequency of BPI in Switzerland. A survey of patients admitted to the University Hospital of Lausanne after trauma

Table 16.1 Aetiology of brachial plexus injuries caused by kinetic displacement (patients seen by the author between 1.1.1965 and 15.5.1988)

		%	Conservative treatment or orthopaedic reconstruction	Operated on their plexus	Operated by other surgeons
Road traffic accidents 669 = 77.4%					
Using motorcycles (125 cc and more)	394	45.6	115	292	7
Using motorcycles (< 125 cc)	76	8.8	33	42	1
Using bicycles	37	4.3	10	27	
Using cars and other vehicles	105	12.2	50	54	1
Pedestrians hit by vehicles	57	6.6	33	24	
Various accidents 195 = 22.6%					
In factories, building sites, forestry, agriculture	59	6.8	41	18	
Sport (mostly skiing)	47	5.4	38	9	
Benign falls (from own height)	78	9.0	77	1	
Severe falls	11	1.3	4	7	
Totals	864	100	401	455	9

† Deceased

Table 16.2   Various plexopathies (referred for diagnosis and treatment between 1.1.1965 and 15.5.1988)

		Conservative treatment or orthopaedic surgery	*Operated on their plexus*	*Operated by other surgeons on the plexus*
Obstetrical palsy	162	141*	19	2
Post-radiation	72	34**	36	2
Iatrogenic (sections, ligatures, crush, drills, etc.)	32	13	18	1
Gunshot wounds	19	10	9	
Various tumours	19	4	15	
Pancoast tumour	8	1	7	
Secondary compressions after trauma (callus, fibrous bands, scar)	12	0	12	
Severe paralytic thoracic outlet syndromes	19	0	17	2
Parsonage–Turner syndromes	19	17	2	
Rucksack palsy or analogous	3	3	0	
Cervical disk hernias	3	0	0	3***
Various radicular syndromes	21	2	2	17***
Various myelopathies and encephalopathies	12	3	0	9***
Probable psychogenic (hysterical palsy)	3	2	1	
Post-vaccination	3	1	0	2***
Idiopathic	5	0	0	5***
Totals	412	231	138	43

* Nine patients are on the waiting list for reconstructive orthopaedic surgery.
** One patient on the waiting list for neurolysis and omentoplasty.
*** Referred elsewhere or no treatment prescribed.

has shown a yearly variation (over 7 years) between 3 and 7.5 per 10 000 cases. A survey of patients admitted to hospital after motorcycle accidents or related vehicles has shown a variation of 2% maximum to 0.7% minimum. This does not include patients coming to polyclinics in the departments of neurology, orthopaedics or plastic and reconstructive surgery; the latter is incorporated in our hospital which is primarily involved with hand surgery.

Diagnosis has evolved over the years because of refinements such as CT scan combined with myelography with hydrosoluble dye, magnetic resonance imaging, evoked sensory and nerve action potentials which have become available. The operative treatment has also involved combining nerve reconstructive measures with old and new orthopaedic operative procedures. The requirements of today's patients with BPI have also changed. Young people with persisting complete palsy do not accept amputations and even refuse orthotic devices because it 'stamps' them as invalids. Therefore these 864 cases of BPI are far from homogenous. However, they provided

the author with ever increasing experience in this field, and in this chapter attempts will be made to convey it to the reader.

Classification of brachial plexus injuries

Traditionally BPIs are divided into supraclavicular and infraclavicular palsies, the former being complete or incomplete, the latter sparing usually the suprascapular nerve and the clavicular portion of pectoralis major. However, experience has shown that this classification does not necessarily correspond to levels of injury. A classification into five levels has been proposed by the author [1]. Level I corresponds to roots, level II to the anterior ramus of the spinal nerve, level III to trunks, level IV to cords and level V to the origins of individual peripheral branches of the BP. This classification has to be applied for each anatomical structure originating from the five roots of the BP. For instance, a common type of injury is a rupture of the upper trunk C5–C6 (level III), a rupture of the anterior branch of C7 (level II) and a root avulsion C8 and T1 (level I). However, the same clinical picture will be produced by a rupture of the suprascapular nerve at the scapular notch (level V), rupture of the divisions leaving the upper and middle trunks (level III–IV) to form the cords and a lower root avulsion C8–T1 (level I). Retro- and infraclavicular lesions often show a distal lesion of the suprascapular nerve, of the whole posterior cord or only of the axillary and possibly radial nerves of the lateral cord or only the musculocutaneous

nerve. Occasionally the origin of the median and ulnar nerves is also affected. In fact, any classification is condemned to have numerous exceptions or subgroups due to the complex anatomical features of the BP. Total loss of function can be explained by five degrees of severity of injury as proposed by Sunderland [2] each having a totally different prognosis and requiring different types of treatment [3].

For example: degree 1 (Seddon's neurapraxia [4] requires rest only, degrees 2 and 3 (axo-

Table 16.3   Radicular avulsions as seen at operation in patients with traction injuries of the brachial plexus ($n = 422$, supraclavicular $n = 219$, more distal $n = 203$)

Roots avulsed	n pat.	n roots	Distribution and n of individual roots					Remarks
			C5	C6	C7	C8	T1	
C5 isolated	1 (PRF)	1	1	0	0	0	0	C5 in a prefixed plexus corresponds actually to C6
C6 isolated	14	14	0	14	0	0	0	
C7 isolated	17 (2 POF)	17	0	0	17	0	0	C7 in a post fixed plexus corresponds to C6
C8 isolated	5 (1 POF)	5	0	0	0	5	0	C8 in a POF corresponds to C7 actually
T1 isolated	2	2	0	0	0	0	2	
C5–C6	6	12	6	6	0	0	0	
C6–C7	9 (2 POF)	18	0	9	9	0	0	C6–C7 in POF correspond actually to C5–C6
C7–C8	4 (1 POF)	8	0	0	4	4	0	C7–C8 correspond to C6–C7
C8–T1	32	64	0	0	0	32	32	
C5–through C7	7	21	7	7	7	0	0	In one case C4 was also avulsed
C6–C8–T1	5 (1 POF)	15	0	5	0	5	5	The POF case corresponds to a C5–C7–C8 avulsion
C7–C8–T1	44	132	0	0	44	44	44	
C6–C7–T1	2	6	0	2	2	0	2	
C5 through C8	3	4	3	3	3	3	0	
C5–C6, C8–T1	2	8	2	2	0	2	2	
C5, C7–C8–T1	2	8	2	0	2	2	2	
C6 through T1	39	156	0	39	39	39	39	
C5 through T1	25	125	25	25	25	25	25	In one case C3 and C4 were also avulsed
Totals	219	624	46	112	152	161	153	
%		52		7.4	17.9	24.4	25.8	24.5	

N.B. In 13 additional cases with root avulsions: two of C6, three of C8, two of T1, three of C6–C7, two of C5–C6–C7 and one of C7–C8–T1 have not been recognized at operation (intraforaminal avulsion or in the spinal canal) and diagnosed much later. This increases to 232 (55%) patients with root avulsions and to 646 the roots avulsed, percentages changing to 18, 4 for C6, the others being hardly affected.

notmesis) requires rest followed by physio-therapy, degrees 4 and 5 (neurotmesis), possible surgery. Five roots, five anterior branches of spinal nerves C5–T1, three trunks, three cords, eleven terminal branches and in 5% of cases the accessory spinal and phrenic nerves, can present with any of these five degrees of severity of injury, including avulsion of roots in various combina-tions. Moreover, traction lesions may extend over a length of the entire plexus which produces a great variety of pathological changes and further confuses a set classification. However, instrumental and surgical explorations of BPI provide us with some information about the fre-quency of some lesions. Table 16.3 shows the distribution of root avulsions. C5 is the least vulnerable, but C6 and in some cases C7 are tethered by fibrous tissue investing their epi-neurium to the rims of the foramen, while C8 and T1 have such an anchorage rendering them more vulnerable to avulsion [5]. Table 16.4 shows the frequency of lesional patterns encountered at sur-gical exploration.

Lesions associated with BPI

Whenever the surgeon is confronted with a trac-tion BPI in the days or weeks after injury present-ing with a partial or total palsy, he has to decide which degrees of injury he is dealing with. Treat-ment will depend on this initial assessment of pathology. Some clues are helpful, such as the evaluation of kinetic deceleration energies caused by the accident. Only violent trauma will rupture or avulse the BP. Such violence will frequently produce regional injuries [6].

Fractures

When associated with BPI, fractures have a sini-ster significance, e.g. fractures of the transverse processes of the lower cervical vertebrae, and fractures or dislocation of the neck of the first and second ribs are consistent with lower root avulsions.

A rupture of the subclavian or axillary artery in young patients is practically always accom-panied by ruptures of nerve trunks, cords, ter-minal branches or root avulsions. In 57 consecutive cases of injury to these vessels, there has been only one case in a young patient in whom portions of the plexus were not ruptured but only elongated (degrees 2 and 3 of severity of injury), therefore not requiring nerve repair. Conversely, two patients aged over 60 years pre-sented with an axillary artery lesion, one after a fall from her own height dislocating the shoulder, the other after receiving a blow to the upper

Table 16.4(a)   Pathology found at operation in 100 consecutive patients with a total BP palsy persisting 2 months or more after the accident

Macroscopical pathology	N	Missed pre- or peroperative diagnosis
Avulsion of C5 through T1	14	2 partial Brown–Séquard syndromes
Rupture of C5 through T1	4	2 avulsions C8–T1 and one C7–T1
Rupture of C5, avulsion C6 through T1	23	
Elongation of C5, avulsion C6 through T1	3	
Rupture of C5–C6, avulsion C7–C8–T1	22	one C6 avulsion
Rupture of C5–C6, various injuries to C7–C8–T1	3	
Avulsion of C5–C6, elongation C7–C8–T1	1	one avulsion of C7
Elongation of C5–C6–C7, avulsion C8–T1	11	one avulsion of C7
Rupture C5–C6–C7, elongation C8–T1	3	
Rupture C5, avulsion C6, rupture C7–C8–T1	2	
Rupture C5, avulsion C6, rupture C7, elongation C8–T1	1	
Rupture C5–C6, elongation C7, avulsion C8–T1	1	
Avulsion C5, rupture C6, avulsion C7–T1	2	
Elongation of all primary trunks	1	
Elongation of cords and terminal branches	2	one avulsion of C7
Rupture of cords and/or terminal branches	6	

In 76 patients there were root avulsions at operation; in 6 they were missed, giving a total of 82 patients with root avulsions.

Table 16.4(b)   Pathology found at operation in 50 consecutive patients with apparently partial supraclavicular BPI persisting 2–12 months after injury

	N	Remarks
Clinical palsy (C4) C5–C6		
Elongation C5–C6 ± suprascapular nerve	4	
Elongation C5–C6, musculocutaneous and axillary nerves	3	2 partial C5–C6 avulsions not recognized
Elongation C5, avulsion C6	1	
Rupture C5, elongation C6 ± suprascapular nerve	2	
Rupture C5–C6	6	
Rupture C5, avulsion C6	2	
Avulsion C5–C6	4	one partial Brown–Séquard syndrome not recognized
Clinical palsy (C4) C5, C6, C7		
Elongation C5–C6–C7	3	one axillary nerve rupture found and repaired
Rupture C5, avulsion C6, elongation C7	1	one axillary and musculo-cutaneous nerve found and repaired
Rupture C5–C6, elongation C7	2	
Rupture C5–C6–C7	5	
Rupture C5, avulsion C6–C7	3	
Avulsion C5–C6, elongation C7	1	
Avulsion C5–C6–C7	4	one partial Brown–Séquard syndrome not recognized
Clinical palsy C7–C8–T1 or C8–T1		
C5–C6 normal, C7 elongation C8–T1 avulsion	1	
C5–C6 normal, avulsion C7–C8–T1	4	one rupture of musculocutaneous nerve found and one of axillary nerve
C5–C6–C7 normal, elongation C8–T1	2	
C5 to C7 normal, avulsion C8–T1	1	
C5–C6 normal, avulsion C7 ⎱		
C8–T1 ruptured ⎰	1	

N.B. In 44% of patients with incomplete supra-clavicular lesions there are root avulsions and in 8% two level injury is present.

chest. The vascular lesion of the brittle artery was similar to a fracture and less like a rupture caused by elongation. Both patients had 2–3 degrees nerve injuries, i.e. without interruption; therefore they did not require nerve repair and the function of their limbs recovered fairly well in $1\frac{1}{2}$ years. The author has seen also three cases of acute thrombosis, one of the axillary and two of the subclavian artery, followed by a complete BP infraclavicular palsy, i.e. without any mechanical trauma. Pathogenesis of BP palsy with 'fractures' of atheromatous arteries after minor trauma could be analogous to the ones seen in thrombosis. Similarly, ulnar artery thrombosis in the Guyon's canal also produces a complete distal ulnar nerve palsy.

Other associated and relatively minor injuries

Table 16.5 give useful information with regards to regional associated lesions seen in BPI. We have studied the frequency of BP in trauma to the cervical spine [7], of the shoulder girdle and arm using the files of Lausanne's University Hospital, and from several main trauma centres in Switzerland. An error varying from 2 to 3% has to be admitted, e.g. shoulder dislocations may present with a suprascapular, an axillary musculo-cutaneous nerve palsy or a mild BP involvement which are not diagnosed during ambulatory treatment or a short stay in hospital. Diagnosis will be made later and will not necessarily appear in the hospital files. In this region with a popu-

Table 16.5 Associated lesions in 300 consecutive patients with traction BPI

| Regional trauma | Complete supraclavicular palsies C5 – T1 n = 168 | | Incomplete supraclavicular palsies | | | | Extended or limited infraclavicular palsies n = 47 | |
| | | | C5–C6 (C7) n = 79 | | (C7)C8–T1 n = 6 | | | |
	n	%	n	%	n	%	n	%
Lateral fractures of cervical spine	9	5.3	2	2.5	1	16.7	0	0
Fractures and dislocations of first rib, and first and second ribs	10	5.9	0	0	2	33.3	0	0
Fractures of the scapula	43	25.6	8	10.1	0	0	4	8.5
Acromio-clavic ⎱ joint or sterno-clavic ⎰ disloc.	10	5.9	3	3.8	1	16.7	2	4.3
Fractures of clavicle	17	10.1	4	5.1	0	0	2	4.3
Proximal humerus fract.	17	10.1	2	2.5	1	16.7	4	8.5
Fract. of scapula and clavicle and/or of proximal humerus	11	6.5	1	1.3	0	0	2	4.3
Ruptures of the rotator cuff	4	2.4	3	3.8	0	0	5	10.6
Disloc. of the shoulder	3	1.8	6	7.6	1	16.7	6	12.8
Multitrauma to upper limb	12	7.1	0	0	0	0	4	8.5
Partial Brown–Séquard syn.	5	3	1	1.3	0	0	0	0
Rupture of subclavian or axillary artery	32	19	3	3.8	1	16.7	6	12.8
Rupture of artery and vein	4	2.4	0	0	0	0	2	4.3
Rupture of the vein alone	1	0.6	0	0	0	0	1	2.1

lation of half a million, the author sees practically all the cases of BPI and the error rate of our hospital statistics could be ascertained. Initially it is very difficult to diagnose a partial BPI or an isolated nerve palsy in a patient with multiple trauma who is possibly unconscious. Even in shoulder dislocation producing acute distress it requires much experience to establish a supra-scapular or an axillary nerve palsy. We have proceeded to routine EMG in traumatic humero-scapular dislocations in 34 consecutive cases before that study was stopped for ethical reasons. In over 70% of cases (25 patients) there were significant alterations in the deltoid (fibrillations, etc.), showing that a partial lesion of the axillary nerve was present. Only five patients in this group presented with a clinical palsy; three required exploration and the nerve was ruptured in two, continuous in one. The latter did not recover satisfactorily after neurolysis, whereas the other two did well after grafting. We should have resected the rosary type lesion in continuity and grafted the defect. This shows that not only the diagnosis is difficult clinically but even the sever-

ity of lesions can be misinterpreted at operation by an experienced surgeon such as the author who has operated on 103 axillary nerves.

Analysis of 994 cases of trauma to the shoulder girdle (Table 16.6) admitted to three hospitals shows clearly that there is a considerable differ-ence regarding nerve injury between cases with lesions to isolated structures of the shoulder girdle and those who have multiple regional or general injuries from a violent accident. One patient out of three with severe cervical shoulder girdle and general trauma will present a BPI or related nerve injury. Fifty-eight percent of these patients were motorcycle riders or passengers. About 1.3% of patients admitted to hospital with significant multiple injuries to the upper limbs (fractures, dislocations, etc.) after a motorcycle accident present a BP or a related nerve injury, while this incidence is 15 times less in occupants of cars. In 115 consecutive cases with fractures of the cervical spine and no spinal cord injury, three patients (2.6%) presented a BPI all associated with fractures of segments C4 to C7 (51 cases); none with fractures of segments C1 to C3 (64

Table 16.6   Incidence of BP and related nerve injuries in shoulder girdle trauma
n = 994 patients admitted to 3 hospitals*

Diagnosis	n *patients*	n *with diagnosed nerve injuries*	%
A. Severe blunt trauma including contused wounds but no dislocations nor fractures	48	2	4.2
One bone or one joint injured	537	7	1.3
Several shoulder girdle structures injured	349	31	8.9
Extended shoulder girdle and general trauma	60	19	31.7
	994	59	5.9
B. 1. any shoulder dislocation	219	24	11
2. proximal humerus fract.	254	8	3.1
3. fract. clavicle	234	7	3
4. AC jt dislocation	105	1	0.97
5. fract. scapula	90	8	8.9
6. fract. scapula and clavicle	18	4	22.2
7. AC dislocation, fract. of proximal humerus	5		
8. shoulder dislocation and fract. prox. humerus	13	2	15.4
9. scapula and shoulder dislocation	8	2	25
10. fract. scapula, shoulder and AC joint dislocation	2	1	50
	946	57	

*I am indebted to Dr. R. Blatter from the General Hospital, Bellinzona, to Professors J. J. Livio and S. Krupp from the University Hospital, Lausanne, and to Professor W. Taillard from the University Hospital Geneva, for making their statistics available.

cases). Conversely in 600 consecutive BPI patients (8.8%) presented with fractures of the cervical spine. There were four at the level of C1 to C3 and 49 (92.5%) at the level from C4 to T1 including the first rib. In particular, fractures of transverse processes are frequent in these cases (32 patients of 49, i.e. 65%) while vertebral bodies were fractured in only 16 patients (32.7%) and articular processes in nine patients (18.4%).

Spontaneous recovery

Bonney [8], Yeoman [9], Wynn Parry [10,11], Sedel [12], Ransford and Hughes [13], and the author have followed a certain number of patients with complete palsies of the upper limb after BPI under conservative treatment observing spontaneous recovery. Though these authors have not always used the same criteria for evaluation, a comparison between these studies has been attempted in Table 16.7. This table shows essentially that after excluding those with neuropraxia approximately 45% of patients with a total palsy persisting a few months will stay that way for ever. A detailed study of our series of 50 patients who were not operated on for various reasons (infection, late referral, operations refused, etc.) though they would have been if it had been possible, shows that there are seven patterns of recovery:

Group 1: 2 patients
All recovered well except those with involvement of C7.
Group 2: 8 patients
C5/6 lesions recovered well; C7 poor recovery and C8/T1 no recovery at all.
Group 3: 4 patients
C5 recovered well; C6 and C7 poor recovery and C8/T1 no recovery at all (myelography carried out in only 2 and avulsion of C8 and T1 nerve roots confirmed).
Group 4: 13 patients
Minimal recovery in C5 and C6 but none elsewhere. All had Horner's syndrome. Myelography was carried out in eight patients and all revealed multiple root avulsions.
Group 5: 3 patients
All had Horner's syndrome. One myelograph performed which showed avulsion of C8 and T1 nerve roots. All three patients showed some recovery in C7 but none elsewhere.
Group 6: 14 patients

Table 16.7 **Spontaneous recovery in complete traumatic brachial plexus injuries**

Authors	n patients	n with recovery	%	Shoulder %		Elbow %		Wrist %		Fingers %	
				Add	Abd	Fl	Ex	Fl	Ex	Fl	Ex
Bonney (4)	19	12	63	63	16	32	32	26	0	21	0
Yeoman (18)	99	53	53	45?	3	50	30	23	7	9	7
Wynn Parry (16)	23*	3	13	13	0	13	0	13	0	13	0
Sedel (12)	65	44	68	?	18	35	25	27	0	23	11
Wynn Parry (17)	several hundred		approx. 67	70	10	50	30	20	?	20	?
Narakas	50	30	60	58	18	30	18	28	4	18	4
	Average percentage of recovery		54	50	11	35	23	23	2	17	4

N.B. External rotation in the shoulder was studied only by Bonney and Narakas, noting recovery respectively in 10.5% and 14%, i.e. an average of 12% of patients.
* 14 amputees in Wynn–Parry series.

All had Horner's syndrome. Myelography carried out in 9; avulsions of lower 3 roots in 4 patients and all roots C6–T1 in the other 5.
Group 7: 6 patients
Some recovery in C8/T1 but none elsewhere. One had Horner's syndrome.

Twenty-three patients in this series which were similar to those reported by Yeoman had marked or severe pain. Thirty-four were involved in a motor cycle accident. The follow-up ranged from 3 to 27 years; mean 5.6 years.

Motor recovery in 50 patients in the non-operative series. Muscle power to M3 [MRC grading (6) = contraction against gravity] or better:

Protective skin sensibility

Eleven patients in groups 1, 2, 3 and 7 recovered protective skin sensibility in the median; and 7 in groups 1, 5 and 7 in the ulnar distribution.

Conclusion

The varied pattern of recovery in this relatively small series of patients who did not undergo operative treatment serves to show the wide area of damage that can be inflicted by traction on the plexus (Table 16.4).

Group 1: C7 involvement

In group 1 there was 1 normal myelogram but a lesion in continuity of the upper and lower trunks and either a rupture of the middle trunk or possible avulsion of C7 nerve root. Isolated rupture of C7 is rare.

The author has seen one case of isolated C7 avulsion without any marked injury to the remaining plexus caused by sudden traction on the arm: a nurse when running down steps was passing her finger along the vertical bars of the rail when her hand got caught. She presented an immediate isolated motor and partially sensory loss of C7 function, with temporary urine retention and transient paraesthesiae in her homolateral lower extremity. Lumbar puncture showed blood in her CSF fluid and twice the normal albumin content. A myelography was refused by the patient whose upper limb recovered almost completely in 2 years. However, she still presents an atrophy of the middle portion of her pectoralis major, upper portion of latissimus dorsi and some weakness of wrist flexion. Power of her grip is diminished by 25% compared to the dominant other hand.

Group 2

Group 2 patients must have had an elongation of the upper trunk, partial rupture of C7 and probably an avulsion of C8–T1 in six patients who had Horner's syndrome (two positive myelographies); a crush injury to the lower trunk in two patients (one normal myelography) with no Horner's syndrome. After 2–3 years their residual palsy was very similar to that of a Klumpke's paralysis.

Group 3

Group 3 patients had an elongation in continuity (degrees 2–3 of Sunderland) of C5, and severe disruptions and/or avulsions of the other roots are even worse.

Group 4

They must have had a degree 3–4 injury to the upper trunk.

Group 5

Group 5 patients probably had a lower root avulsion (all presented with a Horner's syndrome) a rupture of the upper trunk and a degree 3–4 to C7.

Group 6

Group 6 patients had complete either C5–T1 avulsions or rupture of C5, and C6–T1 avulsions.

Group 7

Group 7 had upper root avulsions and/or ruptures, with degrees 2, 3, 4 injury to C8–T1.

Direct operative treatment

Brachial plexus surgery has evolved over the years and there is little sense in detailing what has been done in the past. The indication for operation remains the same: young patients who present with a total palsy after a violent deceleration accident. The operation is then performed as early as the condition of the patient permits, particularly when a vascular injury is present and the limb is well perfused. Vascular and nerve repair are then carried out simultaneously. In cases when vascular repair is urgent the plexus surgeon or any surgeon belonging to his team are called to evaluate the lesions and the arterial reconstruction is performed when possible outside the plexus. Nerve repair is done later when it is not possible as an emergency. Emergency nerve repair is very rarely carried out in traction injuries. It is, however, performed in low velocity missile wounds or lacerations to produce gratifying results even when lesions are close to the foramen or intraforaminal. This confirms that contrary to traction these type of injuries (as iatrogenic sections) do not produce any important retrograde degeneration. In patients with partial palsy (e.g. Erb's type) repeated clinical examinations are carried out including the study of evoked potentials and when possible in the first few days before distal nerve degeneration occurs. Except for C5, which is difficult to test, the level of lesions of C6 and C7 may be determined. When the surgeon is convinced that ruptures and/or root avulsions are present there is no sense in procrastinating with a persisting palsy, and exploration is carried out as early as possible before scarred tissue occurs. Dissection is thereby facilitated. The extent of injury is often devastating; in half of the cases it was worse than expected. Only in two occasions out of more than 400 operations, was no macroscopical lesion found, one in a case of possible hysteria after a deep wound opening the humero-scapular joint, the other presenting with motor loss inconsistent with the sensory loss. Both patients made a complete recovery within a month from surgery when nothing had been done other than to inspect the supra and infraclavicular plexus by a wide exposure and perform peroperative stimulation.

Delayed operation

Patients were observed and operation was delayed when the degree of trauma overall was insufficient to avulse or rupture the brachial plexus; or in the absence of vascular injury, neighbouring fractures and in particular when the sensory loss was less extensive than the motor. When there is incomplete loss of sensation the patient is always treated conservatively and examined at regular intervals; weekly in the first month; then monthly. EMG and conduction tests are performed from the 18th post-trauma day. CT scan, myelography and MRI are confined to those who are candidates for surgery.

Only four patients with incomplete sensory loss corresponding to their involved motor territory had to come to operation because they failed to recover within their expected time, i.e. 6–9 months after injury. They had either partial trunk or cord lesions requiring grafting in three and neurolysis in one.

Correlation between sensory and motor loss

This is a reliable method of evaluating degrees of injury more severe than degree 1 (neurapraxia), bearing in mind that variations of sensory innervation are less precise than motor distribution.

Degree of damage

The importance of distinguishing between neurapraxia, axonotmesis and neurotmesis has to be stressed because at present only neurotmesis requires early repair (degrees 4 and 5, plus root avulsion). We have never seen neurapraxia affecting the entire plexus, although electrocution will produce a clinical state approaching this widespread neurapraxia. In our experience there was apparent total paralysis but further testing revealed M1 function in most muscle groups and incomplete sensory loss. By contrast, numerous cases have been observed of pure neurapraxia of some structures of the BP while others were normal or totally paralysed. Invariably some degree of sensation could be elicited when palsy seemed to be total, but sometimes involuntary defence movements were possible. Without implying psychogenic attitudes, it seems to the author that sensory and motor functions offer basically different mechanisms. Sensation is a passive function imposed to a large extent on an individual by the environment. Motor function, excluding reflexes, requires volition, i.e. active participation. The former is less likely to be suppressed than the latter. So far the author has seen only three cases of so-called hysterical BP palsy, one ending with a subcapital amputation of the upper limb after 5 years of unsuccessful psychi-

atric treatment. The patient, who because of her palsy, had become a total invalid moving about in a wheelchair, resumed walking 1 week after amputation, regained normal behaviour, returned to a successful professional life, became an international swimming champion, married, had children, etc. She cannot explain today why a simple carpal tunnel operation under plexus block caused a total persisting BP palsy. I did explore her plexus 1 year after the surgery, finding no lesions and all muscles responding to peroperative stimulation. Five years later I amputated her arm which was still functional according to electrophysiological investigations. The reader may imagine how difficult it was after exploring the plexus for a second time and finding no lesions to decide to amputate after receiving advice by several psychiatrists who had treated or seen the patient.

Surgical reconstruction

Goals of repair

The restoration and planning of function of a paralysed upper limb depends on the extent of the paralysis weighed against the known results of available reconstructive operations or prosthetic and orthotic devices [14].

There are contradicting patterns in use depending on the parts affected. A patient with a paralytic hand and a normal shoulder and elbow will use his dominant or non-dominant extremity mainly for coarse activities. Conversely, a patient with a paralytic shoulder, a good elbow and a normal hand will restrict the use of his limb to refined activities provided this extremity is dominant. When it is not, the hand will be only a 'helping hand'; it is rare for that hand to be used to initiate an activity followed by the other. The shoulder, which has the highest mobility of all our joints, serves to position the hand, but there are other important functions concerning balance of the body, protecting it, etc. At present the author considers that the shoulder and elbow function have to be favoured when basic requirements of a non-dominant upper limb have to be satisfied, bearing in mind that good hand function cannot be reconstructed in total BP palsies. Basic hand functions (key-pinch, grasp and protective sensation) have a subsidiary role in recon-

Table 16.8(a)   Graphical representation of function gained by direct surgical treatment (sutures, grafts, neurotizations) in total BP palsies with complete interruptions (lesions in continuity excluded): Root avulsions: ●; Ruptures of nerves: //. The criteria of evaluation are given in Table 16.9. The height of each line represents the result achieved in each individual case. Results improve when more than one proximal stump is available to be connected to the periphery

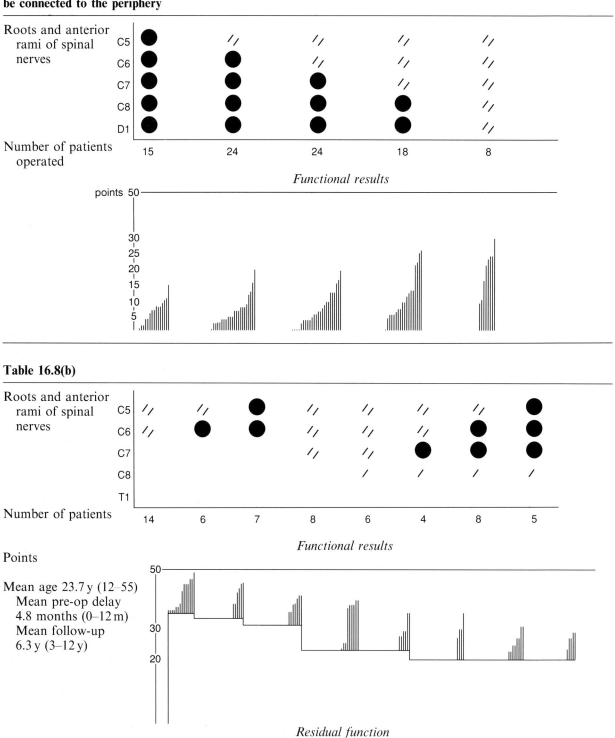

Table 16.8(b)

Table 16.8(c)

Posterior cord ruptures

Pattern of ruptures:	Isolated	+ SS	+ MC	+ SS MC	+ MC MED	+ All term branches
Number of patients operated	6	5	5	4	4	4

Mean age 21.7 y (13–34)
Mean pre-op delay 4.2 mo (15–7)
Mean follow-up 4.8 y (3–10)

Residual function

struction. Therefore, the basic requirements in restoring some function to a totally paralysed upper extremity are as follows :

1. Thoraco-humeral grasp, i.e. adduction of the humerus against the chest, and if possible the opening of the pinching element, i.e. abduction of the humerus with a stable humero-scapular joint and sensation on the thorax and opposite inner aspect of the arm.
2. Elbow flexion and internal rotation of the humerus; when possible, some external rotation to allow opening and closing of the antebrachio-thoracic grasp.
3. and 4. Flexion and extension of the wrist. Active flexion allows opening of the fingers provided they are not totally clawed. Extension, particularly when powerful, allows the reconstruction of grasp or pinch with a paralytic hand. Primitive sensation in the radial fingers is also a prerequisite.
5. Active thumb adduction, possibly abduction, to allow a key pinch and a fair sensation in order to use it.
6. Active finger PIP flexion combined to MP flexion produced by a tenodesis effect.
7. Active MP and PIP extension or obtained by any ancillary function (flexion of the wrist) by a tenodesis effect.
8. The last and ultimate is pollici-digital pulp to pulp pinch with a good sensation, and fourth and fifth finger flexion to obtain a locking effect on objects held in the hand.

Techniques of repair according to pathology

In complete root avulsion C5–T1 the goal is to reconstruct thoraco-brachial grasp, stabilize the shoulder, restore elbow flexion and internal and external rotation of the humerus; to restore sensation to the inner aspect of arm (usually preserved by the injury), outer aspect of forearm and even thumb and index (C5–C6 dermatomes). First of all we need scapulo-thoracic and scapulo-humeral function. The serratus anterior is all important to provide abduction of the arm and flexion (anterior projection) when a scapulo-humeral arthrodesis has been performed. The lower digitations of the serratus anterior are more efficient and they are innervated through C7, partially through C6. But these roots are avulsed. This means that either we reinnervate these digitations using intercostal nerves or we give them up for a modest opening and closing of

Table 16.9   Evolution of basic functions of the upper limb points

Shoulder (max. 13 points)	0	1	2	3	4	5
Abduction and/or forward flexion (any of both better prevailing) (max. 5 points)	0° Flail joint, no active function, humero-scapular dislocation >1 cm	0–30° Stable, humero-scapular dislocation <1 cm	30–60°	60–90° With extended extremity	90–120° (at 60° with 1 kg at least at wrist level on extended limb)	>120° or at 90° with 3 kg at wrist with extended arm
External rotation (max. 4 points)	0° Forearm in passive or active flexion of elbow cannot be brought away from chest	Forearm can be brought by 5–10° away from chest	Forearm (elbow flexed) can be brought by 10–30° away from chest	Forearm (elbow flexed) can be brought by 30–60° (60° means that the forearm is in sagittal plane) from chest	Forearm (elbow flexed) can be more than 60° away from chest (outside sagittal plane) or to sagittal plane against resistance	
Thoraco-brachial grasp, i.e. abduction and/or internal rotation when elbow can be actively flexed (max. 2 points)	Cannot hold anything between arm/forearm and chest wall	Can hold a patient's file under arm	Can hold a bag of 1 kg and more between chest and arm			
Posterior projection (max. 2 points)	None	Wrist with elbow in extension can be brought to lateral aspect of gluteus (slit of pocket)	Wrist can be brought behind plane of glutei or better or patient can push something behind him (e.g. shifting gears of a car)			

External rotation arm in abduction is not evaluated. This basic function would deserve at least 2 points. However this additional score would emphasize external rotation as being a very important basic function deserving 6 points, i.e. 4 points for external rotation in the transverse plane (arm in adduction against the chest) and 2 points in the sagittal plane (arm in abduction). There is no doubt that compared to the points awarded for other functions, this way to evaluate would give an undeserved importance to external rotation.

Table 16.9 (continued)

Elbow (max. 9 points)	*0*	*1*	*2*	*3*	*4*	*5*
Flexion (5 points)	Not possible or insignificant	Hand to pocket or belt	To 90° against gravity	To 90° with 1 kg in hand or 1.5 kg at wrist	To 90° and more with 3 kg in hand or 4.5 kg at wrist	Flexes 90° and more with 5 kg or 7.5 kg at wrist
Extension (4 points)	Not possible	Extends arm in passive abduction and full internal rotation to full passive ROM against gravity	Extends with 1 kg in hand or 1.5 kg at wrist	Extends with 3 kg in hand or 4.5 kg at wrist	Better than 3 kg in hand or 4.5 kg at wrist	
Forearm prono-supination (max. 3 points)	None	Only incomplete pronation or supination	Both functions present totalling 50°	Both functions totalling 100°		
Wrist (max. 8 points)		Against gravity (forearm in supination)	With 1 kg in hand	With 3 kg	Better than 3 kg	
Flexion (4 points)	None					
Extension (4 points)	None	Incomplete against gravity	Complete against gravity	With 1 kg in hand or against strong grasp (5–10 kg/cm²)	More than 1 kg or grasp of over 10 kg/cm²	

The position of weights along the limb plays a definite role because of the lever momentum.
Flexion of elbow at 90° with 3 kg suspended on the upper third of the forearm has not the same meaning as the same flexion with the same weight suspended at the wrist level or held in the hand.

the thoraco-brachial pinch being effected by the trapezius, levator scapulae and rhomboids. A very valuable solution is to reinnervate the suprascapular nerve with a transfer of the distal portion of the accessory nerve; a solution which produces good function of the upper trapezius, sometimes fair function of the middle trapezius because of satellite innervation and an active abduction between scapula and humerus of at least 50°. This will bring the arm almost to 90° away from the thorax provided the scapula can be stabilized against the thorax or rotated outwards due to reinnervation of the lower digitations of the serratus anterior. Internal rotation of the humerus can be obtained by reinnervating the sternal portion of pectoralis major with one intercostal nerve, and flexion of the elbow is obtained using two or three intercostal nerves

Table 16.9 (continued)

Hand (max. 17 points)	0	1	2	3	4	5
Long fingers motor (max. 5 points)	Total palsy (no flexion, no extension). Hand is a passive, flail weight	Passive hook (fingers are flexed in a position either by contracture or active muscle function, an active closure of fist not possible. Patient can hook on something he uses the hand as a kind of shovel or spoon	Active hook by active finger flexion (primitive grasp) from a half open position the long fingers can be brought down to touch the palm. Patient can hold something	Opening and closing of fist. Grasp power less 3 kg/cm^2 (Jamar dyna-mometer)	Good function of long fingers for flexion and extension. Grasp power 3–8 kg/cm^2 (Jamar dyna-mometer)	Fair independence of fingers. Grasp 8 kg (Jamar dyna-mometer)
				One point is subtracted if finger extension (opening) is not possible		
		Adduction or flexion present (key pinch) no opening	Closure and opening of key pinch	Pulp to pulp pinch		
Thumb motor (max. 3 points)	Total palsy		Power up to 1 kg/cm^2	Key pinch over 1 kg/cm^2		
				One point is subtracted if extension of thumb (opening) is not possible.		

It has been admitted, however disputable, that the most primitive function of the hand is to be a 'paper weight' or a kind of spoon or shovel (e.g. arthogrypotic, sclerodermic and other patients with analogous type of deformity). A totally paralytic hand or unstable as in advanced rheumatoid arthritis has not even that function. The next functional step seems to be a hook enabling the patient to carry a bag whether it is produced by stiffness of the joints or active long finger flexor function. This function in daily life seems to be equivalent to a key pinch. Correlation of motor function of the hand seems to be thumb to pulp pinch and independence of finger motion. In brachial plexus injury sophisticated hand function is beyond the possibilities of nerve repair. Therefore it is only grossly evaluated.

transferred onto the lateral cord. Some sensory rami originating from C4 may also be transferred to the lateral cord to provide protective sensation which is initially referred to the shoulder then, after 2–3 years, referred to the antero-lateral aspect of arm, thumb and index; possibly the middle finger. Transfers of intercostal nerves to the lateral cord may sometimes produce an M2 +

Table 16.9 (continued)

	0	*1*	*2*	*3*	*4*	*5*
5th finger motor 1 point	No strong flexion 0	Strong flexion (locking position when a knife or the handle of a tool is held in the hand)	—	—	—	—
Sensory (8 points) median n. area 5 points (pulp of thumb, index and long fingers)	No sensation	Temperature and pain felt, paraesthesias disturbing or not	Touch felt (without disturbing paraesthesias) no dysaesthesia	Light touch felt without paraesthesias gross localisation	Some tactile gnosis Weber above 15 mm	Fair tactile gnosis Weber below 15 mm
Ulnar nerve area 3 points (pulps of 4th and 5th fingers)	No sensation	Temperature and pain felt, paraesthesias disturbing or not	Touch felt (without disturbing paraesthesias) no dysaesthesia	One point is subtracted if dysaesthesia is present, two if hyperpathia is present		

The final result consists of the residual function, the function gained by operation and the function obtained by spontaneous regeneration. In complete paralysis the residual function is nil. When all spinal nerves are interrupted the final result corresponds to the gain obtained by operation. When some nerves are not functional but are not interrupted anatomically (degrees 1 to 3 of Sunderland) recovery by spontaneous regeneration has to be evaluated and subtracted from the final result in order to obtain the gain yielded by surgical nerve reconstruction.
In incomplete paralysis the maximal loss caused by nerve interruption has to be evaluated against the loss caused by degrees 1 to 3 of Sunderland in order to assess the gain obtained by nerve repair of degrees 4 and 5 and root avulsion.

to M3 flexion of the wrist but unfortunately not strong enough to reconstruct a useful key-pinch. The patients ask for it once they have a stable shoulder and M4 elbow flexion.

In C5 rupture and C6 through T1 root avulsion, we use presently the distal spinal accessory nerve to neurotize the suprascapular nerve. Part of C5 is connected to the lateral fascicles of the posterior cord (axillary nerve fibres); the anterior fascicular groups of C5 are connected to fascicles in the lateral cord going to the anterior thoracic nerves for the pectoralis major; the remaining to fascicles innervating the musculo-cutaneous nerve, while one or two intercostal nerves re-innervate the lower digitations of the serratus anterior. Intercostal nerves can be used to reinnervate the anterior and inferior thoracic nerves as an alternative to C5 which will reinnervate the serratus. There is no doubt at present that healthy nerves such as the spinal accessory, deep motor branches from the cervical plexus and intercostals have a potential for reinnervation superior to that of ruptured C5 when C6 through T1 are avulsed. Histological examination of the last slice cut when trimming the proximal stump of C5 has shown that in more than half of the cases 80% of the fibres were damaged, thus demonstrating the ascending character of traction lesions. In C5–C6 ruptures and lower root avulsions a maximum effort of repair is devoted to the shoulder and elbow, but also attempting to obtain some wrist extensor reinnervation; a goal, alas, we fail to reach in many cases. It is easier to reconstruct a grasp with the hand when powerful wrist extensors are available. C5 can, in conjunction with the spinal accessory nerve or on its own, be connected to nerves commanding the shoulder; while C6 is used for elbow and wrist flexion, elbow extension and/or wrist extension. Combined contractions are frequent and can be used for transfer to an antagonist. Intercostals are used on fascicles originating from C7, either its posterior or anterior division. The former choice gives better results than the latter.

In C5–C6–C7 ruptures with lower root avulsion the BP is reconstructed as anatomically as possible using the XIth nerve for the suprascapular and connecting at least the motor fascicles of C8 to the proximal stump of C7 (plexoplexal neurotization). Intercostals have been used to innervate the median or ulnar nerves with poor results.

In total ruptures of the primary trunks repair is carried out in order to reproduce the normal anatomy. It seems worthwhile to reconstruct the lower trunk C8–T1 when one is certain that the corresponding roots have not been avulsed, provided that the defect is not wider than 4 cm. Some function of the flexor carpi ulnaris and deep flexors of the third, fourth and fifth fingers can be expected. In partial BP palsies reconstruction is also performed according to the pathological findings. When C5 is ruptured and C6 avulsed, reconstruction is carried out by uniting the XIth nerve to the suprascapular nerve while grafts connect C5 to posterior and lateral cords. A marked or partial trumpet sign is always obtained, i.e. the patient compulsively flexes the elbow when he abducts the shoulder. He may, however, flex the elbow without abducting the shoulder using his pectoralis major to counterbalance the abductors. He may flex his arm with-

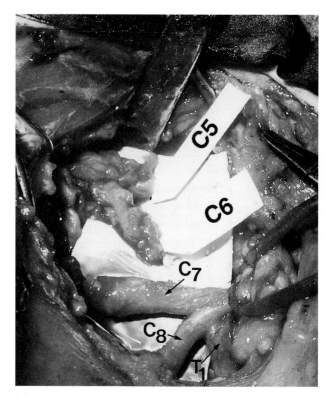

(a)

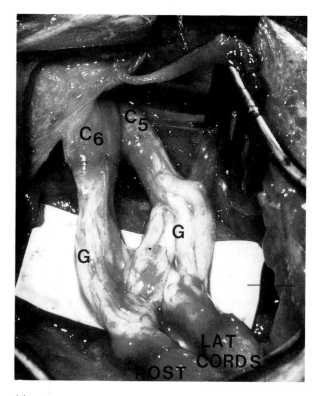

(c)

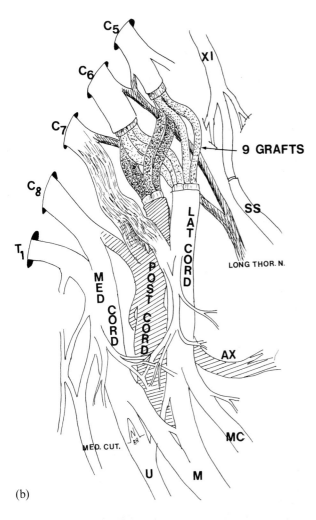

(b)

Fig. 16.1 (a) Lesions seen in a typical Erb's palsy: rupture of C5 and C6, elongation in continuity of C7 while C8 and T1 are normal (left plexus). (b) Drawing showing the repair performed: four grafts cover the proximal stump of C5, five grafts that of C6 while the spinal accessory nerve is used to neurotize the supra-scapular nerve. (c) Repair was performed using fibrin glue and a few stay stitches. The grafts will be spread on their bed (medial scalenus) for better revascularization.
(d) Neurotization of the supra-scapular nerve (SS) with the distal branch of the spinal accessory nerve (XI). The preserved ramus for the upper portion of the trapezius can be seen disappearing under the labels.

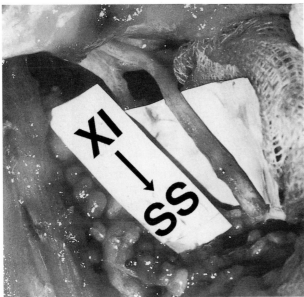

(d)

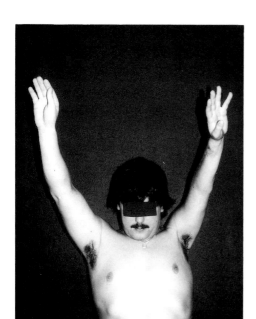

(a)

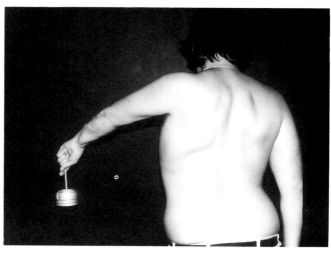

(b)

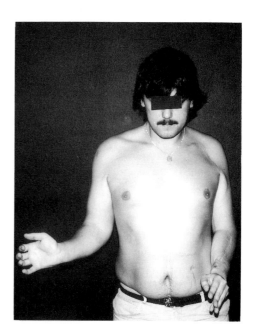

(c)

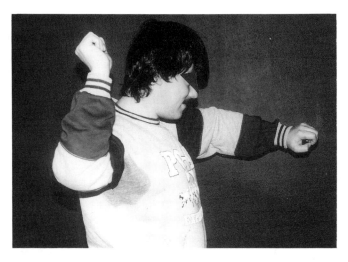

(d)

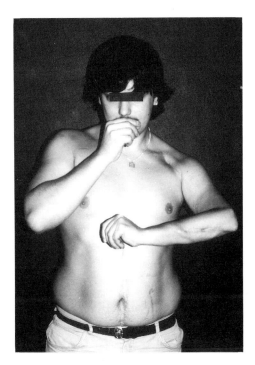

(e)

Fig. 16.2   Result 4 years after the repair illustrated in Fig. 16.1 (b–d). Forward elevation and abduction in the shoulder are good (a). The extremity, however, is in internal rotation (arm and forearm) and the power of abduction not impressive (b) as the patient reaches only 60° of global abduction carrying 2 kg in the hand. Note the paralysis of the lower portion of the trapezius and latissimus dorsi. The forearm is pronated. The lack of external rotation in the transverse and sagittal plane are well demonstrated (c and d). The patient was a victim of a motorcycle accident with multiple lesions. Visible scars relate to a laparotomy for splenic rupture and compound fractures of the forearm with a compartment syndrome (rupture of the subclavian artery). Because of inactivity after the accident he gained 20 kg in weight. The attempt to reach the mouth (e) shows the lack of external rotation of the humerus. Because the patient did not recover digit extension the flexor carpi ulnaris was transferred onto the common extensor of the fingers and onto the long extensor of the thumb with a satisfactory result (a) for the fingers and a poor result for the thumb (a and c). The tendon of the FCU passing over the dorsal aspect of the forearm is clearly visible (e) as well as the hyperactivity of the ulnar nerve (c) which tends to produce a flexion of the MP joints and hyperextension of the DIP joints. Three months later the humeral tendon of teres major was transferred onto the teres minor and infraspinatus tendons with a gain of 20° in external rotation. Note the maintained function of the upper trapezius. The patient can flex the elbow with 5 kg in his hand (not shown on photographs).

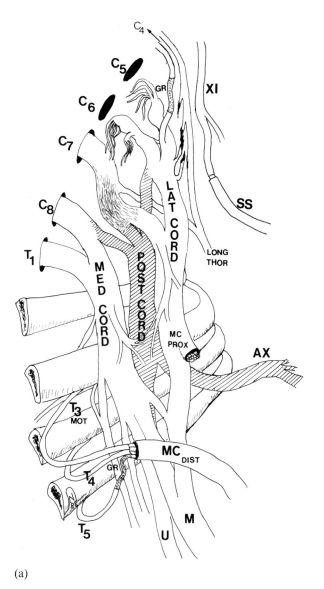

(a)

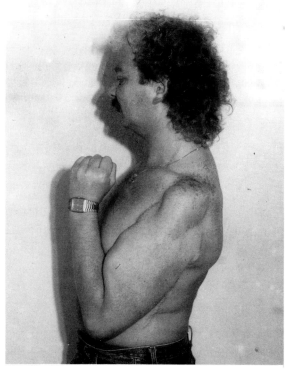

(b)

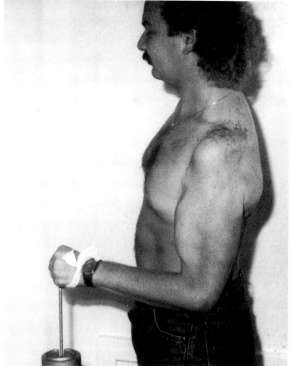

Fig. 16.3   By contrast, a patient with root avulsion C5–C6. The repair performed is shown in (a). Recovery of shoulder function is almost as good as in Fig. 16.2, but elbow flexion was incomplete and weak (M2+). A latissimus dorsi transfer was performed onto the biceps. Flexion is good (b) but the patient cannot lift more than 1.5 kg (c) held in the hand in spite of the impressive bulk of the muscle transferred. Note the partial winging of the scapula caused by a subtotal denervation of serratus anterior; also note the bulk of recovered deltoid.

(c)

out flexing the elbow; however external rotation when obtained is always linked with some abduction of the arm.

In C5–C6 ruptures reconstruction tries to reproduce the normal fascicular distribution, but the author favours the use of the XIth nerve to neurotize the supra-scapular nerve because the abduction between scapula and humerus is essential for acceptable shoulder function. Grafting the suprascapular nerve from C5 rarely gives satisfactory results because the cranial portion of C5 (12 o'clock) is particularly damaged in traction lesions and because simultaneous contractions between the spinati, teres major, subscapularis and pectoralis major are very common.

Reconstruction of cords and individual nerves

The lateral cord is rarely damaged. When it happens care must be taken to reconstruct the anterior thoracic nerves when there is a lower root palsy. Absence of pectoralis major function, usually in conjunction with subscapularis, latissimus dorsi and teres major function is very disturbing; the patient cannot adduct his arm unless he has very powerful biceps and coracobrachialis. He then has the feeling of a flail shoulder.

Lateral cord repair yields good results. The posterior cord is invariably injured in infraclavicular BPI because of its anchorage; isolated injuries to the posterior cord also occur. Reconstruction yields good results except for MP joint extension. The medial cord is rarely injured. Either C8 or T1 is avulsed; rarely, the lower primary trunk is ruptured; or the median, ulnar and medial cutaneous nerves are ruptured close to their origins. It is always worthwhile reconstructing them even if it takes years before recovery is seen in the forearm and hand.

Results of BP repair

In BPI supraclavicular lesions presenting with degrees 4, 5 and root avulsions, normal function of the limb has never been restored even when lesions were limited to C5 and C6. Useful function has often been obtained but when it is not we question our pre- and peroperative diagnosis. Root avulsions have been misdiagnosed several times – occasionally our choices of repair was incorrect. For instance, the role of serratus anterior in shoulder function has only been recognized in the last 3 years, while the importance of the suprascapular nerve has been known for 2 decades. However, a possible rotator cuff rupture present in 3% of supraclavicular BPI has been identified only during the last 7 years. Brown–Sequard's partial syndromes have been missed initially in more than half of the cases; and the use of intercostal nerves in them has led to a partial or total failure. Avulsion of nerves from muscles (suprascapular from spinati, axillary from deltoid, median and radial from muscles in the forearm, musculo-cutaneous from biceps) have been recognized slowly over the years as well as fibrosis of muscles caused by ischaemia in late revascularizations of the limb. Pitfalls in BPI are more often encountered than thought of and the author has to admit many failures in the past caused by his incapacity to observe and identify pathological conditions which are now evident.

Infraclavicular BPI can yield excellent results provided the median and ulnar and to some extent radial nerve fibres have not been severely damaged. A distinction has to be made between mono- or bifunctional nerves such as the long thoracic, suprascapular, axillary and musculocutaneous nerves and the multifunctional nerves such as the radial, particularly ulnar and median nerves which convey impulses to numerous antagonist–agonist muscles and subtle sensory messages. Their normal function cannot be reconstructed satisfactorily whatever the refinement and minuteness of technique. When good or excellent results in their repair are obtained, either there is an anomalous innervation or the result is obtained by chance.

Reporting results of BPI is almost impossible [15–20] due to the complexity of functions in the upper limb. We have attempted together with P. Raimondi and A. Morelli from Legnano, Italy, to create an evaluation which takes into account only the basic functional requirements of the upper extremity (Table 16.8). The results obtained are represented in Table 16.9 and illustrated by Figs 16.1–16.6.

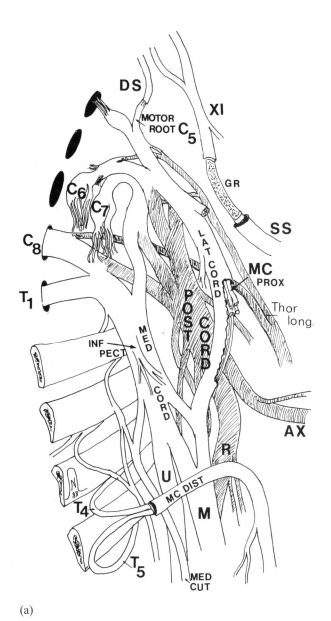

(a)

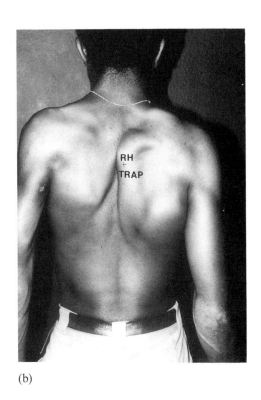

(b)

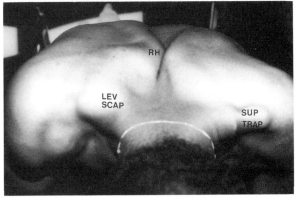

(c)

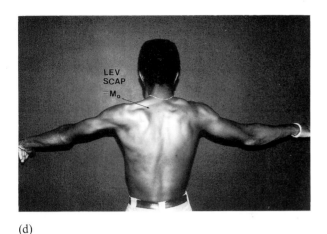

(d)

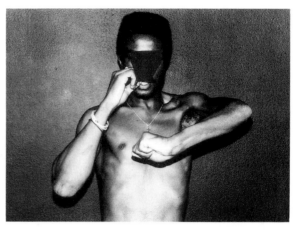

(f)

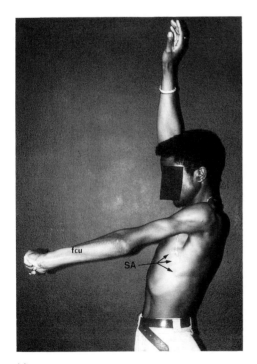

(e)

Fig. 16.4 Patient with root avulsion C5, C6 and C7 and minor stretch injury to C8 after a motorcycle accident operated 3 weeks post-trauma (see (a)). Photographs show the result 3 years and 9 months after operation.
(b) demonstrates the palsy of middle and lower trapezius and of levator scapulae confirmed by the axial view
(c) which demonstrates that the upper trapezius has recovered half of its bulk; (d) and (e) show the abduction and flexion in the shoulder; the recovery of deltoid and serratus anterior (lower digitations) is well demonstrated, also the transferred FCU onto EDC and EPL, while pronator teres was transferred onto ECRB, causing some radial deviation on extension of the wrist. The patient has full extension of the fingers (not shown here). (f) shows an attempt to bring the hand to the mouth; the lack of external rotation of the humerus is quite evident (e). This could be partially corrected by transferring the teres major (which has recovered to M4) tendon onto the external rotators. The biceps is only at M2+. The latissimus dorsi whose superior portion is at M2 and inferior at M4 could be transferred onto the biceps. The patient is, however, well adapted to his handicap and does not wish any further surgery.

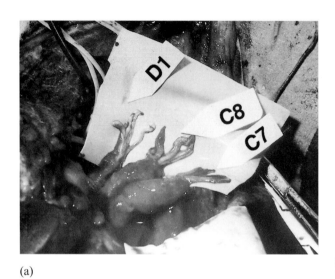

(a)

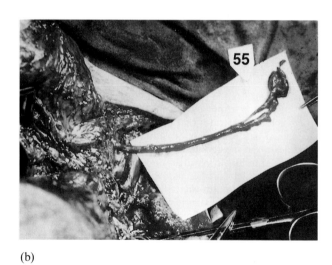

(b)

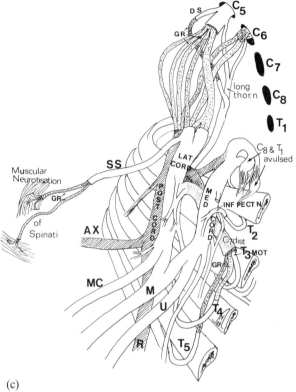

(c)

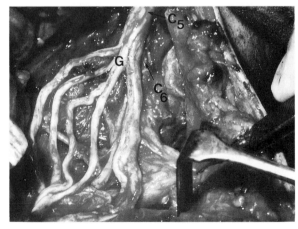

(d)

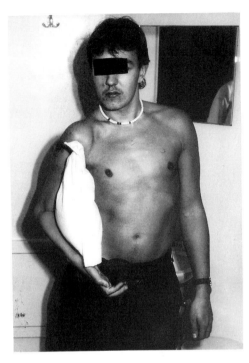

(e)

Fig. 16.5 Rupture of C5 and C6, root avulsion C7, C8 and T1 (a). The suprascapular nerve was avulsed from the spinati (b) and the proximal stump of C6 was poor. The repair was carried out according to drawing (c) and photograph (d). (e) shows the brachio-thoracic grasp (biceps at M3+ and triceps lateral portion at M2 synchronous to biceps, FCR at M2). (f) despite a deltoid at M3 the function of the shoulder is poor (spinati at M2); therefore the humero-scapular angle does not increase on attempted abduction and the scapula is lateralized by a strong serratus anterior (finger of examiner on tip of scapula). This shows the importance of good function of the suprascapular nerve, contrasting with Fig. 16.4.

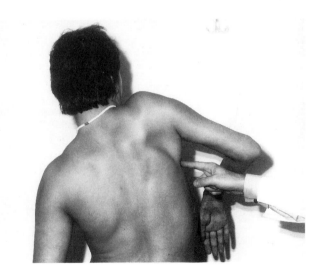

(f)

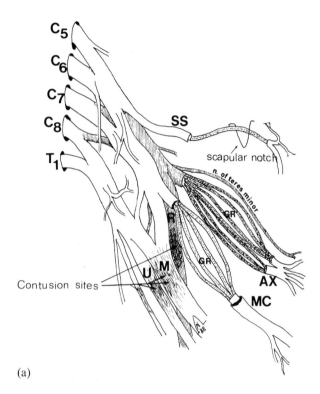

(a)

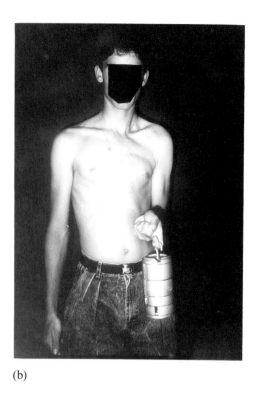

(b)

Fig. 16.6 This patient presented an axillary artery rupture and an extended brachial plexus palsy sparing the pectoralis major, teres major and minor and latissimus dorsi. At operation a suprascapular, axillary and musculo-cutaneous nerve ruptures were found; whereas the radial, median and ulnar nerves were contused but in continuity. Twelve grafts 7 cm long (both sural nerves were harvested) were used for the repair. His shoulder function, not shown here, is complete and powerful except for weak external rotation; the infra-spinatus did not recover for some unknown reason. His biceps is at M4+: he lifts 7 kg easily to 90° with one finger! This result demonstrates the striking contrast between supra-clavicular and more distal lesions with sparing of severe injuries to the ulnar, median and radial nerves.

References

1. Narakas, A. (1977) Indications et résultats du traitement chirurgical direct dans les lésions par élongation du plexus brachial. *Rev. Chir. Orthop. (Paris)*, **63**, 88–106.
2. Sunderland, S. (1951) A classification of peripheral nerve injuries producing loss of function. *Brain*, **74**, 491–516.
3. Medical Research Council (1954) *Peripheral Nerve Injuries*. HMSO, London, p. 4.
4. Seddon, H. J. (1943) Three types of nerve injury. *Brain*, **66**, 17–293.
5. Herzberg, G., Narakas, A., Comtet, J. J. *et al.* (1985) Microsurgical relations of the roots of the brachial plexus. Practical applications (in French and in English). *Ann. Chir. Main.*, **4**, 120–133.
6. Narakas, A. (1977) Les lésions dans les élongations du plexus brachail: différentes possibilités et associations lésionnelles. *Rev. Chir. Orthop. (Paris)*, **63**, 44–54.
7. Narakas, A. (1985) The treatment of brachial plexus injuries. *Int. Orthop. (SICOT)*, **9**, 29–36.
8. Bonney, G. (1959) Prognosis in traction lesions of the brachial plexus. *J. Bone Joint Surg.*, **41B**, 4–35.
9. Yeoman, P. M. (1975) *Traction Injuries of the Brachial Plexus.* Thesis for doctorate of Medicine, Cambridge (unpublished). Data in Seddon, H. J. (1975) *Surgical Disorders of the Peripheral Nerves*, 2nd edn. Churchill Livingstone, Edinburgh, p. 194.
10. Wynn Parry, C. B. (1974) The management of injuries to the brachial plexus. *Proc. R. Soc. Med. (London)*, **67**, 488–490.
11. Wynn Parry, C. B. (1978) Management of peripheral nerve injuries and traction lesions of the brachial plexus. *Int. Rehabil. Med.*, **1**, 9–20.